MW01120375

Metal-based Neurodegeneration:
From Molecular Mechanisms
to Therapeutic Strategies

Metal-based Neurodegeneration:
From Molecular Mechanisms to Therapeutic Strategies

Robert R. Crichton & Roberta J. Ward
Université Catholique de Louvain, Belgium

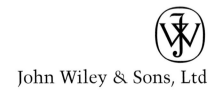

John Wiley & Sons, Ltd

Other Wiley Editorial Offices

John Wiley & Sons Inc., 111 River Street, Hoboken, NJ 07030, USA

Jossey-Bass, 989 Market Street, San Francisco, CA 94103-1741, USA

Wiley-VCH Verlag GmbH, Boschstr. 12, D-69469 Weinheim, Germany

John Wiley & Sons Australia Ltd, 42 McDougall Street, Milton, Queensland 4064, Australia

John Wiley & Sons (Asia) Pte Ltd, 2 Clementi Loop #02-01, Jin Xing Distripark, Singapore 129809

John Wiley & Sons Canada Ltd, 22 Worcester Road, Etobicoke, Ontario, Canada M9W 1L1

Wiley also publishes its books in a variety of electronic formats. Some content that appears in print may not be
available in electronic books.

Library of Congress Cataloguing-in-Publication Data
Crichton, Robert R.
    Metal-based neurodegeneration: from molecular mechanisms to therapeutic strategies/Robert R. Crichton &
Roberta J. Ward.
        p. ; cm.
    Includes bibliographical references and index.
    ISBN-13: 978-0-470-02255-9 (cloth : alk. paper)
    ISBN-10: 0-470-02255-8 (cloth : alk. paper)
    1. Nervous system – Degeneration – Etiology. 2. Brain – Pathophysiology. 3. Oxidative stress.
    4. Metals – Health aspects.
        [DNLM: 1. Neurodegenerative Diseases – etiology. 2. Brain – physiology. 3. Metals – adverse effects.
    4. Oxidative Stress. WL 359 C928m 2006]. I. Ward, Roberta J. II. Title.
RC365.C75 2006
616.8'0471–dc22   2005023372

British Library Cataloguing-in-Publication Data

A catalogue record for this book is available from the British Library

    ISBN-13 978-0-470-02255-9
    ISBN-10 0-470-02255-8

Typeset in 10/12pt Times by Thomson Press (India) Limited, New Delhi, India
Printed and bound in Spain by Grafos S.A. Barcelona
This book is printed on acid-free paper responsibly manufactured from sustainable forestry
in which at least two trees are planted for each one used for paper production.

Contents

Preface

As actuaries confront life insurance companies in the developed world with their tables of life expectancy over the next decades, some very important positive and negative points emerge from their projections. One of the most striking, is that our children's children will live to be centenarians. Bravo, what enormous progress we have made in extending the longevity of the human race! But this progress has been won at what cost? Given the present correlation between the incidence of debilitating neurodegenerative diseases, like Alzheimer's and Parkinson's diseases, with increasing age, how can we contemplate a situation, where we have only extended our life expectancy, in order to confront the probability that we will be struck down by diseases which will virtually reduce our existence to little more than an advanced vegetative state. In stark terms, what this means is that we must be just as concerned about the quality of life of our ageing population as about their life expectancy. The recent statistics published in the Archives of Neurology of estimates of the incidence of Alzheimer's disease in the US population do not make encouraging reading. They suggest that from around 4-5 million at present, this will increase to around 13 million by the year 2050, much higher than previous estimates. This is essentially due to the rapid ageing of the American population. We can anticipate that, while the rise will also be important in Europe, it will be less pronounced, because the European population is already much older than that of the US. One only needs to talk with a 'carer' for someone with advanced debilitating neurodegenerative disease, to realize that the consequences extend far beyond the individual affected patient.

What this means in concrete terms, is that we must pursue, with the greatest urgency the following three objectives: (i) endeavour to find out what are the causes of these age-related neurodegenerative diseases, (ii) seek to find therapeutic measures which will slow down the onset of these disorders and (iii) ultimately, find ways and means of preventing them – to quote the Chinese proverb 'poor doctor cures, good doctor prevents'.

In this book our objective has been to give an overview of many of the neurodegenerative diseases which currently plague humankind. We have tried in most cases to define the biochemical actors in the disease (proteins or peptides), and to describe their normal, and where possible, their pathological conformations. Then, we have outlined the characteristics of the disease, with frequent emphasis on the role of metal-induced oxidative stress (Table 1) in the disease process, often resulting in the production of intracellular aggregates of the target proteins or peptides. These latter are often characterized by their accumulation in morphologically characteristic inclusion bodies containing proteins, specific to the particular disease. These include β-amyloid plaques and neurofibrillary tangles in Alzheimer's disease, Lewy bodies in Parkinson's disease, prion protein (PrP) plaques in prion diseases and

Table 1: Some neurodegenerative disorders with possible metal-associated pathology

Disorder	implicated Metal	implicated Metalloproteins or enzymes
Alzheimer's disease	Copper, iron, zinc	Aβ, APP
Parkinson's disease	Iron	α-synuclein, neuromelanin, lactoferrin, ferritin, melanotransferrin, ceruloplasmin, divalent cation transporter
Creutzfeldt-Jakob disease	Copper, iron	Prion protein
Familial amyotrophic lateral sclerosis	Copper, zinc deficiency	Superoxide dismutase 1
Friedreich's ataxia	Iron	Frataxin, aconitase, mitochondrial proteins
Multiple sclerosis	Iron	Not known
Wilson's disease	Copper	Ceruloplasmin deficiency, Wilson's protein
Hallervorden-Spatz syndrome	Iron	Vitamin B5 metabolism
Huntington's disease	Iron, calcium	Huntingtin

nuclear inclusions in Huntington's as well as in other neurodegenerative diseases. The formation and subsequent accumulation of these insoluble protein aggregates in neurons must in some way reflect an incapacity of the cell to correctly respond to their formation and to eliminate them. The degradation of cellular proteins takes place by one of two pathways. They may degraded by proteolytic enzymes within the intracellular compartments known as lysosomes – this appears to be a relatively non-selective process. However there is a second, cytosolic-based and energy (ATP)-dependent proteolytic system which is independent of the lysosomal system. Proteins that are selected for destruction by this are first marked by covalently linking them to ubiquitin, a small protein that is both ubiquitous and abundant in eukaryotes, indeed it is the most highly conserved protein known. The ubiquinated protein is degraded in an energy-dependent process within a large multiprotein complex, known as the proteosome. And it is this process which seems to be dysfunctional in many neurodegenerative diseases.

Finally we discuss the progress that is being made in understanding the pathogenesis of the diseases and the identification of targets for their treatment. As a recent article has pointed out, the pharmaceutical industry is frequently in the process of looking for Cinderella after the ball – in other words, they have a glass slipper (a low molecular weight molecule) which exerts an enormous effect on a disease process (the unfortunate Prince), but they do not know to which cellular protein (the glass slipper) it fits. As we gain a greater understanding of the mechanisms which are involved in the oxidative and other stress factors that provoke degeneration of nervous tissue and the often debilitating diseases that are their consequence, we will hopefully also find effective therapeutic approaches, which will not only improve their treatment once they have been diagnosed, but also enable the effective delay of their onset.

Robert R. Crichton
Roberta J. Ward

1

Metals in Brain, Metal Transport, Storage and Homeostasis

1.1 INTRODUCTION – THE IMPORTANCE OF METAL IONS IN BRAIN FUNCTION

There can be little doubt that purely organic molecules, such as amino acids, fatty acids and lipids, carbohydrates, purines and pyrimidine bases and the polymers made out of them, proteins, polysaccharides and the nucleic acids RNA and DNA, are extremely important for living organisms. However, in order to fulfil a series of important functions, such as energy production, and, in higher organisms, for example, nerve transmission, muscle contraction and oxygen transport, metal ions are also absolutely essential. They include spectroscopically silent metal ions like potassium, sodium, calcium, magnesium and zinc together with the more spectroscopically accessible iron, copper, manganese, cobalt, molybdenum, vanadium and a few others. The role of some of these metal ion in brain function is particularly important, and has led to the introduction of the term metalloneurochemistry to describe the study of metal ions in the brain and the nervous system at the molecular level (Burdette and Lippard, 2003).

The alkali metal ions Na^+ and K^+ play a crucial role in the transmission of nervous impulses both within the brain and from the brain to other parts of the body. The opening and closing of ion channels generates electrochemical gradients across the plasma membranes of neurons. A nerve impulse is constituted by a wave of transient depolarization/ re-polarization of membranes which traverses the nerve cell, and is designated as an action potential. As was shown by Hodgkin and Huxley (1953) a microelectrode implanted into an axon (the long process emanating from the body of a nerve cell) will record an action potential (**Figure 1.1a**). This results from a rapid and transient increase in Na^+ permeability followed by a more prolonged increase in K^+ permeability (**Figure 1.1b**). The opening and closing of ion channels across cellular membranes creates the electrochemical gradients (action potentials) across these membranes, which transmits information and also regulates cellular function. The determination of the X-ray structure of the K^+ ion channel has allowed us to understand how it selectively filters completely dehydrated K^+ ions, but not the smaller Na^+ ions. Not only does this molecular filter select the ions to be transported, but the

Metal-based Neurodegeneration: From Molecular Mechanisms to Therapeutic Strategies R. R. Crichton and R. J. Ward
© 2006 John Wiley & Sons, Ltd

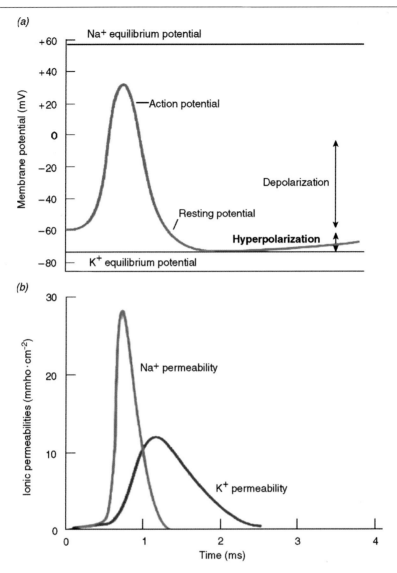

Figure 1.1: The time course of an action potential. (a) The axon membrane undergoes rapid depolarization followed by a nearly as rapid hyperpolarization and then a slow recovery to its resting potential. (b) The depolarization is caused by a transient increase in Na^+ permeability (conductance), whereas the hyperpolarization results from a more prolonged increase in K^+ permeability that begins a fraction of a millisecond later. From Voet and Voet, 1995.

electrostatic repulsion between K^+ ions, which pass through this molecular filter in Indian file provides the force to drive the K^+ ions rapidly through the channel at a rate of 10^7 to 10^8 per second.

Within cells, including nerve cells, fluxes of Ca^{2+} ions play an important role in signal transduction*. When intracellular Ca^{2+} increases, the ubiquitous eukaryotic Ca^{2+}-binding

---

* For a superb and entertaining review of calcium signalling see Carafoli, 2002.

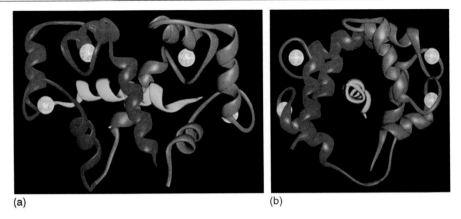

(a)   (b)

Figure 1.2: Ribbon diagrams showing the NMR structure of $(Ca^{2+})_4$-calmodulin from the fruit fly *Drosophila melanogaster* in complex with its 26-residue target polypeptide from rabbit sketelal muscle myosin light chain kinase. The N-terminal domain of calmodulin is on the left, the C-terminal domain on the right, the target peptide in the middle and the Ca^{2+} ions represented as spheres. (**a**) A view of the complex with the N-terminus of the target peptide on the right. (**b**) A perpendicular view as seen from the right side of (a). From Voet and Voet, 1995.

protein calmodulin binds Ca^{2+} ions, thereby exposing a previously buried hydrophobic patch, which in its turn can bind to a large number of target enzymes and modify their activity. The structure of the complex between $(Ca^{2+})_4$-calmodulin and a target polypeptide is shown in **Figure 1.2**. Evidence has been presented for a role for Ca^{2+}-dependent translocation of calmodulin in neuronal nuclei in both rapid signalling and memory formation (Mermelstein et al., 2001). A target protein for calmodulin in mammalian brain is calcineurin, a heterodimeric phosphatase, which has both a calmodulin binding domain in its catalytic subunit and a subunit which binds Ca^{2+} (Olson and Williams, 2000). Calcineurin seems to be involved in some way in synaptic plasticity (Arambura et al., 2001). It may be involved in an oestrogen-dependent pathway in the hippocampus, the memory and learning centre of the brain (Sharrow et al., 2002), which could have implications in hormone replacement therapy for improving memory. Another family of Ca^{2+}-binding proteins, called synaptotagmins, have been localized on the membranes of synaptic vesicles (Sudhoff, 2002), where they seem to be involved in the release of neurotransmitters (Augustine, 2001; Koh and Bellen, 2003). While the mechanism by which synaptotagmins are involved in Ca^{2+}-mediated synaptic transmission remains unclear, it appears likely that the neurotoxicity of heavy metals such as Pb may be due to a higher affinity of synaptotagmins for Pb^{2+} than for Ca^{2+} (Godwin, 2001).

Highly enriched in brain tissue, and present throughout the body, the Ca^{2+}/calmodulin-dependent protein kinase CaMKII plays a central role in Ca^{2+} signal transduction (Hudmon and Schulman, 2002). CaMKII accounts for about 2% of total hippocampal protein and around 0.25% of total brain protein (Erunda and Kennedy, 1985), and is the most abundant protein in the postsynaptic density. This is a region of the postsynaptic membrane which is physically connected to the ion channels which mediate synaptic transmission. The structural modification of synaptic proteins is thought to be the molecular event which is involved in the memory storage process. The unique biochemical properties of CaMKII have made it one of the paradigms of the long sought after '**memory molecule**'. Binding of Ca^{2+}/calmodulin to CaMKII allows autophosphorylation together with complex changes in

CaMKII's sensitivity to Ca^{2+}/calmodulin, which confer a kind of molecular memory to its autoregulation and activity (Hudmon and Schulman, 2002; Cammarota et al., 2002). In addition, the central role of CaMKII as a sensor of Ca^{2+} signals generated by activation of NMDA receptors after the induction of long-term plastic changes, has underlined its role in synaptic plasticity (Cammarota et al., 2002).

Another metal ion that has been implicated in brain function is Zn^{2+}. Around 10% of total brain zinc is found distributed throughout the CNS in synaptic vesicles of glutamatergic neurones, although the function of vesicular zinc is poorly understood. It has been suggested from microdialysis studies that zinc enhances GABA release via potentiation of α-amino-3-hydroxy-5-methyl-4-isoxalolepropionate (AMPA)/kainate receptors in the CA3 region of the hippocampus, followed by a decrease in presynaptic glutamate release in the same region (Takeda et al., 2004). In both the CA1 and CA3 regions of the hippocampus, zinc seems to be an inhibitory neuromodulator of glutamate release (Takeda et al., 2003, 2004). When hippocampal fibres are stimulated, large amounts of Zn are co-released with glutamate, and it has been suggested that this synaptic pool of Zn functions as a neuromodulator. However, *Znt-3*-null mice exhibit no characteristic phenotype, which would indicate either that Zn does not play an important role, or that the lack of vesicular Zn is compensated in another way.

We have, clearly not by accident, left until the last in this overview the redox metal ions iron, copper, manganese. Metalloenzymes containing these metals play extremely important roles in a number of key metabolic pathways within nervous tissues, They are, for example, involved in neurotransmitter synthesis (the Fe enzyme, tyrosine hydroxylase in the formation of dopa from tyrosine, the Cu enzyme dopamine β-hydroxylase which transforms dopamine to nor-adrenaline) and in neuroprotection (the Cu/Zn superoxide dismutase in cytosol and the Mn superoxide dismutase in mitochondria). However, as we will see in later chapters, the presence of any of these redox-active metals in excess within localized regions of the CNS frequently spells disaster, with associated neurodegeneration.

1.2 METAL ION TRANSPORT AND STORAGE – IRON

Iron is normally transported in plasma and other extracellular fluids bound to transferrin, a bilobal protein which can bind two Fe^{3+} ions, in octahedral coordination, with four protein ligands and a bidentate carbonate anion (Crichton, 2001). It is taken up by cells via the transferrin-to cell cycle (**Figure 1.3**), which begins with the binding of the holo(diferric)-transferrin molecule (HOLO-TF) to transferrin receptors at the cell surface. The complexes localize to clathrin-coated pits, which pinch off from the membrane to form coated vesicles, initiating the process of endocytosis. After budding is complete, the clathrin coat is removed, and smooth-surfaced endosomes are formed. The pH of the endosome is acidified by the action of an ATP-dependent proton pump. At the acidic pH, the holotransferrin undergoes a conformational change, releasing iron from transferrin as Fe^{3+}, presumably accompanied by protonation of the bound carbonate. Acidification facilitates proton-coupled transport of iron transport out of the endosomes through the action of the divalent metal transporter, DMT1, a member of the SLC11 family of H^+-coupled metal ion transporters (McKenzie and Hediger, 2004). However, the ferric reductase, which is assumed to reduce the iron, prior to its transport out of the endosome by DMT1, has not yet been identified. Apotransferrin (APO-TF) bound to its receptor, returns to the plasma membrane, where, at neutral pH, the complex dissociates. The two proteins can then participate in further

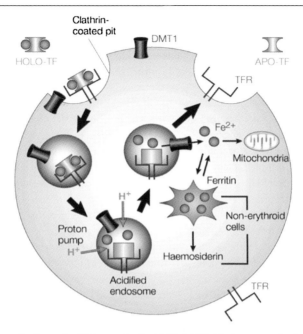

Figure 1.3: The transferrin cycle. Holotransferrin (HOLO-TF) binds to transferrin receptors (TFR) at the cell surface. The complexes localize to clathrin-coated pits, which invaginate to initiate endocytosis. Specialized endosomes form, and are acidified by a proton pump. At the acidic pH, iron is released from transferrin and is co-transported with protons out of the endosomes by the divalent metal ion transporter DCT1. Apotransferrin (APO-TF) bound to TFR is returned to the cell membrane, where, at neutral pH they dissociate to participate in further rounds of iron delivery. In non-erythroid cells, iron is stored as ferritin and haemosiderin. From Zecca et al., 2004. Reproduced by permission of Nature Reviews Neuroscience.

rounds of iron delivery. This transferrin to cell cycle ensures iron uptake by cells that have transferrin receptors.

The Iron Regulatory Protein 1, IREG1, (also known as ferroportin) is thought to be involved in iron export at the plasma membrane in macrophages: mutations in this protein are associated with iron accumulation within macrophages. IREG1 is also implicated as the iron transporter at the basolateral membrane of gastrointestinal enterocytes.

During evolution, mammalian species appear to have developed extensive mechanisms for iron uptake into parenchymal cells but have not developed corresponding pathways for its removal. This is in marked contrast to reticuloendothelial cells which can both take up iron and release it by utilization of IREG1.

Within the cell, the 'labile iron pool' (LIP) in the cytoplasm is used for the synthesis of haem and Fe-S cluster iron-containing proteins within the mitochondria, or is stored in the cytosol as ferritin. When large amounts of iron accumulate, haemosiderin is formed, due to the breakdown of ferritin within lysosomes. Haemosiderin was in fact the first iron-containing protein to be detected histologically by the intense Prussian blue reaction that it gave with potassium ferrocyanide by Perls (1867), a detection technique that is still used today. Haemosiderin is present in tissues when iron concentration increases 10 to 20 fold, e.g. liver and spleen, and has been characterized by a variety of biophysical and electron microscopic techniques, e.g. Mossbauer, EXAFS (Ward et al., 1994). However brain haemosiderin has not been characterized, and may not actually occur, since L-ferritin, its precursor, is not necessarily increased in many of the neurodegenerative diseases, as we shall discuss. Ferritin is a hollow protein shell made up of 24-subunits of two types, namely H (heavy) and L (light) within which substantial amounts of iron (up to 4,500 atoms/molecule) can be stored in a soluble, non-toxic yet bio-available form. In mammals this iron core is relatively well ordered and corresponds to the mineral phase ferrihydrite (Crichton, 2001). The two ferritin subunits have different functions and are encoded on different chromosomes. The H subunit catalyses the oxidation of Fe^{2+} to Fe^{3+} at di-iron sites known as ferroxidase centres. Indeed, H-chain ferritins are members of a superfamily of (μ-carboxylato)diiron proteins, which include methane monooxygenase, ribonucleotide reductase, stearoyl-acyl carrier protein desaturase and hemerythrin. In contrast, the L subunit contains a site within the protein shell to which iron from the ferroxidase site migrates, which allows nucleation of the ferrihydrite core.

In mitochondria, iron is utilized by ferrochelatase for haem synthesis, and for the assembly of Fe-S clusters. It has become apparent recently that the mitochondrial protein frataxin may function as a kind of iron chaperone which delivers iron both to ferrochelatase (Lesuisse et al., 2003; He et al., 2004) and to the scaffold proteins which assemble the Fe-S clusters (Muhlenhoff et al., 2002). Indeed, as we will see later in Chapter 5, defective production of frataxin is the cause of Friedreich's ataxia, and results in massive mitochondrial iron accumulation.

The brain is unique among all the organs of the body, hidden behind a relatively poorly permeable vascular barrier, which limits its access to plasma nutrients, such as iron (**Figure 1.4**). Iron transport into the brain mostly involves the transferrin to cell cycle, using

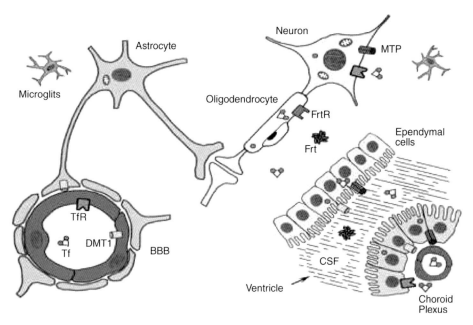

Figure 1.4: Diagrammatic portrayal of the blood-brain barrier and the iron transport proteins thought to be involved in iron movement into brain. DMT1, divalent metal transporter; Tf, transferrin; TfR, transferrin receptor; Frt, ferritin; FrtR, ferritin receptor; MTP, metal transport protein (or IREG1, or ferroportin) BBB Blood-Brain Barrier. From Beard, 2003. Reproduced by permission of the American Society for Nutritional Sciences.

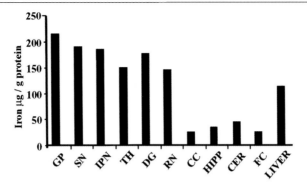

Figure 1.5: Distribution of iron in human brain. GP, globus pallidus; SN, substantia nigra; IPN, interpeduncular nucleus; TH, thalamus; DG, dentate gyrus; RN red nucleus; CC, cerebral cortex; HIPP, hippocampus; CER, cerebellum; FC, frontal cortex. From Götz et al., 2004.

transferrin receptors within epithelial cells lining the blood-brain barrier, although the precise mechanism of iron transfer is still uncertain (Connor, 2003). Iron content within the brain varies greatly from one region to another. Significantly greater iron concentrations, as high as 150–200 µg/g protein, are found in the substantia nigra and the globus palidus than in liver (Götz et al., 2004), and other brain regions with high concentrations are the dentate gyrus, interpeduncular nucleus, thalamus, ventral pallidus, nucleus basilis and red nucleus (**Figure 1.5**). Regions of the brain associated with motor functions tend to have more iron than non-motor related regions (Koeppen, 1995). This may explain why movement disorders are often associated with iron loading. In early studies (Connor et al., 1994) the iron in oligodendrocytes was reported to be bound to both H- and L-chain ferritin, in microglia to L-ferritin, while neurons had mostly neuromelanin with a little H-ferritin, and astrocytes contained hardly any ferritin. Since H-ferritin and L-ferritin have different functions their specific locations might indicate specific biological roles, one predominantly involved with iron storage (L-ferritin) and the other associated with responses to stress as well as catalysing the oxidation of Fe^{2+} to Fe^{3+} via the ferroxidase centre (H-ferritin). Large amounts of iron are sequestered in substantia nigra and in locus coerulus in neuromelanin, particularly in dopaminergic neurons (Zecca et al., 2003). Transferrin is thought to transport iron within the brain, although there is some evidence to suggest that other transport pathways may also be present, involving NTBI, non-transferrin-bound iron (Qian and Shen, 2001). The latter may include various forms of iron, as ferritin, and/or low-molecular weight iron. There appear to be at least two receptors in the brain for iron uptake, namely transferrin receptors, expressed exclusively in grey matter, and ferritin receptors present only in white matter (Hulet et al., 1999).

Evidence has been recently found for the presence of DMT1 and IREG1 in brain cells (Siddappa et al., 2002; Jiang et al., 2002), suggesting that they play an active role in both iron uptake and iron export pathways within the CNS.

1.3 METAL ION TRANSPORT AND STORAGE – COPPER

Ceruloplasmin contains 95% of the copper found in serum (Harris and Gitlin, 1996), and was assumed for many years to be the principal copper transport protein, although this

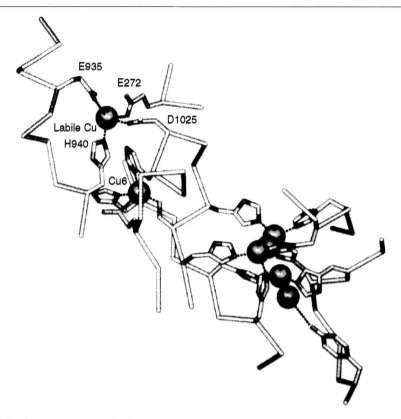

Figure 1.6: The putative metal binding site in the vicinity of the domain 6 copper atom (Cu_6) of human ceruloplasmin. The trinuclear copper cluster is located at the interface between domains 1 and 6 (bottom right of figure, copper atoms in green, water molecules in red). The green sphere at the top left of the figure represents a labile metal ion binding site (copper or iron), surrounded by His 940 and three negatively charged residues, E272 from domain 1 and E935 and D1025 from domain 6: the distance from the mononuclear copper centre is about 0.75 nm (centre of figure). The negatively charged residues Asp 1025, Glu 272 and Glu 935 could bind to a ferrous ion prior to its oxidation to the ferric state and the transfer of an electron via His 940 and the mononuclear copper towards the trinuclear centre. Adapted from Lindley (1996); figure kindly provided by Peter Lindley.

now seems improbable (see below). There are six atoms of Cu in ceruloplasmin, three mononuclear centres and one trinuclear centre (Zaitseva et al., 1996). The latter, together with the closest mononuclear site, is organized in a similar manner to that in other multi-copper oxidases (**Figure 1.6**), like ascorbate oxidase (Messerschmidt et al., 1992), suggesting that ceruloplasmin could also have oxidase activity. There is a labile metal binding site close to the mononuclear site, which could be a site for binding and oxidation of Fe^{2+} to Fe^{3+}. Ceruloplasmin has long been thought to be a ferroxidase (Osaki and Johnson, 1969), and it has been proposed (Lindley, 1996) that ceruloplasmin has a custodial role *in vivo*, ensuring that Fe^{2+} released from cells is oxidized to the potentially less toxic Fe^{3+} prior to its incorporation into apotransferrin. The neurodegenerative disease aceruloplasminaemia (Chapter 9) is associated with the absence of Cu-ceruloplasmin due to the presence of inherited mutations within the ceruloplasmin gene. This condition results in disruption of iron homeostasis, with extensive iron accumulation in a number of tissues such as brain and liver. However, in these patients, as in aceruloplasminaemic mice (Meyer et al., 2001), both copper transport and metabolism are normal, providing strong evidence against the role of ceruloplasmin as a major copper transporter (for a review see Nittis and Gitlin, 2002). It is most likely that copper is transported in serum bound to albumin.

Much of what we know about many of the component proteins which play a role in copper metabolism has been gleaned from studies in the baker's yeast, *Saccharomyces cerevisiae* (De Freitas et al., 2003) and from our increased understanding of the molecular basis of Cu-related genetic diseases (Shim and Harris, 2003). Mutations in one of two genes encoding Cu transporting P-type ATPases are responsible for Menkes and Wilson diseases in humans (Di Donato and Sarkar, 1997; Schaeffer and Gitlin, 1999). Menkes patients have a defect in intestinal Cu absorption, accumulate Cu in intestinal cells, and have Cu deficiency reflected in defects in the activity of Cu-containing enzymes. In Wilson's disease, Cu accumulates in the liver, resulting in liver cirrhosis and subsequent 'copper leakage' from the liver results in Cu deposition in the brain, provoking neurodegeneration. Characteristic Kayser-Fleischer rings arise in a similar manner from Cu deposition in the cornea of the eye.

Cu is imported across the plasma membrane of mammalian cells by a transport system that certainly requires the product of the Ctr1 gene (**Figure 1.7**), which was first identified in yeast as one of a number of high affinity Cu transporters. Yeast cells lacking high-affinity Cu transporters have defective Cu and Fe uptake, which can be restored by complementation of yeast Ctr mutants by the human Ctr1 gene (Zhou and Gitschier, 1997). Mammalian Ctr1 mRNA is expressed in all tissues examined with higher levels in liver and kidney and lower levels in brain and spleen. Ctr1 is a 190 amino acid residue protein predicted to have three

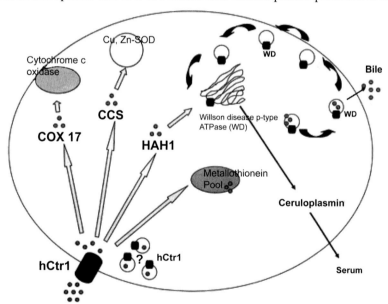

Figure 1.7: Model of copper trafficking in a hepatocyte; Cu, bound either to albumin or histidine, enters the cell via the copper transport protein Ctr1, which can be localized to the plasma membrane and to an intracellular vesicular compartment. Once inside the hepatocyte, Cu can be incorporated into the Cu/metallothionein pool, transfer to the mitochondria bound to COX17, to the cyosol bound to CCS, transfer to the Golgi compartment bound to HAH1. COX17, CCS and HAH1 are all members of the copper chaperone family. Reproduced with permission from Shim and Harris, 2003. Copyright (2003) American Society for Nutritional Sciences.

transmembrane-spanning domains (Lee et al., 2002), which can be localized to the plasma membrane and, in certain cell lines, to an intracellular vesicular compartment (Klomp et al., 2002). The role of mouse Ctr1 protein has been studied using Ctr1 gene knock-out mice (Kuo et al., 2001; Lee et al., 2001). Homozygotes die *in utero*, while heterozygotes are indistinguishable from wild-type littermates, but have a severely reduced brain Cu content. This underlines the crucial role for Ctr1 for Cu uptake, notably in brain, as well as for Cu homeostasis and embryonic development. An additional human gene, hCTR2, similar to hCTR1 and like it located in chromosome 9q31/32 has been identified in a data-base search (Zhou and Gitschier, 1997), but its role in Cu transport remains unknown. However, it shows greater homology to the yeast Ctr2 protein, which is located in the vacuole, suggesting that its role in human cells may be the release of Cu from internal compartments (Petris, 2004).

Once inside the cell (**Figure 1.7**) copper can suffer one of four possible fates: (i) it can directly enter the Cu-metallothionein storage pool, (ii) it can be transported to the mitochondria for incorporation into the terminal oxidase of the respiratory chain, cytochrome c oxidase, (iii) it can be incorporated into cytoplasmic Cu/Zn superoxide dismutase or (iv) it can be transported to the Wilson disease P-type ATPase in the *trans*-Golgi network for subsequent incorporation into the multicopper oxidase of serum, ceruloplasmin. The last three of these processes require the Cu to be transported to the target acceptor protein by specific copper chaperones (for a review see Huffman and O'Halloran, 2001). Cox17 transports copper to its site of incorporation into cytochrome c oxidase in the mitochondrion, CCS to superoxide dismutase in the cytosol, and HAH1 to the P-type ATPase and to the key enzyme in neurotransmitter synthesis, tyrosinase, in the secretory pathway (Petris, 2004). The copper chaperones are a ubiquitous family of proteins which have been identified in species from bacteria to man. They have very similar protein folds, an open-faced β-sandwich consisting of four β-strands forming an antiparallel β-sheet, situated below two α-helices, illustrated for CopZp in **Figure 1.8**. The metal-binding sequence motif –CxxxC–, occurs on the mobile loop between the first β-strand and the first α-helix. Like the Cu transporter Ctr1, they are adapted to bind Cu^+ rather than Cu^{2+}. Since Cu is transported in extracellular fluids bound to albumin or to histidine (most likely as Cu^{2+}), the question which remains is whether Cu is transported across the plasma membrane in mammals in this form by the divalent cation transporter DMT1, or whether a reductase system coupled to the Ctr1 gene product, is involved. It also remains to be established whether the transport of Cu across the intestinal tract and within brain cells may also involve the divalent metal ion transporter DMT1 or a reductase associated with an apical membrane Ctr1 protein.

Metallothioneins are ubiquitous, low molecular weight, thiol-rich proteins which have a selective capacity to bind metal ions, such as zinc, cadmium, mercury and copper. Mammalian metallothioneins are made up of 4 major isoforms designated MT-1 to MT-4. MT-1 and MT-2 are expressed in most tissues, including brain while MT-3 is predominantly expressed in the CNS, and is thought to be involved in neuromodulatory events (Hidalgo et al., 2001).

1.4 METAL ION TRANSPORT AND STORAGE – ZINC

Zinc is a ubiquitous metal ion, which plays an important role both in catalysis and in the stabilization of the structure of many proteins, including a number of so-called zinc-finger

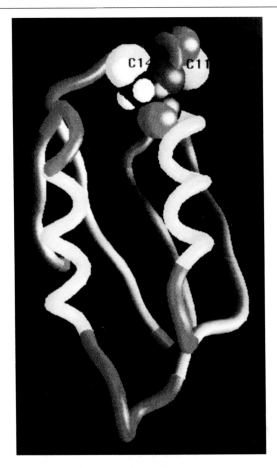

Figure 1.8: NMR structure of the reduced copper chaperone CopZ from *Enterococcus hirae*. Reprinted from Harrison et al., Copyright 2000, with permission fron Elsevier.

proteins, many of which bind to DNA promoter sites. Several mammalian Zn transporters have been identified recently (for recent reviews see Eide, 2004; Palmiter and Huang, 2004), and the number of candidate genes is growing rapidly. They can be classified into two families. The first, the SLC39 transporters (Eide, 2004), are found across the entire phylogenetic spectrum and are members of the ZIP family of metal ion transporters. This designates Zrt-, Irt-like proteins, reflecting the first members of the family to be identified, namely Zrt1 and Zrt2, the primary Zn uptake transporters in the yeast *Saccharomyces cerevisiae*, and Irt1, the major iron uptake transporter into the roots of the plant *Arabadopsis thaliana*. There are more than 90 members of the ZIP family (Gaither and Eide, 2001) which transport metal ions into the cytosol, mostly across the plasma membrane, although some, like Zrt3 in yeast, transport Zn out of intracellular compartments (the lysosome-like storage vacuole). The human genome encodes 14 SLC39-related proteins, of which so far only a few (Zip1, Zip2, Zip4) have been shown to be involved in Zn transport (**Figure 1.9**). Zip1 is widely distributed in mammalian tissues, localizes to plasma membrane and endoplasmic reticulum and seems to be regulated by Zn status. Zip2 is expressed at low levels and only in a few tissues, which however include cervical epithelium and optic nerve: this expression,

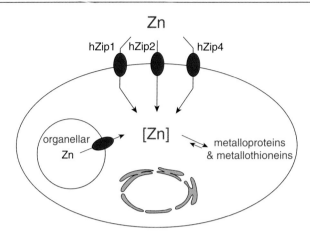

Figure 1.9: Roles of SLC39 proteins in metal metabolism. Available evidence indicates that hZip1, hZip2 and hZip4 are responsible for Zn uptake in cells where they are expressed. Based on their similarity to yeast ZIP proteins, it is possible that human SLC39 proteins transport metal ions out of intracellular compartments. Some SLC39 proteins may transport other metal ions than Zn (eg. Fe, Mn). From Eide (2004). Reproduced with kind permission of Springer Science and Business Media.

like Zip1, appears to be regulated by Zn (Cao et al., 2001). Zip4 is clearly involved in the uptake of dietary Zn into intestinal enterocytes, and mutations in Zip4 have been found in patients with acrodermatitis enteropathica, a recessive disorder of Zn absorption which results in Zn deficiency.

The second, the SLC30 family of transporters (Palmiter and Huang, 2004), was previously called the CDF (cation diffusion facilitator) family and all of the members are thought to be involved in the efflux of Zn from the cytosol, either out of the cell across the plasma membrane or into intracellular compartments, like endosomes, secretory granules, synaptic vesicles, or the Golgi apparatus. Nine members of the ZnT family have been identified in mammals (**Figure 1.10**). ZnT-1 is widely expressed in tissues, including brain, and is the only member of the family to locate to the plasma membrane where it is assumed to function as a Zn efflux transporter (Palmiter and Findley, 1995). Its expression is regulated by Zn, and loss of function of mouse *Znt1* is embryonic lethal. ZnT-2 is found in the membrane of an acidic endosomal/lysosomal compartment and may play a role in zinc sequestration (Palmiter et al., 1996a). The mRNA of ZnT-3 is expressed particularly in brain and testis, although the protein is not found in testis. ZnT-3 is most abundant in the neurons of the hippocampus and the cerebral cortex, and is localized to synaptic vesicles of glutaminergic neurons which sequester Zn, suggestive that ZnT-3 transports zinc into this compartment (Palmiter et al., 1996b). Loss of mouse *Znt-3* prevents Zn accumulation in these synaptic vesicles.

It is possible that in humans Zn can also be transported across membranes by other proteins, like the SLC11 gene family of metal ion transporters which are energized by H^+ electrochemical gradients (for a review see McKenzie and Hediger, 2004). This family has two members, DMT1 and NRAMP1. DMT1 is involved in the transport of dietary iron and perhaps zinc across the brush border membrane of the intestine and the transport of iron out of the endosomal compartment in the transferrin-cell cycle described above. NRAMP1

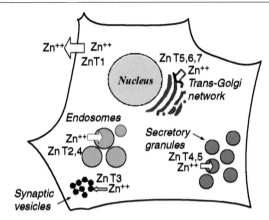

Figure 1.10: Cellular localization of SLC30 class of Zn efflux transporters. ZnT1 is targeted to the plasma membrane where it facilitates Zn efflux from cells: all the other members facilitate Zn transport into various intracellular compartments. From Palmiter and Huang (2004). Reproduced with kind permission of Springer Science and Business Media.

(natural resistance-associated macrophage protein-1) confers resistance to microbial infection, and functions at the phagolysosomal membrane of macrophages and neutrophils, either by extruding essential metal ions (including Mn^{2+} and possibly Fe^{2+}) from the phagolysosome, or alternatively, by concentrating metal ions like Fe^{2+} within the phagolysosome, resulting in the generation of toxic free radicals.

Zn metabolism itself seems to be regulated essentially through Zn-dependent control of transcription, translation and intracellular trafficking of transporters as well as its storage, like copper, in metallothionein. It is likely that Zn homeostasis in humans requires the coordinated activity of members of several Zn transporter families, particularly those involved in Zn ingress and egress from cells and organelles.

1.5 METAL ION TRANSPORT AND STORAGE – OTHER METALS

While specific transporters in animal cells for iron, copper and zinc have been described, there are other important metal ions which must also be accumulated, like manganese, a key component of mitochondrial superoxide dismutase, cobalt, with its important role as a cofactor in cobalamine (vitamin B12) enzymes, and molybdenum, present for example in xanthine oxidase. It is likely that some of the systems mentioned previously for Zn and Fe transport are also used by other divalent transition metal ions, like Mn and Co. This is most notably the case for the SLC11 and for the SLC39 gene families, which are, by definition, divalent metal ion transporters. Of the SLC11 family, DMT1, is widely expressed in human tissues, including brain, and accepts a broad range of metal ions, including Mn^{2+} and Co^{2+}, and NRAMP1 (see above), which is clearly involved in transporting Mn out of the phagolysosome in activated macrophages. Among the members of the SLC39 family, the Atx2 protein seems to transport Mn out of the Golgi apparatus in yeast (Lin and Culotta, 1996). The role of these families of proteins in the transport of Mn and Co in human cells is still not clear, while for Mo we have virtually no information.

1.6 METALS AND THEIR HOMEOSTASIS (WITH PARTICULAR REFERENCE TO IRON AND COPPER)

Cellular iron homeostasis is regulated at the level of translation of pre-existing mRNAs into protein by the ribosomal protein synthesizing machinery. These systems have been characterized both *in vitro* in cell lines as well as *in vivo* in tissues after iron loading and depletion. However, iron homeostasis in neurons, astrocytes and microglia has received little attention.

Iron Responsive Elements (IREs) are RNA-hairpin structures which are found in the 3'-untranslated region of transferrin receptor mRNA, and in the 5'-untranslated region of ferritin subunits (**Figure 1.11**). The regulation of the translation of these mRNAs involves cytosolic IRE-binding proteins, called Iron Responsive Proteins (IRP), which in conditions of iron deficency bind to the IREs, permitting synthesis of transferrin receptor, and preventing ferritin synthesis. In iron overload, the IRPs do not bind to the mRNAs, and as a consequence, ferritin is synthesized and transferrin receptor mRNA is degraded (Crichton, 1991). This ensures that when iron is in short supply, transferrin receptors are expressed allowing the cell to take up iron from circulating transferrin, while blocking synthesis of the un-required storage protein. When the cellular levels of iron are adequate, the potentially toxic iron excedent in the LIP can be stored in ferritin, while in the absence of IRP protection, the transferrin receptor mRNA is subjected to nuclease digestion, and destroyed.

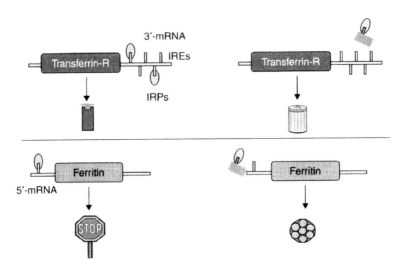

Figure 1.11: Production of transferrin receptor and of ferritin are regulated at the level of mRNA. Iron Responsive Elements (IREs) in mRNA of the transferrin receptor (TfR) are localized in the 3'mRNA region, and in mRNA of ferritin in the 5'mRNA promotor region. The system is designed to allow the cells to procure iron from the plasma, by expressing more transferrin receptors, if they need iron for production of proteins, and to protect cells against potentially toxic iron by expressing ferritin molecules, able to hide Fe(III) within its core. The system is regulated by Iron Responsive Protein 1 (IRP). In iron deficiency IRP inhibits RNase attack of TfR mRNA, and inhibits production of ferritin while sitting on an IRE in the 5'mRNA region. If the LIP contains abundant amounts of iron, modified IRP has no affinity for IRE, resulting in destruction of TfR mRNA. At the same time free IRE on ferritin mRNA allows sufficient expression of ferritin. From Crichton, 2001.

There are two closely related Iron Responsive Proteins, designated IRP-1 and IRP-2 in many mammalian cell types, which act as iron sensors by existing in two different conformations. When iron is in short supply, both IRPs can bind with high affinity to the IREs. Both IRP-1 and IRP-2 are induced in iron-deficient cells but lose their IRE-binding capacity after iron administration (**Figure 1.12**). Both IRP-1 and IRP-2 have been identified in perinatal rat brain (Siddappa et al., 2002). Immunolocalization studies show a quite distinct distribution of the two IRPs in mouse brain (Liebold et al., 2001), which may be indicative of distinct roles for IRP-1 and IRP-2 in the regulation of iron homeostasis. It is suggested that IRP1 may provide a maintenance function whereas IRP-2 could participate in modulating central autonomic network functions, including cardiopulmonary, gustatory and fine motor control. Targeted deletion of IRP-2 in mice leads to misregulation of iron metabolism in the intestinal mucosa and the CNS, which leads to neurodegenerative disease associated with a movement disorder in adulthood, characterized by ataxia, bradykinesia and tremor (La Vaute et al., 2001). Iron accumulates in the cytosol of neurons and oligoden-drocytes in distinctive brain regions. Abnormal accumulations of ferritin colocalize with iron accumulations in populations of neurons that degenerate, and iron-loaded oligodendrocytes

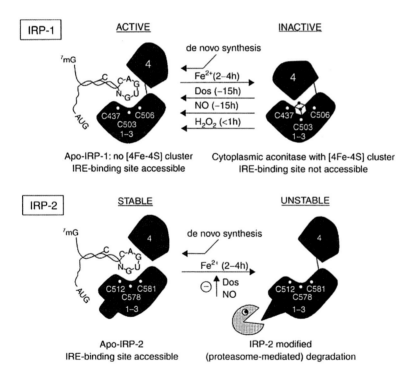

Figure 1.12: Regulation of IRP-1 and IRP-2. The two IRPs are shown as homologous four domain proteins that bind to IREs (*Left*) In iron-replete cells, IRP-1 assembles a cubane Fe-S cluster that is liganded via cysteines 437, 503 and 506. Similar cysteines are conserved in IRP-2 (Cys 512, 578 and 581), but it is unresolved whether they also coordinate an Fe-S cluster. (*Right*) In iron-replete cells, IRP-2 is targeted for destruction via a specific region (shaded in black), whereas IRP-1, with a 4Fe-4S cluster, is stable and active as a cytoplasmic aconitase. Multiple signals induce IRE-binding by IRP-1 with distinct kinetics. Whether or not NO and H_2O_2 induce IRP-1 by apoprotein formation remains to be addressed directly. From Hentze and Kühn, Copyright (1996) National Academy of Sciences, USA.

accumulate ubiquitin-positive inclusions. Mice which are homozygous for targeted deletion of IRP-2 and in addition heterozygous for targeted deletion of IRP-1 develop a much more severe form of neurodegeneration with extensive axonopathy in white matter tracts associated with marked increases in ferritin and ferric iron, and eventually vacuolization, notably in the substantia nigra (Smith et al., 2004). Axonal degeneration is apparent before evidence for abnormalities or loss of neuronal cell bodies can be detected. At a later stage, neuronal cell bodies degenerate in the substantia nigra and other vulnerable areas, microglia are activated and vacuoles appear. Gait and motor impairment are seen when axonopathy is pronounced but loss of neuronal cell bodies is minimal. A high resolution magnetic resonance imaging (MRI) study has been carried out on mice which are homozygous for targeted deletion of IRP-2 (Grabill et al., 2003) and a distinctive MRI pattern was found, reflecting both ferritin accumulation in areas known to accumulate ferritin iron in this animal model, but also increased water content in several areas of the brain, including the substantia nigra and superior colliculus. Subsequent histological examination showed the presence of relatively small, previously unappreciated vacuoles in these brain regions. If this high resolution technique can be applied to human subjects, it could represent a very significant advance in both the diagnosis and therapeutic monitoring of human neurological diseases. Iron homeostasis in neurons, astrocytes and microglia has received little attention. Whether these cells behave like parenchymal or RE cells is unknown. Studies of an *in vitro* iron-loaded immortalized microglial cell line, showed similar results to that of the inflammatory processes identified in the iron-loaded macrophage, i.e. a reduction in iNOS (Ward and Ledeque, unpublished results).

IRP-1 is expressed in all vertebrate tissues, whereas IRP-2 is less abundant than IRP-1 in most cells, but is highly expressed in intestine and brain. IRP-1 is a monomeric 889 amino acid protein with an amino acid sequence which shows extensive homology to mitochondrial and bacterial aconitases. These 4Fe-4S cluster enzymes convert citrate to isocitrate, and IRP-1 has three of the cysteine residues (Cys 437, 503 and 506) which anchor the iron-sulphur cluster into the mitochondrial and bacterial enzymes (Hirling et al., 1994). Their mutagenesis to Ser converts IRP-1 to a form which constitutively binds to IREs. When iron supply to cells is increased, the IRE binding capacity of IRP-1 is lost, by incorporation of the 4Fe-4S cluster (**Figure 1.12**).

Human IRP-2 shares 57% homology with human IRP-1, but is slightly larger than IRP-1, due to the presence of a 73-residue inclusion. IRP-2 has no aconitase activity, although three cysteine residues similar to those that coordinate the iron-sulphur cluster in IRP-1 are conserved (Cys 512, 578 and 581). IRP-2 binds to IREs like IRP-1, however, in iron-replete cells, IRP-2 is degraded (**Figure 1.12**). This degradation is mediated through the inclusion domain (Iwai et al., 1995), and is prevented by inhibitors which block proteosome formation, but not by inhibitors of lysosomal proteases or calpain (Iwai et al., 1995; Guo et al., 1995). It seems likely that the proteosome (and also ubiquitinylation) is involved in IRP-2 degradation. IRP-2 is sensitive to iron status and can compensate for loss of IRP-1 by increasing its binding activity in animals. Therefore IRP-2 dominates post-transcriptional regulation of iron metabolism.

Since this mode of protein degradation will be relevant for later Chapters on the formation of aggregated protein inclusion bodies in many neurodegenerative diseases, we present here a brief summary of the operation of this important protein degradation mechanism. Eukaryotic cells have two systems for protein degradation, lysosomal mechanisms and ATP-dependent cytosol localized mechanisms. The lysosomal compartment fuses with autophagic vesicles, consisting of membrane-enclosed bits of cytosol, and the

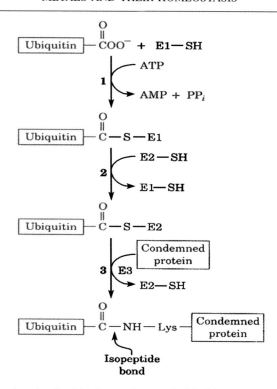

Figure 1.13: The reactions involved in the attachment of ubiquitin to a protein. In the first part the carboxyl group of ubiquitin is coupled to E_1 by a thioether linkage in a reaction driven by ATP hydrolysis. The activated ubiquitin is subsequently transferred to a sulphydryl group of E_2 and then in a reaction catalysed by E_3 to the ε-amino group of a Lys residue on a condemned protein, thereby flagging the protein for proteolytic degradation by the 26S proteosome. From Voet and Voet, 1995.

contents are degraded to their basic building blocks which are recycled in a non-selective manner.

Reticulocytes, which do not contain lysosomes, nonetheless degrade abnormal proteins. This observation led to the discovery of the ATP-dependent ubiquitin system for protein degradation, which also involves the 26S proteosome (**Figure 1.13**). Proteins that have been marked out for degradation are identified by covalent coupling to **ubiquitin**, a 76-residue protein which is both ubiquitous and abundant in eukarotes. Ubiquitin is very highly conserved–identical in human, fish, frogs and fruit fly (*Drosophila*) and with only 3 residues different between human and baker's yeast. The attachment of the ubiquitin tag to the condemned protein involves three steps, as described in **Figure 1.13**. In the first step, ubiquitin is bound by its carboxyl terminus to **ubiquitin-activating enzyme**, E_1 in an ATP-dependent process. Most organisms, including humans, have only one E_1. Ubiquitin is then transferred to the thiol group of one of a number of **ubiquitin-conjugating enzymes**, E_2s, of which there are over 20 in mammals. Then, the **ubiquitin-protein ligase** (E_3) transfers the ubiquitin from E_2 to the amino group of a Lys residue of its target protein, forming an isopeptide bond. Mammalian cells contain a large number of E_3s, each mediating the ubiquitination of a specific set of proteins. Ubiquinated proteins are subsequently proteo-lytically degraded by the large (2000kD) multisubunit protein complex known as the 26S

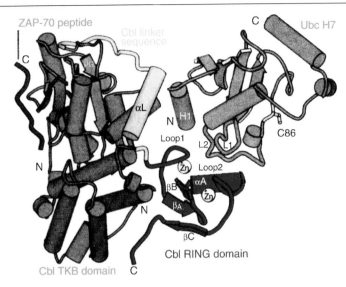

Figure 1.14: The structure of the ternary complex, consisting of an E_2 ubiquitin-conjugating enzyme, an E_3 RING finger ubiquitin ligase and the target protein's ubiquitination domain. From Voet and Voet, 2004.

proteosome. In this process, the ubiquitin molecules are not degraded, but are returned to the cell for reutilization.

An important family of E_3 ubiquitin-protein ligases are members of the so-called **RING finger** (RING for *R*eally *I*nteresting *N*ew *G*ene) protein family. They all contain a RING finger, a 40- to 60-residue motif which binds two Zn^{2+} ions in a characteristic consensus sequence (like the zinc-finger motif in certain DNA-binding proteins). The RING finger interacts with both the ubiquitin-conjugating E_2 and with the domain of the condemned protein containing the Lys residue to be ubiquinated (**Figure 1.14**). A number of post-transcriptional modifications in condemned proteins have been described, including phosphorylation, proline hydroxylation and glycosylation as recognition signals for E_3. We might point out here that **parkin**, the product of a gene linked to Parkinson's disease, is a RING finger E_3 ubiquitin-protein ligase (Shimura et al., 2000). Recently (Yamanaka et al., 2003) the RING finger protein **HOIL-1** has been shown to act as an E_3 ligase for oxidized IRP-2, suggesting that oxidation is the specific recognition signal for ubiquination. In iron-rich cells oxidation of IRP-2 is generated by haem and by oxygen, which might indicate that iron sensing by IRP-2 depends on haem synthesis and availability.

REFERENCES

Arambura, J., Rao, A. and Klee, C.B. (2001) *Curr. Top. Cell Regul.*, **36**, 237–295.
Augustine, G.J. (2001) *Curr. Opin. Chem. Biol.*, **5**, 223–227.
Beard, J. (2003) *J. Nutr.*, **133**, 1468S–1472S.
Burdette, S.C. and Lippard, S.J. (2003) *Proc. Natl. Acad. Sci. USA*, **100**, 3605–3610.
Cammarota, M., Bevilaqua, L.R., Viola, H., Kerr, D.S. *et al.* (2002) *Cell. Mol. Neurobiol.*, **22**, 259–267.
Cao, J., Bobo, J.A., Liuzzi, J.P. and Cousins, R.J. (2001) *J. Leucocyt. Biol.*, **70**, 559–566.

Carafoli, E. (2002) *Proc. Natl. Acad. Sci. USA*, **99**, 1115–1122.

Connor, J.R. (2003) *J. Neurol. Sci.*, **207**, 112–113.

Connor, J.R., Boeshore, K.L. and Benkovic, S.A. (1994) *J. Neurosci., Res.*, **37**, 461–465.

Crichton, R.R. (2001) *Inorganic Biochemistry of Iron Metabolism From Molecular Mechanisms to Clinical Consequences.* John Wiley & Sons, Chichester.

De Freitas, J., Wintz, H., Kim., J.H., Poynton, H. *et al.* (2003) *Biometals*, **16**, 185–197.

Di Donato, M. and Sarkar, B. (1997) *Biochim. Biophys. Acta*, **1360**, 3–16.

Eide, D.J. (2004) *Pflugers Arch.*, **447**, 796–800.

Erunda, N.E. and Kennedy, M.B. (1985) *J. Neurosci.*, **5**, 3270–3277.

Gaither, L.A. and Eide, D. (2001) *Biometals*, **14**, 251–270.

Godwin, H.A. (2001) *Curr. Opin. Neurobiol.*, **11**, 320–326.

Götz, M., Double, K., Gerlach, M., Youdim, M.B.H. and Riederer, P. (2004) *Ann. N. Y. Acad. Sci.*, **1012**, 193–208.

Grabill, C., Silva, A.C., Smith, S.S., Koretsky, A.P. and Rouault, T.A. (2003) *Brain Res.*, **971**, 95–106.

Guo, B., Phillips, J.D., Yu, Y. and Leibold, E.A. (1995) *J. Biol. Chem.*, **270**, 21645–21651.

Harris, Z.L. and Gitlin, J.D. (1996) *Am. J. Clin. Nutr.*, **63**, 836S–841S.

Harrison, M.D., Jones, C.E., Solioz, M. and Dameron, C.T. (2000) *TIBS*, **25**, 29–32.

He, Y., Alam, S.L., Proteasa, S.V., Zhang, Y. *et al.* (2004) *Biochem.*, **43**, 16254–16262.

Hentze, M.W. and Kühn, L.C. (1996) *Proc. Natl. Acad. Sci. USA*, **93**, 8175–8182.

Hidalgo, J., Aschner, M., Zatta, P. and Vasak, M. (2001) *Brain Res. Bull.*, **55**, 133–145.

Hirling, H., Henderson, B.R. and Kühn, L.C. (1994) *EMBO J.*, **13**, 453–461.

Hodgkin, A.L. and Huxley, A.F. (1953) *J. Physiol.*, **117**, 530–.

Hudmon, A. and Schulman, H. (2002) *Annnu. Rev. Biochem.*, **71**, 473–510.

Huffmann, D.L. and O'Halloran, T.V. (2001) *Annnu. Rev. Biochem.*, **70**, 677–701.

Hulet, S.W., Powers, S. and Connor, J.R. (1999) *J. Neurol. Sci.*, **165**, 48–55.

Iwai, K., Klausner, R.D. and Rouault, T.A. (1995) *EMBO J.*, **14**, 5350–5357.

Jiang, D.H., Ke, Y., Cheng, Y.Z., Ho, K.P. and Qian, Z.M. (2002) *Dev. Neurosci.*, **24**, 94–98.

Klomp, A.E.M., Tops, B.B.J., Van Den Berg, I.E.T., Berger, R. *et al.* (2002) *Biochem. J.*, **364**, 497–505.

Koeppen, A.H. (1995) *J Neurol. Sci.*, **134**, Suppl. 1–9.

Koh, T.-W. and Bellen, H.J. (2003) *TRENDS Neurosc.*, **26**, 413–422.

Kuo, Y.M., Zhou, B., Cosco, D. and Gitschier, J. (2001) *Proc. Natl. Acad. Sci. USA*, **98**, 6836–6841.

La Vaute, T., Smith, S., Cooperman, S., Iwai, K. *et al.* (2001) *Nat. Genet.*, **27**, 209–214.

Lee, J., Pena, M.M.O., Nose, Y. and Thiele, D.J. (2002) *J. Biol. Chem.*, **277**, 4380–4387.

Lee, J., Prohaska, J.R. and Thiele, D.J. (2001) *Proc. Natl. Acad. Sci. USA*, **98**, 6842–6847.

Lesuisse, E., Santos, R., Matzanke, B.F., Knight, S.A. *et al.* (2003) *Hum. Mol. Genet.*, **12**, 879–889.

Liebold, E.A., Gahring, L.C. and Rogers, S.W. (2001) *Histochem. Cell Biol.*, **115**, 195–203.

Lin, S.J. and Culotta, V.C. (1996) *Mol. Cell Biol.*, **16**, 6303–6312.

Lindley, P.F. (1996) *Rep. Prog. Phys.*, **59**, 867–893.

McKenzie, B. and Hediger, M.A. (2004) *Pflugers Arch.*, **447**, 571–579.

Mermelstein, P.G., Deissenroth, K., Dasgupta, N., Isaksen, A.L. *et al.* (2001) *Proc. Natl. Acad. Sci. USA*, **98**, 15342–15347.

Meyer, L.A., Durley, A.P., Prohaska, J.R. and Harris, Z.L. (2001) *J. Biol. Chem.*, **276**, 36857–36861.

Messerschmidt, A., Steigemann, W., Huber, R., Lang, G. *et al.* (1992) *Eur. J. Biochem.*, **209**, 597–602.

Muhlenhoff, U., Richhardt, N., Ristow, M., Kispal, G. and Lill, R. (2002) *Hum. Mol. Genet.*, **11**, 2025–2036.

Nittis, T. and Gitlin, J.D. (2002) *Semin. Hematol.*, **39**, 282–289.

Osaki, S. and Johnson, D.A. (1969) *J. Biol. Chem.*, **244**, 5757–5758.

Olson, E.N. and Williams, R.S. (2000) *BioEssays*, **22**, 510–519.

Palmiter, R.D. and Findley, S.D. (1995) *EMBO J.*, **14**, 639–649.

Palmiter, R.D., Cole, T.B. and Findley, S.D. (1996a) *EMBO J.*, **15**, 1781–1791.

Palmiter, R.D., Cole, T.B., Quaife, C.J. and Findley, S.D. (1996b) *Proc. Natl. Acad. Sci. USA*, **93**, 14934–14939.

Palmiter, R.D. and Huang, L. (2004) *Pflugers Arch.*, **447**, 744–751.

Perls, M. (1867) *Virchows Arch. A*, **39**, 44–48.

Petris, M.J. (2004) *Pflugers Arch.*, **447**, 752–755.

Qian, Z.M. and Shen, X. (2001) *Trends Mol. Med.*, **7**, 103–108.

Schaeffer, M. and Gitlin, J.D. (1999) *Am. J. Physiol.*, **276**, G311–G316.

Sharrow, K.M., Kumar, A. and Foster, T.C. (2002) *Neuroscience*, **113**, 89–97.

Shimura, H., Hattori, N., Kubo, S., Mizuno, Y. *et al.* (2000) *Nat. Genet.*, **25**, 302–305.

Siddappa, A.J., Rao, R.B., Wobken, J.D., Leibold, E.A. *et al.* (2002) *J. Neurosci. Res.*, **68**, 761–775.

Shim, H. and Harris, Z.L. (2003) *J. Nutr.*, **133**, 1527S–1531S.

Smith, S.R., Cooperman, S., La Vaute, T., Tresser, N. *et al.* (2004) *Ann. N. Y. Acad. Sci.*, **1012**, 65–83.

Sudhoff, T.C. (2002) *J. Biol. Chem.*, **277**, 7629–7632.

Takeda, A., Minami, A., Seki, Y. and Oku, N. (2003) *Epliepsy Res.*, **57**, 169–174.

Takeda, A., Minami, A., Seki, Y. and Oku, N. (2004) *J. Neurosci. Res.*, **75**, 225–229.

Voet, D. and Voet, J.G. (1995) *Biochemistry 2nd edition*, John Wiley & Sons, Chichester.

Voet, D. and Voet, J.G. (2004) *Biochemistry 3rd edition*, John Wiley & Sons, Chichester.

Ward, R.J., Ramsey, M., Dickson, D.P., Hunt, C. *et al.* (1994) *Eur. J. Biochem.*, **225**, 187–194.

Yamanaka, K., Ishikawa, H., Megumi, Y., Tokunaga, F. *et al.* (2003) *Nat. Cell Biol.*, **5**, 336–340.

Zaitseva, I., Zaitsev, V., Card, G., Moshkov, K. *et al.* (1996) *J. Biol. Inorg. Chem.*, **1**, 15–23.

Zecca, L., Youdim, M.B., Riederer, P., Connor, J.R. and Crichton, R.R. (2004) *Nature Rev. Neurosci.*, **5**, 863–873.

Zecca L., Zucca, F.A., Wilms, H. and Sulzer, D. (2003) *Trends Neurosci.*, **26**, 578–580 (2003).

Zhou, B. and Gitschier, J. (1997) *Proc. Natl. Acad. Sci. USA*, **94**, 7481–7486.

2

Oxidative Stress and Redox-Active Metal Ions

2.1 INTRODUCTION – THE OXYGEN PARADOX

It can be argued that one of the most momentous events in the evolution of our now green planet was the appearance about 2.7×10^9 years ago of cyanobacteria which were capable of using solar energy to split water molecules and evolve molecular dioxygen. This progressively transformed the previously essentially reducing atmosphere of earth into the oxidizing atmosphere that we have today. In the space of a relatively short time, at least as measured on a geological time scale, oxygen become a dominant chemical entity. One of the consequences, clearly visible in the Precambrian deposits of red ferric oxides laid down in the geological strata at that time, was that iron, freely available in its reduced Fe^{2+} form, became much less so, as the product of its oxidation, Fe^{3+}, hydrolysed, polymerized and precipitated. At the same time, copper, poorly available in its reduced Cu^+ form became much more accessible as the more water soluble Cu^{2+}.

The positive side of the arrival of oxygen was that organisms which developed respiratory chains were able to extract almost 20 times more energy from metabolism than was available using redox-balanced fermentations. However, as we will see in what follows, the downside was that molecular oxygen proved to be toxic, particularly in the presence of redox-active metal ions like iron and copper. Since we live in an oxygen-rich environment, the consequence is that we continuously produce oxygen-derived free radicals, so-called Reactive Oxygen Species (ROS). The most potentially dangerous of ROS is the hydroxyl ion, $OH^\bullet$, a short-lived but highly reactive free radical, which causes enormous damage to biological molecules. In addition to ROS, reactive nitrogen species (RNS) are also generated, notably $NO^\bullet$. Under normal conditions, such free radicals will be rapidly detoxified by the body's defence systems described below. However, as we will see, under certain circumstances, greater amounts of ROS and RNS are produced, which end up by overwhelming the cellular defence mechanisms. This is the so-called oxygen paradox – oxygen is an absolute necessity for our energy-economical aerobic life style, yet it is a potential toxin.

Metal-based Neurodegeneration: From Molecular Mechanisms to Therapeutic Strategies   R. R. Crichton and R. J. Ward
© 2006 John Wiley & Sons, Ltd

2.2 REACTIVE OXYGEN SPECIES (ROS)

Most atoms and molecules have their electrons arranged in pairs, each of which has opposite intrinsic spin angular momentum. Molecules which have one or more unpaired electrons are termed free radicals, and are generally very reactive. Free radicals are produced in the normal course of intermediary metabolism, but are usually contained within the confines of enzyme active sites. An example is the transformation of methylmalonyl-CoA to succinyl-CoA by methylmalonyl-CoA mutase **(Figure 2.1)**. This reaction is important in the metabolism of fatty acids with an odd number of carbon atoms. Among other important biochemical reactions which require free radical intermediates is the transformation of ribonucleotides into deoxyribonucleotides, catalysed by ribonucleotide reductases.

The dioxygen molecule prefers to accept electrons one at a time, and since transition metals like iron and copper can accept and donate single electrons, they greatly facilitate the reduction of O_2. The chemistry of iron with oxygen and its two-electron reduction product, hydrogen peroxide is outlined in **Figure 2.2** (Crichton and Pierre, 2001). The first oxyradical, or Reactive Oxygen Species (ROS) to be formed from O_2, by autoxidation of metal complexes, is the superoxide radical, O_2^-. Superoxide is not itself particularly reactive, but it is the precursor of much more reactive radicals. Addition of a second electron to O_2^-

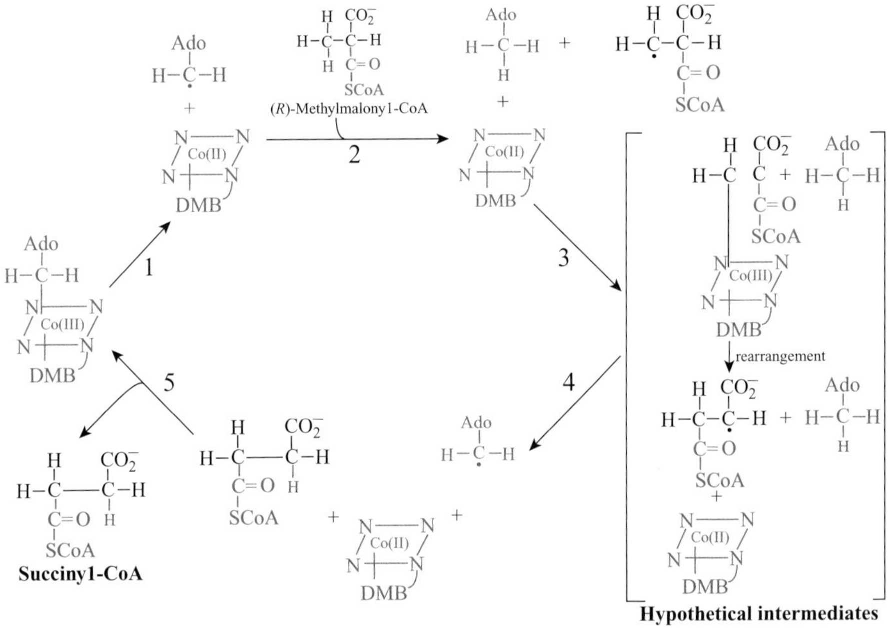

Figure 2.1: The proposed mechanism of methylmalonyl-CoA mutase: **(1)** The homolytic cleavage of the C-Co(III) bond yielding a $5'$-deoxyadanosyl radical and cobalamin in its Co(II) oxidation state. **(2)** Abstraction of a hydrogen atom from the methylmalonyl-CoA molecule, generating a methylmalonyl-CoA radical. **(3)** Hypothetical formation of a C–Co bond between the methylmalonyl-CoA radical and the coenzyme, followed by carbon skeleton rearrangement to form a succinyl-CoA radical. **(4)** Abstraction of a hydrogen atom from $5'$-deoxyadanosine by the succinyl-CoA radical to regenerate the $5'$-deoxyadanosyl radical. **(5)** Release of succinyl-CoA and reformation of the coenzyme. From Voet and Voet (1995).

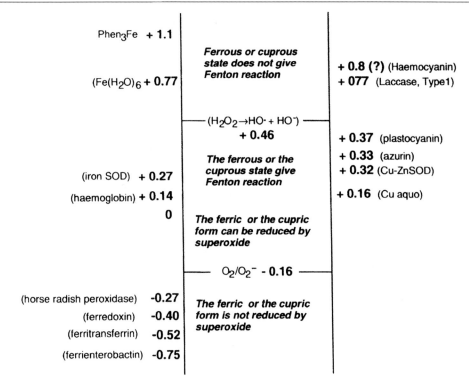

Figure 2.2: Iron-oxygen chemistry (multi-bridged species have been omitted). Copper can carry out many of the same reactions, with Cu^I and Cu^{II} replacing Fe^{II} and Fe^{III}, although the Cu^{III} state is probably not biologically relevant. From Crichton and Pierre (2001).

gives the peroxide ion O_2^{2-}, which is not a free radical. At neutral pH values, O_2^{2-} will be protonated to give hydrogen peroxide, H_2O_2. The one-electron reduction of H_2O_2, the well known Fenton reaction (Fenton, 1894), gives the hydroxyl radical, $OH^\bullet$ [1], one of the most reactive free radical species known, which can react with a wide number of cellular constituents.

$$Fe^{2+} + H_2O_2 \rightarrow Fe^{3+} + OH^\bullet + OH^- \qquad [1]$$

It has been suggested that superoxide can then reduce Fe^{3+} to molecular oxygen and Fe^{2+}. The sum of this reaction [2] plus the Fenton reaction [1] leads to the production of molecular oxygen plus hydroxyl radical and hydroxyl anion from superoxide and hydrogen peroxide [3] in the presence of catalytic amounts of iron –the Haber-Weiss reaction described by Haber and Weiss (1934), but which cannot function in the absence of trace amounts of iron.

$$Fe^{3+} + O_2^- \rightarrow Fe^{2+} + O_2 \qquad [2]$$
$$O_2^- + H_2O_2 \rightarrow O_2 + OH^\bullet + OH^- \qquad [3]$$

As has been pointed out (Pierre et al., 2002) one must be careful to avoid the pitfalls of using standard redox potentials under equilibrium conditions, conditions which are certainly not met within cells. This implies that in physiological conditions it may not be so easy to carry out reaction [2], particularly in competition with the rapid dismutase reaction.

A number of iron-dependent enzymes (catalases, peroxidases and monooxygenases) generate high-valent Fe(**IV**) or Fe(**V**) reactive intermediates in their catalytic cycle. Copper can carry out many of the same reactions with oxygen as iron, with Cu(**I**) and Cu(**II**) replacing Fe(**II**) and Fe(**III**), although the Cu(**III**) state is probably not biologically relevant (Crichton and Pierre, 2001).

ROS are produced in the course of normal metabolism by some enzyme-catalysed reactions, such as xanthine oxidase, cyclooxygenases and the cytochrome P45Os. However, it has become clear that the most important cellular source of free radicals (including ROS) is the electron transport chain in the mitochondria (Cadenas, 2004), as is discussed below.

ROS play an important role in signal transduction and gene expression, through the activation of nuclear transcription factors. However, there are some cells in the body which use the cytotoxicity of ROS to attack and kill invading microorganisms. When macrophages and neutrophils encounter a bacterium or other foreign particle, they ingest it and internalize it within an intracellular compartment known as a phagosome (**Figure 2.3**). The multi-component enzyme, NADPH oxidase is then assembled within the membrane of the phagosome (**Figure 2.3**). This enzyme then generates superoxide inside the phagosome, which undergoes dismutation to hydrogen peroxide, and leads to Fe^{2+}-catalysed hydroxyl

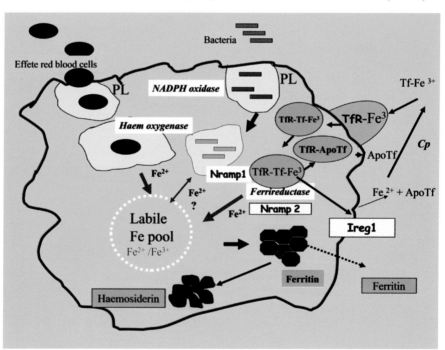

Figure 2.3: Iron homeostasis and immune functioning of the macrophage. Effete red blood cells or bacteria are phagocytosed by the macrophage and incorporated into a phagolysosome, PL. Transferrin-bound iron ($Tf-Fe^{3+}$) is endocytosed by the transferrin receptor (TfR), released into the cytosol as Fe^{2+} by the combined action of a ferrireductase and the transporter, Nramp2. Apotransferrin (ApoTf) is returned to the circulation where it can take up iron with the assistance of ceruloplasmin (Cp). Reproduced with permission from Crichton and Pierre, 'Old Iron, Young Copper...', in *Biometals*, Vol 14. Copyright (2001) Kluwer. With kind permission of Springer Science and Business Media.

radical formation. In neutrophils the presence of myeloperoxidase allows the production of hypochlorous acid from the reaction between hydrogen peroxide and choride ions.

$$H_2O_2 + Cl^- \rightarrow HOCl + OH^-$$

In the presence of Fe^{2+}, hypochlorous acid can also generate hydroxyl radicals.

$$Fe^{2+} + HOCl \rightarrow OH^\bullet + Cl^- + Fe^{3+}$$

These activated killer cells also produce reactive nitrogen species (RNS) in response to infection and inflammation, as described next.

2.3 REACTIVE NITROGEN SPECIES (RNS)

Reactive nitrogen species also play an important role as messengers in cells. The first to be discovered, nitric oxide ($NO^\bullet$), is produced by the enzyme nitric oxide synthase (NOS), which generates $NO^\bullet$ and citrulline from arginine in a 5-electron oxidation reaction (**Figure 2.4**). Several $NO^\bullet$ synthases are known, nNOS (neuronal NOS), eNOS, (endothelial

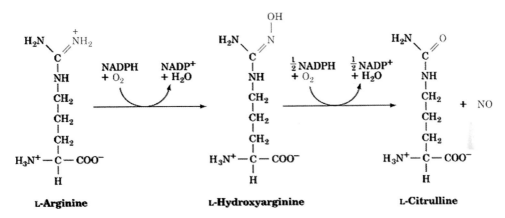

Figure 2.4: The NO synthase (NOS) reaction. The hydroxyarginine intermediate is tightly bound to the enzyme. From Voet and Voet (1995).

NOS) and iNOS (inducible NOS). They all show around 50% identity in amino acid sequence and have significant sequence homology with mammalian cytochrome P_{450} reductase, an enzyme involved in detoxification reactions. Both eNOS and nNOS are expressed constitutively, and both are rapidly activated by Ca^{2+} through their interaction with Ca^{2+}-calmodulin; however, the $NO^\bullet$ output is transient and its concentration low (in the nanomolar range). At this level, $NO^\bullet$ is mainly involved in homeostatic processes such as neurotransmission and blood pressure regulation. In contrast to the two constitutive forms, iNOS is calmodulin-independent. When macrophages and neutrophils are exposed to cytokines or to endotoxins (bacterial cell wall lipopolysaccharides which elicit an inflammatory response) iNOS is transcriptionally induced. Under these conditions, $NO^\bullet$ is produced continuously as a cytotoxic agent and at much higher levels (micromolar concentrations) often for periods of up to days or weeks. Stimulated macrophages attain steady state levels of NO$^\bullet$ of up to 4×10^6 molecules/cell/sec (Lewis et al., 1995). It seems that many cell types can be activated to express iNOS in the presence of the appropriate cocktail of cytokines. In addition to the three NOSs described above, there is also a mitochondrial NOS (Riobo et al., 2002). NO$^\bullet$ diffuses very rapidly through water and across cell membranes, so NO$^\bullet$ can easily diffuse from one cell to the next. At physiological concentrations, NO$^\bullet$ is relatively unreactive, and most of its physiological actions are mediated through its binding to the ferrous iron in haemoproteins, notably soluble guanylate cyclase. Guanylate cyclase forms cyclic GMP (cGMP), an intracellular second messenger, which causes smooth muscle relaxation. When NO$^\bullet$ reacts with guanylate cyclase to form nitrosohaem, the enzyme activity is increased some 50 fold. NO$^\bullet$ can also cause vasodilation of cerebral arteries; nerve impulses cause an increase in $[Ca^{2+}]$ in nerve terminals, stimulating nNOS. The NO$^\bullet$ generated diffuses to neighbouring smooth muscle cells and acts on guanylate cyclase as described above.

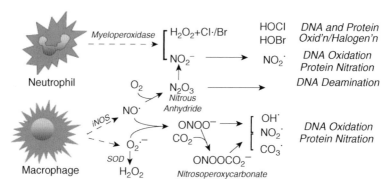

Figure 2.5: Reactive nitrogen and oxygen species (RNS and ROS) produced during inflammation. Reprinted from Dedon and Tannenbaum, Copyright 2004, with permission from Elsevier.

Once it has been formed, NO$^\bullet$ can diffuse and exert its effects on other cells, but it can also react to form other RNS (**Figure 2.5**) such as peroxynitrite, ONOO$^-$, NO$_2^\bullet$ and nitrous anhydride, N$_2$O$_3$ (Chen and Deen, 2001). The latter is formed by the autoxidation of NO$^\bullet$ by molecular oxygen, and is a powerful nitrosating agent, thought to be the principal RNS responsible for nitrosative deamination of nucleobases in DNA (Lewis et al., 1995). Another nitrogen dioxide radical, NO$_2^\bullet$ is thought to be the agent responsible for nitration of proteins and lipids. Neutrophils produce and secrete the enzyme myeloperoxidase and it has been proposed that myeloperoxodase can convert nitrite and peroxides to a nitrating agent for lipids and proteins (reviewed in Dedon and Tannenbaum, 2004).

Activated macrophages not only generate large fluxes of NO$^\bullet$ by induction of iNOS, they also concurrently produce O$_2^-$. While neither of these is particularly reactive, they will rapidly combine to form the much more reactive peroxynitrite, ONOO$^-$. Peroxynitrite is not itself a radical product, and is highly toxic to cells.

$$NO^\bullet + O_2^- \rightarrow ONOO^-$$

The rate constant for this reaction is 3–8 times greater than the rate of O$_2^-$ decomposition by superoxide dismutase (SOD), which would imply that if high fluxes of NO$^\bullet$ are generated, ONOO$^-$ formation can compete with O$_2^-$ scavenging by SOD. ONOO$^-$ is both cytotoxic and mutagenic, but its oxidation reactions remain controversial. At physiological pH, $ONOO^-$ protonates to peroxynitrous acid (ONOOH) which disappears within a few seconds, the end product being largely nitrate. The chemistry of peroxynitrite/peroxynitrous acid is extremely complex, although addition of $ONOO^\bullet$ to cells and tissues leads to oxidation and nitration of proteins, DNA and lipids with a reactivity that is comparable to that of the hydroxyl radical. It has been suggested that in the absence of CO_2, $ONOO^-$ rapidly decomposes to hydroxyl ($OH^\bullet$) and $NO_2^\bullet$ radicals (Halfpenny and Robinson, 1952a,b), with about two-thirds of the radicals degrading to NO_3^- while the remaining one-third become free radicals capable of oxidation reactions (Pryor and Squadrino, 1995; Gerasimov and Lymar, 1999).

2.4 THE TARGETS OF ROS AND RNS

There is considerable evidence, as we will see in later Chapters, that both ROS and RNS are involved in a number of neurodegenerative pathologies. These reactive species can potentially damage all biomolecules, and oxidative damage to lipids, proteins and nucleic acids can have particularly deleterious effects causing tissue injury, frequently associated with cell death either by necrosis or by apoptosis (Dalle-Donne et al., 2003). However, an additional element in these pathophysiologies is the production of unstable, reactive aldehyde intermediates from lipid peroxidation, from glucose-protein or glucose-lipid interactions (glycation) or from oxidative modification of amino acids in proteins (amino acid oxidation). These aldehydes can then form covalent links, both intramolecular and intermolecular, with proteins and phospholipids (Uchida, 2000).

When radical species, like the hydroxyl radical, are formed in the proximity of the polyunsaturated fatty acids (PUFA) present in membrane phospholipids, cholesterol esters and triglycerides they can cause peroxidative degradation. Lipid peroxidation proceeds by a free radical chain reaction mechanism which yields lipid hydroperoxides as major initial reaction products. A characteristic feature of lipid peroxidation is the subsequent breakdown of the C_{18} and C_{20} fatty acids such as linoleic and arachadonic acids to give a broad array of smaller fragments, three to nine carbons in length, including aldehydes, which can be classified into three families: 2-alkenals, 4-hydroxy-2-alkenals and ketoaldehydes (**Figure 2.6a**). The 2-alkenals are highly reactive and electrophilic, the most common, acrolein and its methyl homologue, crotonaldehyde, are not only found in cigarette smoke, but are also produced by lipid peroxidation (**Figure 2.6b**). The most prominent aldehydes produced by lipid peroxidation are the 4-hydroxy-2-alkenals, and of these the major aldehyde produced during peroxidation of ω6 PUFS such as linoleic and arachadonic acids (**Figure 2.6b**) is 4-hydroxy-2-nonenal (HNE). In membranes exposed to oxidative insult, concentrations of HNE from $10\,\mu M$ to $5\,mM$ have been reported. As we will see later, HNE is not only a product, but also a mediator of oxidative stress (Uchida, 2003). Among the ketoaldehydes (**Figure 2.6b**), malondialdehyde (MDA) is the most abundant lipid peroxidation-specific aldehyde and its determination by 2-thiobarbituric acid is commonly used as a measure of lipid peroxidation (although it can be more reliably assayed by HPLC). MDA can form a variety of adducts with amino groups both in proteins and in the amine-containing head-groups of membrane phospholipids. As we shall describe, products of lipid peroxidation are present in specific brain regions of many of the neurodegenerative diseases.

Direct oxidation by ROS of certain amino acid side chains in proteins (proline, arginine, lysine and threonine) or oxidative cleavage of the protein backbone (Berlett and Stadtman, 1997) can lead to the formation of protein carbonyl derivatives (**Figure 2.7**). Such protein

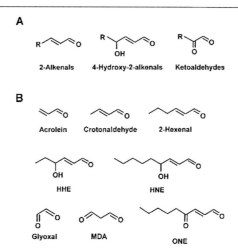

Figure 2.6: Structures of reactive aldehydes (**A**) and lipid peroxidation-specific aldehydes (**B**). Reprinted from Uchida, Copyright 2003, with permission from Elsevier.

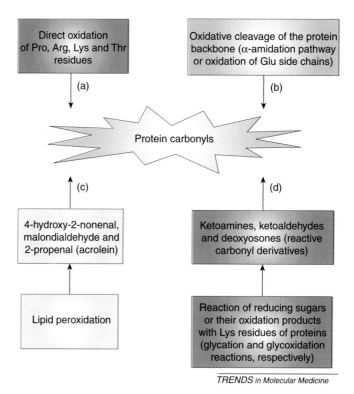

Figure 2.7: Production of protein carbonyls. Reprinted from Dalle-Donne et al., Copyright 2003, with permission from Elsevier.

carbonyls can also be formed by Michael addition reactions of α,β-unsaturated aldehydes like HNE, malondialdehyde and acrolein with either the sulphydryl group of cysteine, the imidazole group of histidine or the amino group of lysine in proteins (**Figure 2.8**) – this results in so-called advanced lipoxidation end-products. Carbonyl groups can also be

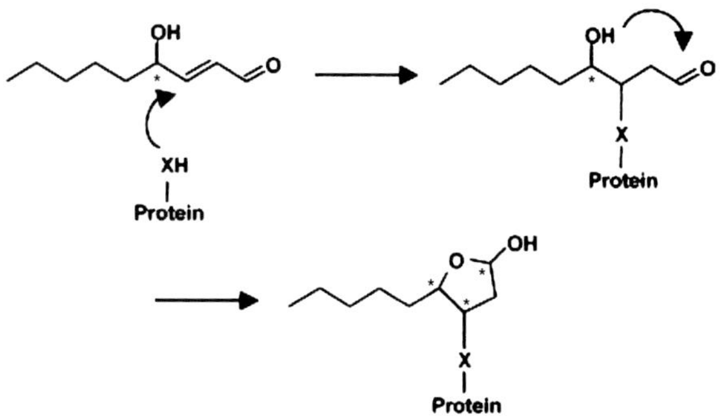

Figure 2.8: The Michael type addition of HNE to proteins. X: the sulphydryl group of cysteine, the imidazole group of histidine or the amino group of lysine. Reprinted from Uchida, Copyright 2003, with permission from Elsevier.

introduced into proteins by addition of reactive carbonyl compounds (ketoamines, ketoaldehydes and deoxyosones) produced by a complex series of reactions between reducing sugars or their oxidation products with the amino groups of lysine residues in proteins, by mechanisms known as glycation and glyoxidation (**Figure 2.7**). These protein carbonyl derivatives are known as advanced glycation end products.

Protein carbonyl (PCO) content is an excellent and reliable marker of protein oxidation, and is by far the most commonly used marker of protein oxidation in neurodegenerative diseases (Berlett and Stadtman, 1997; Schacter, 2000; Beal, 2002). It has the considerable advantage over lipid peroxidation products as a marker of oxidative stress that oxidized proteins are generally more stable. PCOs form early, circulate in the blood for longer periods than other parameters of oxidative stress, like glutathione disulphide and malondialdehyde, and sensitive biochemical and immunological methods have been developed for their determination.

RNS can also cause modifications to proteins, by nitration of tyrosine and by S-nitrosylation of cysteine thiol groups (Greenacre and Ischiropoulos, 2001; Foster et al., 2003), with increasing evidence that the products of these reactions can play important roles in human health and disease.

Last, but certainly not least, among the targets for oxidative stress are nucleic acids. More than 10^4 DNA lesions occur in each mammalian cell every day from spontaneous decay, replication errors and cellular metabolism alone (Lindahl, 1993). Clearly, additional DNA damage is induced by oxidative stress through the production of ROS in many neurodegenerative diseases. These involve damage to DNA bases, to the sugar-phosphates as well as cleavage of phosphodiester linkages in either one or both DNA strands (single- or double-strand breaks). Single-strand breaks can be converted to double-strand breaks in the course of replication. Damage to DNA bases can cause mutations and/or be cytotoxic, while double-strand breaks are lethal (Pfeiffer et al., 2000), so that repair mechanisms abound, involving at least 130 repair genes in man (Wood et al., 2001). More than 20 different type of base damage can be caused by ROS, and some examples are given in **Figure 2.9**. The most common damage to purine bases is the formation of 8-oxoguanine where the hydrogen at position 8 on guanine is replaced by an –OH group. It can be released from DNA by acidic hydrolysis. If enzymatic hydrolysis is used instead, 8-OHG may be released still attached to the 2-deoxyribose sugar. This product is called 8-hydroxy-2′deoxyguanosine (8-OHdG). This latter compound has gained popularity as a putative index of oxidative DNA damage. HPLC methods with electrochemical detections for analysis of 8OHdG are widely used – an

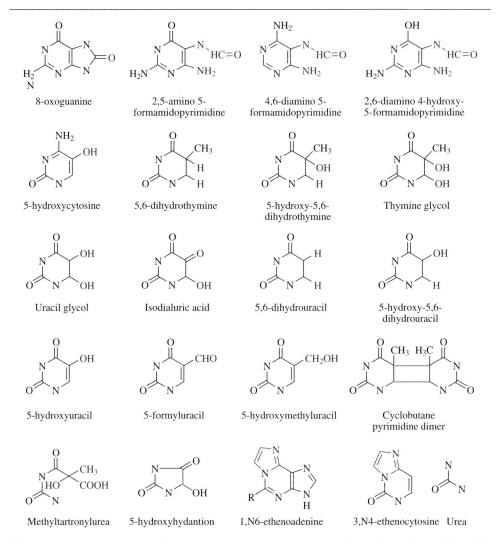

Figure 2.9: A number of the different oxidized and ring-fragmented nitrogen bases formed by ROS. Reprinted from Slupphaug et al., Copyright 2003, with permission from Elsevier.

increase in its amounts may indicate increased oxidative damage but also decreased repair as well. Thymine glycol is the most common product of damage to pyrimidine bases. A discussion of the mechanisms of DNA repair is beyond the scope of this book, but a recent review can be found in Slupphaug et al., 2003.

2.5 CYTOPROTECTION AGAINST OXIDATIVE DAMAGE

As a necessary consequence of the production of ROS and RNS, aerobic organisms, from man to microbe, have developed an elaborate system of cytoprotection against oxidative stress. This includes both enzymes, which react directly with some of the reactive oxidants,

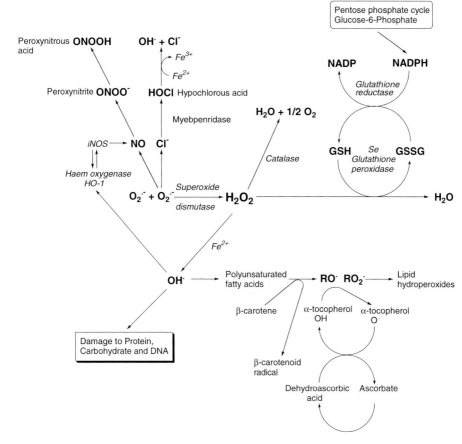

Figure 2.10: The battlefield of oxidative stress with both protagonists drawn up in horizontal and vertical lines. This could also be called the cascade of cytoprotective defense mechanisms which protect cells against the products of oxidative stress. Both defense and attack cohorts are indicated. Adapted from Crichton, 2001.

as well as a number of antioxidant molecules present within the cell. These cytoprotective enzymes and antioxidants do not act independently of one another to scavenge ROS and RNS, but function in a co-operative manner as a cascade, as is illustrated in **Figure 2.10**. We begin by consideration of the enzymes (and proteins) which can react with either the ROS and RNS, themselves, or their products, and then consider the non-enzymatic molecules which are involved in protection against oxidative damage.

At the very first step of the oxygen reduction pathway, superoxide dismutases (SOD) intervene to transform two molecules of superoxide anion into one each of hydrogen peroxide and oxygen:

$$O_2^- + O_2^- + 2H^+ \rightarrow H_2O_2 + O_2$$

In mammalian cells three distinct superoxide dismutases, each unique and highly compartmentalized have been identified, and characterized (Zelko et al., 2002). The first,

SOD-1, commonly known as Cu/Zn-SOD, is a copper- and zinc-containing homodimer, which is found almost exclusively in the cytosol of human cells (Crapo et al., 1992), although its presence in nuclear compartments and lysosomes of rat liver has also been reported (Liou et al., 1993). The synthesis of SOD-1 is increased by metal ions through a metal responsive element on the SOD-1 gene (Yoo et al., 1999). Mutations in SOD-1 are found in familial ALS. SOD-2, or Mn-SOD, is a tetrameric manganese-containing enzyme, synthesized with a leader peptide which targets it exclusively to the mitochondria. The transcription of the SOD-2 gene is induced by a large number of compounds, including cytokines, lipopolysaccharides and interferon-γ (Zelko et al., 2002). SOD-3, the most recently characterized SOD, is a copper- and zinc-containing tetramer, synthesized with a signal peptide which directs it exclusively to extracellular spaces, including cerebrospinal fluid. SOD-3 seems to play an important protective role in blood vessel walls, and its level is markedly increased by factors which increase blood pressure (Stralin and Marklund, 2001). A single amino acid mutation in human SOD-3, which impairs its affinity for endothelial cell surfaces, is associated with a 10 to 30 fold increase in serum SOD-3 levels.

The product of the two electron reduction of molecular oxygen, and of superoxide dismutation, hydrogen peroxide, can be metabolized to non-toxic products by catalase and by glutathione peroxidase. Catalase, a haem enzyme which is localized within the intracellular compartment known as the peroxisome, uses H_2O_2 both as an electron donor and as an electron acceptor:

$$H_2O_2 + H_2O_2 \rightarrow 2H_2O + O_2$$

A key role in controlling the redox state within the cell is played by the redox couple formed by reduced and oxidized glutathione, GSH/GSSG. Glutathione is the tripeptide γ-glutamylcysteinylglycine, which in its oxidized form consists of two GSH molecules linked by a disulphide bridge. It is one of the most important cellular antioxidants since it supplies the electrons for the reduction of peroxides, including H_2O_2, by the enzyme glutathione peroxidase, which contains a selenocysteine at its active site: this is successively oxidized and then reduced during catalytic cycles.

$$H_2O_2 + 2GSH \rightarrow GSSH + 2H_2O$$

Hydrogen peroxide can react with double bonds in membrane fatty acid residues to form organic hydroperoxides and, in principle, glutathione peroxidase can terminate the chain reaction of lipid peroxidation by removing these lipid hydroperoxides from the cell membrane:

$$2GSH + ROOH \rightarrow GSSG + ROH + H_2O$$

There are four members of the selenium-containing glutathione peroxidase (GPx) family (Imai and Nakagawa, 2003): however, three of them, the cytoplasmic forms GPx1 and GPx2 and the extracellular form, GPx3, while able to reduce H_2O_2 and relatively polar organic hydroperoxides, cannot metabolize fatty acid hydroperoxides in membrane phospholipids (Grossmann and Wendel, 1983). The fourth, GPx4, can not only react with hydrogen peroxide and a wide range of lipid hydroperoxides, but can directly reduce phospholipid hydroperoxides, and so it can protect membranes against oxidative damage (Thomas et al., 1990). GPx4 is present in the cytosol, nuclei and endoplasmic reticulum, and is also synthesized with a leader peptide which targets it to the mitochondria (Arai et al., 1999).

Cytoplasmic GPxs can also function as peroxynitrite reductases, thereby scavenging this potentially toxic RNS (Sies and Arteel 2000).

$$ONOO^- + 2GSH \rightarrow ONO^- + GSSG$$

In their removal of peroxides, glutathione peroxidases convert reduced glutathione to oxidized glutathione. The oxidized GSSH formed in this reaction is then regenerated by the NADPH-dependent flavoprotein glutathione reductase:

$$GSSG + NADPH + H^+ \rightarrow 2GSH + NADP^+$$

The activities of some of these cytoprotective enzymes and antioxidants are altered in many of the neurodegenerative diseases.

In an analogous manner to this glutathione system, the thioredoxin (Trx) system can also contribute to the maintenance of the redox status of the cell. Thioredoxins (Trx) are small ubiquitous proteins with a pair of adjacent cysteine residues located on a molecular protrusion (**Figure 2.11**) which can undergo reversible oxidation to form a disulphide bond. Once oxidized by H_2O_2 in a reaction catalysed by thioredoxin peroxidase, thioredoxin reductase regenerates the reduced thiol of Txr at the expense of NADPH.

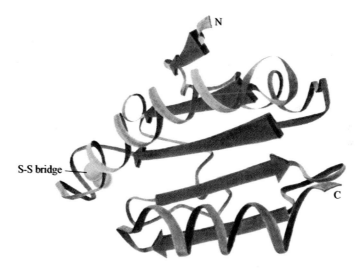

Figure 2.11: The X-ray structure of thioredoxin in its oxidized (disulphide) state. From Voet and Voet (1995).

It follows that a steady supply of NADPH is necessary to protect cells against oxidative stress. In mammalian cells the source of NADPH is the pentose phosphate pathway. This is why congenital defects in glucose-6-phosphate dehydrogenase (G6PD), the first enzyme of this pathway, result in increased sensitivity to oxidative stress. Both the synthesis of intracellular GSH and of pentose phosphate pathway enzymes are increased under conditions of oxidative stress, and the effectiveness of this response will, to a large extent, determine the capacity of the cell to protect itself from ROS toxicity.

Glutathione is present within cells at millimolar concentrations mainly in the reduced form, GSH. Absolute concentrations vary considerably from tissue to tissue (Ward et al.,

1994), with six times higher values for example in liver than in brain. The same is true of the cytoprotective enzymes, which are all present at much lower levels in brain than in most other tissues, except anaerobic muscle. The brain, although it only constitutes 2% of adult body mass, is responsible for 20% of resting oxygen consumption (even when we are asleep). This is on account of its high demand for ATP production, around 50% of which is used to power the plasma membrane ($Na^+ - K^+$)-ATPase, which maintains the membrane potential required for transmission of nerve impulses. The high oxygen consumption together with the decreased antioxidant status makes the brain more susceptible than many other tissues to oxidative stress.

Haem oxygenase catalyses the oxygenation of haem to Fe^{2+}, carbon monoxide and biliverdin, which is converted into bilirubin. The enzyme requires large amounts of reducing equivalents, in the form of NADPH, and O_2. There are two haem oxygenases in man, both of which are thought to be cytoprotective (Baranano and Snyder, 2001), despite their production of Fe^{2+}, potentially capable of participating in Fenton chemistry to produce hydroxyl radical. HO1 is found at high levels in spleen, where senescent and abnormal red blood cells are destroyed, and in liver its transcription can be induced by transition metal ions and by oxidative stress. In contrast, HO2 is constitutively expressed at high levels in some regions of the brain, where the bilirubin and biliverdin so formed could exert a neuroprotective effect. Like NO, the CO produced by neuronal HO2 can stimulate guanylate cyclase and cause smooth muscle relaxation. CO is a neurotransmitter in the brain and in the peripheral autonomic nervous system (Baranano and Snyder, 2001). In order to function as a gaseous neurotransmitter, CO must be synthesized rapidly following neuronal depolarization. It has been shown that this can be achieved by the activation of HO2 during neuronal stimulation by Ca^{2+}-dependent phosphorylation by CK2 in several model systems (Boehning et al., 2003).

Among the antioxidant proteins (not in **Figure 2.10**) we can also include ferritin, which plays the important role (outlined in Chapter 1) of removing 'free' iron from the cytoplasm, and storing it in a soluble, non-toxic, mineral form.

Finally we have a number of low-molecular weight antioxidants, which can react directly with some of the products of oxidative damage. In the front line, combating lipid peroxidation, we find the antioxidant vitamins A, C and E, whose rise in popular esteem and consumption must mark them down as prime candidates for the in vogue appellation of 'nutriceutical'[1]. Both β-carotene (precursor of vitamin A) and α-tocopherol (vitamin E) can prevent the oxidation of polyunsaturated fatty acids in membrane phospholipids. The former can react with lipid hydroperoxides. Care should be taken in the use of β-carotene as a beneficial nutrient supplement, since recent multi-centre, population-based case-control studies indicated an association between carotene intake and prostate (Vogt et al., 2002) and lung (Black, 2004) cancers. The antioxidant, α-tocopherol, reacts more rapidly with peroxyl and alkoxyl radicals in membrane lipid bilayers than with adjacent PUFAs (Halliwell, 1989), thereby sparing them from oxidation, and acts as a chain-breaking antioxidant. This interrupts the chain reaction of lipid peroxidation. In contrast to these two hydrophobic vitamins, which are found in proximity to membranes, ascorbate (vitamin C) is water soluble, and is thought to be capable of regenerating α-tocopherol (McCay, 1985) from its radical form (**Figure 2.10**). There are a number of other molecules which have been reported

[1] The word nutriceutical has entered our vocabulary from the junk food world of couch potatoes. If this does not make much sense, then please accept this succinct definition. It is a substance which, on account of its absence from the diet of people eating not particularly healthy food, needs to be supplied as a dietary supplement in the 'junk food'.

to have antioxidant properties, including bilirubin and biliverdin derived from haem break-down, uric acid, the end product of the degradation of nucleic acid purine bases, and many more.

2.6 MITOCHONDRIA, FREE RADICALS AND SIGNALLING

Mitochondria, the powerhouses of ATP production in aerobic tissues like brain and heart muscle, are now recognized to be the most important source of both ROS and RNS within cells (reviewed in Cadenas, 2004). They are also the main target for the regulatory and toxic actions of free radicals as well as being the source of signalling molecules which control the cell cycle, proliferation and apoptosis. Superoxide radicals and nitric oxide are produced and metabolized in the mitochondrial matrix (**Figure 2.12**). Several sites of O_2^- generation in the mitochondrial respiratory chain have been identified, and their relative contribution varies from organ to organ, and also depends on whether the mitochondria are respiring actively, or whether the respiratory chain is highly reduced. In heart and lung, Complex III seems to be responsible for most of the O_2^- production (Turrens et al., 1982, 1985), via auto-oxidation by molecular O_2 of the semiquinone form of Coenzyme Q (Boveris et al., 1976). However, in brain, the primary source of O_2^- under normal conditions seems to be Complex I (Barja and Herrero, 1998), with the site of production being one of the iron-sulphur clusters (Genova et al., 2001; Kushnareva et al., 2002). Complex I is the principal source of ROS in the ageing process as well as a number of pathological conditions including Parkinson's disease (reviewed in Turrens, 2003). Nitric oxide is produced in mitochondria by mtNOS: intra-mitochondrial concentrations of the substrates are in the range needed for enzymatic activity. Most of the O_2^- is converted to H_2O_2 by the mitochondrial Mn SOD and to $ONOO^-$ by reaction with nitric oxide (**Figure 2.12**). The major effects of nitric oxide generated within the mitochondrial matrix are inhibition of electron transfer in complexes III and IV, resulting

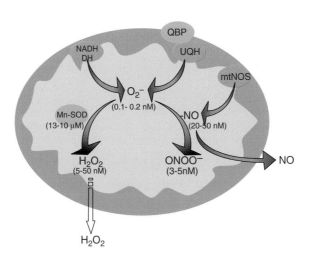

Figure 2.12: Metabolism of superoxide and nitric oxide in the mitochondrial matrix. The numbers below the symbols indicate physiological steady state concentrations for mammalian organs. NADH-DH: NADH dehydrogenase; QBP: ubiquinone binding protein; UQH; ubisemiquinone. Reprinted from Cadenas, Copyright 2004, with permission from Elsevier.

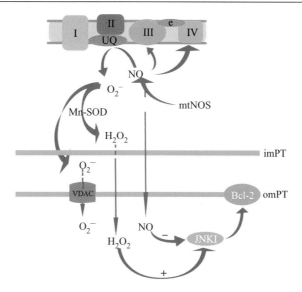

Figure 2.13: Mitochondrion-dependent apoptosis and MAPK signalling. The three major actions of nitric oxide generated in mitochondria are shown. The fates of O_2^-, H_2O_2 and NO are indicated together with their release into the cytosol (the former through voltage-dependent anion channels). Modulation of the MAPK (stimulated by H_2O_2 and inhibited by NO) is indicated. JNK phosphorylates Bcl-2. Reprinted from Cadenas, Copyright 2004, with permission from Elsevier.

in increased oxidation of Coenzyme Q to give O_2^- (**Figure 2.13**). H_2O_2 and NO can diffuse out of the mitochondria, into the cytosol, where they are thought to modulate mitogen-activated protein kinases (MAPK) (Torres and Forman, 2003). The MAPKs are a widely distributed family of protein kinases which are integral components of intracellular phosphorylation MAP kinase signalling cascades (**Figure 2.14a**) in mammalian cells. Each MAP kinase cascade consists of an MKKK (MAP kinase kinase kinase) an MKK (MAP kinase kinase) and an MAPK. Various external stimuli can activate one or more MKKKs which in turn activate one or more MKKs. The MKKs are relatively specific for their target MAPKs. Once activated the MAPKs phosphorylate specific transcription factors as well as specific kinases, and the resulting activated transcription factors induce cellular responses, such as proliferation, differentiation, survival or programmed cellular death (apoptosis – see **2.7**). The MAP kinase cascade can be returned to its resting state by the actions of a series of protein phosphatases. The target of H_2O_2 and NO in the MAP kinase cascade is JNKI, the activity of which is stimulated by H_2O_2 and inhibited by NO (**Figure 2.14a**).

2.7 CYCLIN-DEPENDENT KINASES

Kinases that are activated by cyclin family members, (Cdks), play a critical role in orchestrating transitions through cell cycles in a variety of species. Cdk1 is a critical regulator of cell division while Cdk2 and Cdk4 control the timing of DNA replication. Most Cdk family members are activated upon association with regulatory subunits called cyclins.

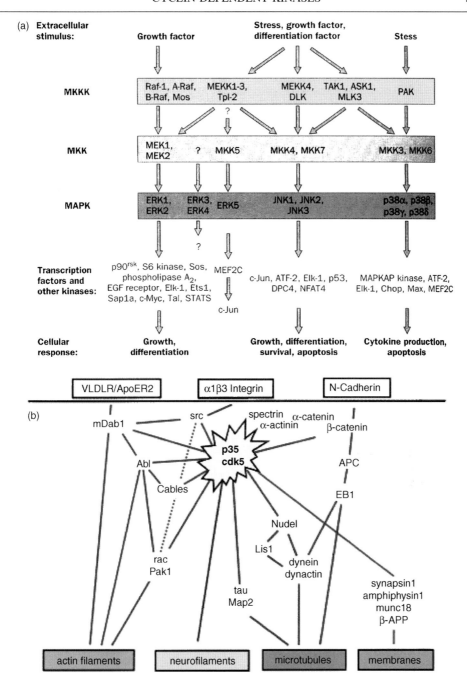

Figure 2.14: (a) MAP kinase cascades in mammalian cells. From Voet and Voet, 2004. **(b)** Cdk5 and its activating partner, p35, may be a point of integration for extracellular signals regulating neuronal migration. In this model, *lines* indicate published interactions between proteins and connect signaling pathways to known downstream events involving cytoskeletal or membrane systems. These or other potential pathways may lead to changes in gene expression, but this is not a well-studied area and has not been included in the model. From Smith et al., 2001. Reproduced by permission of the American Association for Cancer Research.

When activated, Cdks phosphorylate serine and threonine residues in a proline directed fashion.

Cdk5 shows the highest level of expression in postmitotic neurons in developing and adult nervous system. However, Cdk5 is not activated by cyclins, but requires association with one or two brain-specific regulatory subunits, p35 and p39. Cdk5 plays an important role in regulating neuronal migration, as well as axonal growth and synaptic function. **Figure 2.14b**, shows several signalling pathways influenced by Cdk5 activity and points to the effector systems regulated by these pathways. Deregulation of Cdk5 activity is neurotoxic, and leads to neuronal apoptosis (Gong et al., 2003) which has been linked to neurodegenerative diseases such as Alzheimer's disease. *In vitro* studies suggest that aberrant activation of Cdk5 by an endogenous truncated version, p25, might be a key event in the process of neurodegeneration. One enzyme responsible for cleavage of p35 to form p25 is calpain, a calcium-activated protease, that has been shown to be involved in neuronal cell death (Guo, 2003). Furthermore hyperactivation and redistribution of Cdk5 by p25 plays an essential role in the phosphorylation of 'pathological' substrates (e.g. tau) and the cell death of neurons in models of Parkinson's and Alzheimer's diseases. Elucidating the mechanisms of Cdk5 regulation and its downstream signalling may prove to be crucial in the therapeutic treatment of neurodegenerative diseases.

The p25-Cdk5 pathway could cause neuronal death via various signalling pathways which include apoptosis, ischemic damage and tau phosphorylation. Caspase-3 and apoptotic cell death upstream of mitochondrial function can be induced by p25-cdk5.

2.8 APOPTOSIS[2] – PROGRAMMED CELL DEATH

Apoptosis is a phenomenon which was first described in the late 1960s as a normal part of development: for example the conveniently transparent nematode worm, *C. elegans*, loses precisely 131 of its 1090 somatic cells by apoptosis to form the normal adult organism. Unless the cells of multicellular organisms continuously receive hormonal and neurological signals not to commit suicide, they will do so. A number of morphological changes occur in the previously apparently normal and healthy apoptotic cell. The distinct morphological changes of the cell undergoing apoptosis are that the cell begins to shrink and pull away from other cells, bubble-like formations appear at its surface, and chromatin (chromosomal DNA and protein) in the cell's nucleus condenses. Eventually, the cell disintegrates into numerous membrane-enclosed **apoptotic bodies**, which are phagocytosed by neighbouring cells and by roving macrophages without spilling the cell contents and inducing an inflammatory response. This is in marked contrast to the 'explosion' of cells undergoing **necrosis**, the type of cell death caused by trauma, such as lack of oxygen, extremes of temperature and mechanical injury. Inappropriate apoptosis has been implicated in a number of neurological disorders including Parkinson's, Alzheimer's and Huntington's diseases.

Apoptosis of a given cell can be initiated by cell surface receptors (the **extrinsic pathway**) or by the mitochondria (the **intrinsic pathway**). In the extrinsic pathway

---

[2] **Apoptosis** (Greek: falling off, as leaves from a tree), otherwise known as **programmed cell death**, is different from **necrosis**, and is a genetically programmed event which can be set in motion by a variety of internal or external stimuli. In adult humans, of the roughly 10^{14} cells, around 10^{11} cells are eliminated each day by apoptosis (this closely matches the number of cells which are replaced by cellular division).

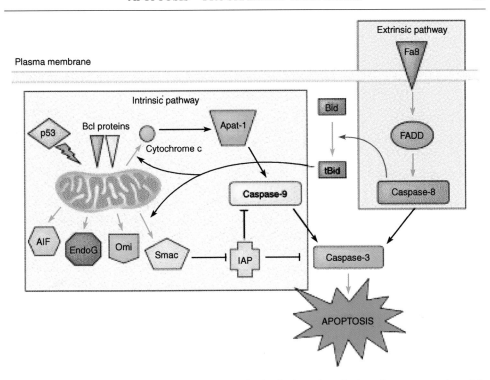

Figure 2.15: The two major apoptotic pathways. The intrinsic and extrinsic pathways are activated in response to internal and external apoptotic stimuli, respectively. Mitochondria contain several pro-apoptotic proteins that have key roles in apoptosis. The intrinsic pathway leads to the release of cytochrome c and Smac from mitochondria into the cytoplasm. Cytochrome c directly binds to and activates Apaf-1, which then facilitates the activation of caspase-9. Caspase-9 activates caspase-3. By contrast, Smac removes the inhibition of caspase-3 and caspase-9 by inhibitor of apoptosis proteins (IAPs). The extrinsic pathway leads to the activation of caspase-8, which activates caspase-3. Thus, both pathways converge at caspase-3 activation. The extrinsic pathway can crosstalk with the intrinsic pathway through caspase-8-mediated cleavage of Bid (red arrow). Truncated Bid (tBid) then induces the release of mitochondrial proteins. Green arrows indicate signal flow. Black arrowheads and perpendicular lines indicate activation and inhibition, respectively. Other proteins, such as apoptosis-inducing factor (AIF), EndoG and Omi (also known as HtrA2), are also released from mitochondria into the cytoplasm to facilitate cell death during apoptosis. Reprinted from Shiozaki and Shi, Copyright 2004, with permission from Elsevier.

(**Figure 2.15**), the process is initiated by the association of the cell selected to undergo apoptosis with a cell which has selected it. The condemned cell has a **death receptor, Fas** in its plasma membrane, which is recognized by a protein projecting from the plasma membrane of the inducing cell, called the **death ligand, FasL**. The outcome, as described in more detail for the intrinsic pathway, is that a family of cysteine proteases (caspases) are activated, resulting in apoptosis.

The mitochondria-mediated (intrinsic) pathway of apoptosis occurs in response to a wide range of death stimuli, including activation of tumour suppressor proteins (like p53), and oncogenes (eg. c-Myc), DNA damage, therapeutic agents, serum starvation and UV radiation. It is clear that this pathway must be switched off in all cancer cells. Apoptosis is executed by the initiator and effector caspases[3], a family of proteases which are produced as catalytically inactive procaspases, and must be proteolytically processed to become active proteases. Six caspases participate exclusively in apoptosis in man – caspases-8, -9 and -10 are initiator caspases, while caspases-3, -6 and -7 are effector caspases. Over 60 cellular proteins have been identified as caspase substrates, including cytoskeletal proteins, proteins involved in cell cycle regulation, in DNA replication, transcription factors and proteins involved in signal transduction. How the cleavage of these proteins causes the morphological changes observed in apoptosis is not known. Induction of apoptosis also involves rapid degradation of chromosomal DNA.

The intrinsic pathway is controlled by proteins of the Bcl-2 family (so-called because the first member, Bcl-2 was characterized as a gene involved in *B* cell lymphoma). More than 20 members of this family have been identified in humans, which can be divided into two subgroups, proteins that suppress apoptosis, like Bcl-2, Bcl-x_L and proteins that promote apoptosis like Bax, Bad, Bid (Adams and Cory, 1998). When an apoptotic stimulus (**Figure 2.15**) is received, cytochrome c is released from the intermembrane space into the cytoplasm in a process regulated by members of the Bcl-2 family. The process is induced by activated pro-apoptotic Bcl-2 family members and is inhibited by anti-apoptotic Bcl-2 family members, and is thought to involve formation of a channel in the outer mitochondrial membrane. Once in the cytosol, cytochrome c binds to Apaf-1 (apoptotic protease activating factor-1). The binary complex of Apaf-1 and cytochrome c then binds dATP or ATP to form a complex called the apoptosome, which recruits and facilitates activation of the initiator procaspase-9. Apaf-1 has an N-terminal caspase recruitment domain (CARD), to which procaspase-9 binds. The primary target of caspase-9 is procaspase-3, one of the most deleterious of the effector caspases (executioner caspases), which then carry out the proteolysis of a wide variety of cellular proteins, resulting in apoptosis.

The way in which the intrinsic apoptotic pathway is regulated is not yet clearly established. In normal cells which have not received an apoptotic stimulus, members of the inhibitor of apoptosis (IAP) family can interact with, and inhibit the enzymatic activity of mature caspases. This is achieved through an 80-residue BIR domain folded around a zinc atom. For example, the human XIAP protein has three BIR domains: the third BIR domain potently inhibits the activity of processed caspase-9, whereas the linker region between domains 2 and 3 selectively targets active caspase-3; **Figure 2.16** illustrates the inhibition of caspase-7 by an XIAP fragment. In cells signalled to undergo apoptosis, this inhibitory effect must be suppressed, and this is mediated by another mitochondrial protein called Smac (second mitochondria-derived activator of caspases). Smac is released from mitochondria into the cytoplasm, together with cytochrome c. Its effect is to interact with the BIR domains of IAPs and to block their inhibitory effects on both initiator and effector caspases.

During the first, and still reversible phase of apoptosis, the release of H_2O_2 and NO into the cytosol results in the activation of JNK1 which in turn leads to the phosphorylation of Bcl-2 and Bcl-x_L and of intramitochondrial proteins (Schroeter et al., 2003). The second, and irreversible phase of the intrinsic pathway of apoptosis is initiated by release of cytochrome c and Ca^{2+} to the cytosol, accompanied by opening of voltage-dependent anion channels,

---

[3] **Caspases** (for c*ysteinyl asp*artate prote*ases*) are a family of cysteine proteases that cleave peptide bonds after an aspartate residue. There are eleven caspases in humans of which six participate exclusively in apoptosis. There are the so-called **initiator caspases (caspases-8, -9 and -10)** which, in their pro-form, are targeted to scaffolding proteins, which promote their autoactivation. The **effector caspases (caspases -3, -6 and -7)** are activated by the initiator caspases. They are often referred to as **executioner caspases**, cleaving a wide variety of cellular proteins, and bringing about apoptosis.

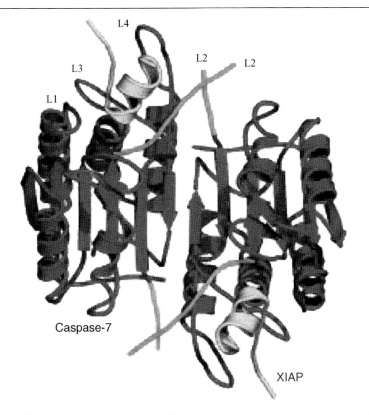

Figure 2.16: Inhibition of caspase-7 by an XIAP fragment. Reprinted from Shiozaki and Shi, Copyright 2004, with permission from Elsevier.

which release O_2^- to the cytosol. The subsequent steps in the cell death programme (apoptosome assembly and caspase activation) are totally independent of mitochondrial intervention.

2.9 ROS, RNS AND SIGNAL TRANSDUCTION

We can define oxidative stress as an imbalance between the level of production of reactive oxygen and nitrogen species and of antioxidant protection. As is illustrated by **Figure 2.17**, oxidative stress can elicit biological responses which can vary enormously (Forman and Torres, 2001). Severe levels of oxidative stress can pose a threat to cell function and viability, and are characterized by the activation of cellular repair mechanisms, and may

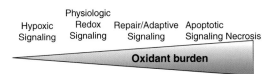

Figure 2.17: The relationship between oxidant burden and biological response. Reprinted from Forman and Torres, Copyright 2001, with permission from Elsevier.

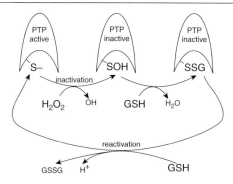

Figure 2.18: Inactivation-reactivation of a protein tyrosine phosphatase. Reprinted from Forman and Torres, Copyright 2001, with permission from Elsevier.

ultimately lead to apoptosis (programmed cell death) or necrosis. Non-damaging levels of oxidative stress are associated with signalling, which is often referred to as 'redox-sensitive signalling'. For ROS and RNS to be designated as second messengers in signalling pathways they need to have four basic characteristics: (i) they are generated enzymatically, (ii) they are degraded enzymatically, (iii) their concentration rises and falls within a short period, (iv) they act at specific sites (Forman and Torres, 2001). Of the ROS and RNS described in the section above, only superoxide, hydrogen peroxide and peroxynitrite fulfil these requirements.

We can illustrate the potential role of H_2O_2 as a second messenger in cell signalling by the following example (Forman and Torres, 2001). In protein tyrosine phosphatase (PTP) the active site thiol can react with H_2O_2 to form a sulphenic acid, which is inactive (**Figure 2.18**). The sulphenic acid can be easily reduced by GSH to form a mixed disulphide. The mixed disulphide can then react with another GSH to form GSSG and restore the active form of the PTP. The role of glutathione peroxidase in decreasing the concentration of H_2O_2 then functions as the turn-off component of redox signalling.

Transcription factors were the first signalling proteins to be identified as redox-sensitive, and for some of them like Sp1, their DNA binding activity is indeed regulated through specific cysteine residues which need to be reduced for activity. However, the prototype of redox-sensitive transcription factors is nuclear factor κB, which is present in nearly all animal cells. Substantial evidence supports the view that NFκB is a powerful suppressor of apoptosis, through the induction of the expression of a number of anti-apoptotic factors, including the inhibitor of apoptosis proteins (IAP[4]) as well as members of the Bcl2 family (Karin and Lin, 2002). In unstimulated cells, the family of NFκB proteins are sequestered in the cytoplasm by virtue of their association with a member of the IκB family of inhibitory proteins (**Figure 2.19**). IκB makes multiple contacts with NFκB, masking the nuclear localization sequence of NFκB and interfering with sequences necessary for DNA binding. The activation of NFκB is induced by ROS, and by a large number of other factors, and results in the expression of various genes in different target cells which have important roles in immune responses, stress responses, cell survival and development. It was originally thought that NFκB activation was due to the production of ROS (Schreck et al., 1991), but later studies have shown that, *in vivo*, NFκB activation by exogenous H_2O_2 was cell-specific and that the requirement to generate ROS intracellularly was not universal, but cell- and stimulus-specific (Bowie and O'Neill, 2000).

---

[4] **IAPs** are part of the elaborate systems that prevent cells from undergoing inadvertent apoptosis. Just as the anti-apoptotic members of the Bcl-2 family keep their pro-apoptotic cousins under control, the members of the IAP family specifically bind to, and inhibit, caspases.

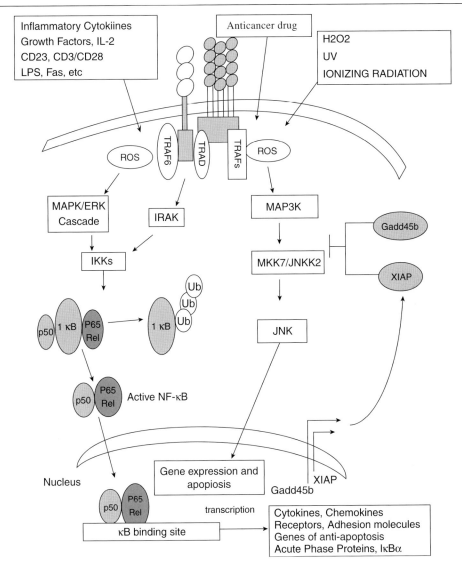

Figure 2.19: NFκB activation in stress conditions. Reprinted from Wang et al., Copyright 2002, with permission from Elsevier.

Activation of NFκB appears to involve the rapid phosphorylation of its inhibitory subunit, IκB by specific IκB kinases. This results in the release of IκB from NFκB itself, and its targeting for ubiquitination and degradation by the proteosome. NFκB is subsequently translocated to the nucleus where it mediates transcriptional initiation by binding to 10 base-pair κB DNA segments (**Figure 2.20**) with an appropriate consensus sequence. Additional specificity may be achieved by synergistic interaction of NFκB with other transcription factors such as Sp1. The activation process is brought to a halt since the most common IκB protein, IκBα is induced by binding of NFκB to the κB sites in this gene's promoter. The newly synthesized IκB enters the nucleus, binds to NFκB, releasing it from its DNA binding sites and directing its export back to the cytoplasm.

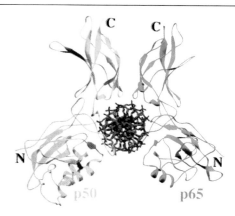

Figure 2.20: X-ray structure of NFκB p50–p65 heterodimer bound to a 12-base-pair κB DNA. From Voet and Voet (2004).

A signalling role for the ROS produced by the respiratory burst in macrophages has also been proposed (Forman and Torres, 2001). The resident immune cells of the central nervous system are the microglia, which resemble peripheral tissue macrophages, and are the primary mediators of neuroinflammation (Kreutzberg, 1996). They exist in a quiescent state in healthy adult brain, with a small cell body, ramified processes and minimal expression of surface antigens. When injury is inflicted on the central nervous system, e.g. neurodegenerative diseases, stroke and traumatic brain injuries (Nakamura, 2002), the microglia are rapidly activated and act on the surrounding neurons and microglia (astrocytes and oligodendrocytes) by releasing cytotoxic and inflammatory molecules, such as oxygen radicals, NO, glutamate, cytokines and prostaglandins (Kreutzberg, 1996; Hanisch, 2002). It seems that their activation also involves NFκB, and that this may involve neurone-microglial interactions (Kaltschmidt and Kaltschmidt, 2000). Microglia have been implicated in many neurological diseases (Kreutzberg, 1996; McGeer and McGeer, 1999).

2.10 MOLECULES INVOLVED IN THE INFLAMMATORY PATHWAY

Glutamate is the principal excitatory neurotransmitter. Cerebral glutamate is derived solely from endogenous sources; mainly from α-ketoglutarate, which is a product of the Krebs cycle (citric acid cycle, TCA cycle). The processing and transport of glutamate within the neuron are highly organized and involve coordinated interactions among multiple cytoplasmic organelles, **Figure 2.21a**. Glutamate is initially synthesized by the endoplasmic reticulum and then transported to the Golgi apparatus where it is enclosed within vesicular (bilipid) membrane, via an uptake system (VGLUT), **Figure 2.21b**. Three VGLUTs have been identified, VGLUT1, VGLUT2 and VGLUT3. Their affinity for glutamate is 100–1000 fold lower than that of EAATs (see below). VGLUT1 and VGLUT2 are expressed in the terminals of all glutamatergic synapses; Compounds such as amino acid analogues, dye compounds related to glutamate structure and bromocriptine will inhibit VGLUT- mediated glutamate uptake.

Vescicles containing glutamate are transported down the axon via a complex system of microtubules, which on reaching the axonal tip, merge with the presynaptic membrane to

(a)

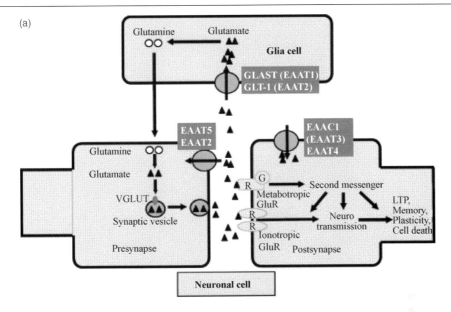

(b)

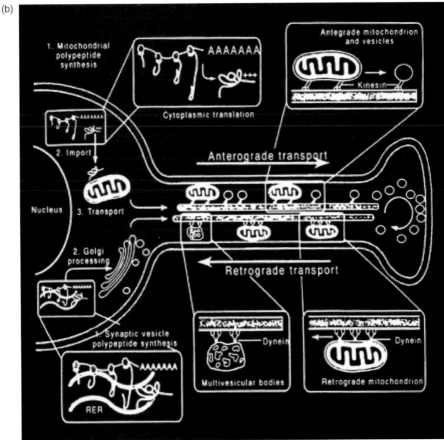

Figure 2.21: (*Continued*)

(c)

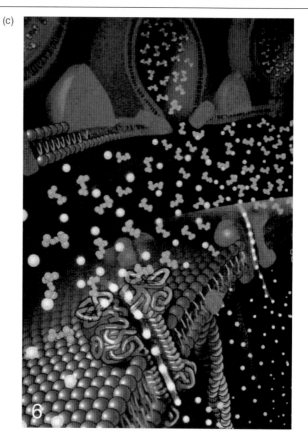

Figure 2.21: (**a**) Mechanisms of excitatory neurotransmission in the mammalian central nervous system. Reprinted from Shigeri et al., Copyright 2004, with permission from Elsevier. (**b**) Neuronal glutamate processing and transport. Glutamate is processed by the endoplasmic reticulum and Golgi apparatus in preparation for fast axonal transport, which requires other transport proteins and mitochondria. When glutamate emerges from the trans face of the Golgi apparatus, it is encapsulated inside a neurosecretory vesicle which is transported down the axon along microtubule tracks to be deposited at the tip of the axon near the presynaptic membrane. Waves of axonal membrane depolarization will trigger the release of glutamate into the synaptic space by exocytosis. From Mark et al., 2001. Reproduced by permission of the American Journal of Neuroradiology. (**c**) Pictorial display of the neurotransmitter glutamate (*orange*) released into the synaptic space and docking with the glutamate receptor site on the postsynaptic membrane. The activation of the glutamate receptor then opens the ion channel coupled to the receptor, allowing the passage of extracellular calcium (*yellow*) into the intracellular cytosol, which in turn triggers a series of biochemical events. From Mark et al., 2001. Reproduced by permission of the American Journal of Neuroradiology.

release the glutamate into the synaptic space between neurons, **Figure 2.21c**. The key process that triggers the entire excitotoxic cascade is the excessive accumulation of glutamate in the synaptic space caused by alteration in normal cycling of intracranial glutamate, an increased glutamate release into the extracellular space, decreased glutamate uptake/transport from the synaptic space, or its release from damaged neurons. The synaptic glutamate will then interact with specific receptor sites on the postsynaptic membrane of the adjacent neuron to initiate an important cascade of molecular events.

There are two main types of glutamate receptors for synaptic glutamate, the ionotropic, (NMDA (N-methyl-D-aspartate), AMPA (α-amino-3-hydroxy-5-methyl-4-isoxazolepro-pionate), and kainite) which are directly coupled to membrane ion channels and the metabotropic receptors. Metabotropic glutamate receptors (mGluRs), a group of seven-transmembrane-domain proteins that couple to G-proteins, have become of interest for studies of neuropathology. Group I mGluRs control the levels of second messengers, such as inositol 1,4,5-triphosphate (IP3), Ca^{2+} ions and cAMP. They elicit the release of arachidonic acid via intracellular Ca^{2+} mobilization from intracellular stores such as mitochondria and endo-plasmic reticulum. mGluRs regulate neuronal injury and survival, possibly through a series of downstream protein kinase and cysteine protease signaling pathways that affect mito-chondrially mediated programmed cell death. They also play a role in glutamate-induced neuronal death by facilitating Ca^{2+} mobilization, resulting in membrane depolarization, which can also activate voltage-dependent calcium channels. These receptors may represent a pharmacological pathway to a relatively subtle amelioration of neurotoxicity because they serve a modulatory rather than a direct role in excitatory glutamatergic transmission.

Sodium – dependent glutamate transporters, EAATs, are located on the plasma membrane of neurons and glial cells and rapidly terminate the action of glutamate in order to avoid excitotoxicity which will occur when the extracellular concentration is high. Glutamate is taken up by glial cells, metabolized to glutamine, which is transported back to the neurons. Various subtypes of EAAT have been identified, EAAT1; EAAT2 and EAAT3, EAAT4 and EAAT5. EAAT3 and EAAT4 are located predominantly outside the synapse; in the perisynapic membrane in contact with glial cells and may influence the time scale of synaptic events. Furthermore EAATs located on glial cell membranes take up the majority of synaptic glutamate, approximately 90%. Therefore any proteins which interact with EAATs to alter their expression on the plasma membrane, localization or clustering, could affect synaptic transmission.

Interestingly in the spinal cord of the transgenic mutant SOD-1 mouse of ALS, the expression levels of all 5 EAARS splice variants are altered indicating that functional regulation of EAAT2 may be related to the pathology of ALS. EAATs, are also regulated by a number of endogenous factors including protein kinases, growth factors and second messengers. A variety of molecules have been designed and synthesized to alter EAATs, e.g. AMPA, kainite, derivatives of pyrrolidine dicarboxylate serine and aspartate.

While apoptosis plays a role in glutamate-mediated toxicity, the mechanisms underlying this process have yet to be completely determined. Recent evidence has shown that exposure to excitatory amino acids regulates the expression of the antiapoptotic protein, Bcl-2, and the proapoptotic protein, Bax, in neurons. The ratio of Bax to Bcl-2 is an important determinant of neuronal survival, the reciprocal regulation of these Bcl-2 family proteins may play a role in the neurotoxicity mediated by glutamate (Schelman et al., 2004).

The cycloxygenases, COX-1 and COX-2 (previously referred to as prostaglandin H_2 synthase, PGH_2 synthase) catalyse the first step of prostaglandin synthesis from arachidonic acid, (**Figure 2.22a**). PGE_2 a principal prostaglandin product of COX-2 enzymatic activity, exerts its downstream effects by signalling through a class of four distinct G-protein coupled E-prostanoid receptors, EP1, EP2, EP3 and EP4, that have divergent effects on cAMP and phospho-inositol turnover. EP2 receptor subtype is abundantly expressed in the cerebral cortex, striatum and hippocampus and is positively coupled to cAMP production (McCullough et al., 2004). COX-1 is primarily involved in the production of prostanoids relevant to physiological processes whereas COX-2 is mainly responsible for the production of prostanoids linked to pathological events.

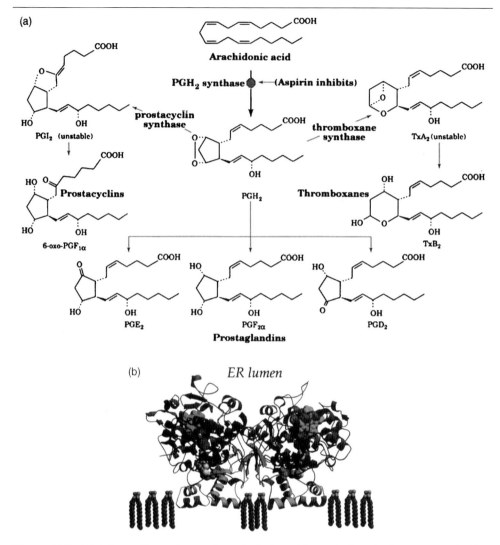

Figure 2.22: (a) The cyclic pathway of arachadonic acid metabolism leads to prostaglandins, prostacycins and thromboxanes. The inhibition of the synthesis of prostaglandins is the target for the analgesic, anti-pyretic and anti-inflammatory properties of aspirin, and for many other non-steroidal anti-inflammatory drugs. (From Voet and Voet, 1995). (b) X-ray structure of PGH synthase in complex with the non-steroid anti-inflammatory drug flurbiprofen. (c) The hydrophobic channel (blue dots) leading to the cyclooxygenase active site below the haem (orange). (From Voet and Voet, 2004).

COX-2 is rapidly upregulated in neurons after NMDA receptor dependent synaptic activation as well as by inflammation leading to elevated levels of PGE_2 and a cascade of deleterious events which will cause neurodegeneration. The pharmaceutical industry has seized on the small, but significant differences between their active site channel (**Figure 2.22b, c**), to develop inhibitors which can enter the COX-2 channel, but are excluded from that of COX-1, and are therefore effective anti-inflammatories, which lack the major side effects of the non-specific inhibitors of both COX isoforms.

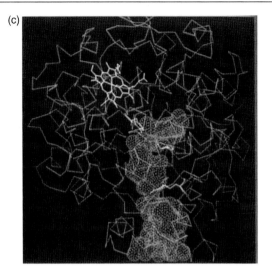

(c)

Figure 2.22: (*Continued*)

Table 2.1: A summary of the main amyloidoses and the proteins or peptides involved[a]

Clinical syndrome	Fibril component
Alzheimer's disease	*Aβ peptides (1–40, 1–41, 1–42, 1–43); Tau*
Spongiform encephalopathies	*Prion protein (full-length or fragments)*
Parkinson's disease	*α-synuclein (wild type or mutant)*
Fronto-temporal dementias	*Tau (wild type or mutant)*
Familial Danish dementia	*ADan peptide*
Familial British dementia	*ABri peptide*
Hereditary cerebral haemorrhage with amyloidoses	*Cystatin C (minus a 10-residue fragment); Aβ peptides*
Amyotrophic lateral sclerosis	*Superoxide dismutase (wild type or mutant)*
Dentatorubro-pallido-Luysian atrophy	*Atrophin 1 (polyQ expansion)*
Huntington disease	*Huntingtin (polyQ expansion)*
Cerebellar ataxias	*Ataxins (polyQ expansion)*
Kennedy disease	*Androgen receptor (polyQ expansion)*
Spino cerebellar ataxia 17	*TATA box-binding protein (polyQ expansion)*
Primary systemic amyloidosis	Ig light chains (full-length or fragments)
Secondary systemic amyloidosis	Serum amyloid A (fragments)
Familial Mediterranean fever	Serum amyloid A (fragments)
Senile systemic amyloidosis	Transthyretin (wild-type or fragments thereof)
Familial amyloidotic polyneuropathy I	Transthyretin (over 45 variants or fragments thereof)
Hemodialysis-related amyloidosis	β2-microglobulin
Familial amyloid polyneuropathy III	Apolipoprotein A-1 (fragments)
Finnish hereditary systemic amyloidosis	Gelsolin (fragments of the mutant protein)
Type II diabetes	Pro-islet amyloid polypeptide (fragments)
Medullary carcinoma of the thyroid	Procalcitonin (full-length or fragment)
Atrial amyloidosis	Atrial natriuretic factor
Lysozyme systemic amyloidosis	Lysozyme (full-length, mutant)
Insulin-related amyloid	Insulin (full-length)
Fibrinogen α-chain amyloidosis	Fibrinogen (α-chain variants and fragments)

[a] Conditions affecting the central nervous system are written in italic.

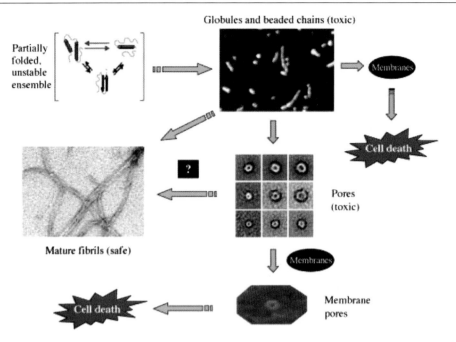

Figure 2.23: The heterogeneous population of pre-fibrillar aggregates comprises globular assemblies further organizing into beaded chains and doughnut-shaped entities currently associated with cytotoxicity due to their ability to interact with cell membranes. In particular, the pore-like assemblies may impair membrane permeability altering metal ion distribution between intracellular and extracellular media as well as among intracellular compartments triggering cell apoptosis. The question mark indicates that it is not known whether amyloid pores (when formed) are on the pathway or are dead end intermediates of fibril formation. Reprinted from Stefani, Copyright 2004, with permission from Elsevier.

A common hallmark of many neurodegenerative diseases is the presence of protein-containing deposits in the affected tissues and organs, which, in some cases, are believed to be the main causative agents of the clinical symptoms. About twenty protein deposition diseases, frequently referred to as amyloidoses, are characterized by deposits of fibrillar aggregates found as intracellular inclusions or extracellular plaques (amyloid[5]). The main component of the amyloid is a specific peptide or protein, which is different in the many neurological diseases (**Table 2.1**). However, despite the considerable differences between their protein constituents, amyloid fibres are remarkably similar, both in their morphological appearance, in their structure (with an increased content of beta structure) and in their capacity to bind dyes. Typically, amyloid fibres are straight, unbranched, 6-12 nm wide (larger in some cases) formed by a variable number of elementary filaments (protofibrils),

---

[5] The term "amyloid" was originally used to describe protein-rich aggregates associated with a number of diseases such as Alzheimer's, Parkinson's, Huntington's, because some of their properties resemble amylose, a component of starch. The traditional test for amyloid involves the red shift in the light absorption of the dye Congo red, and a characteristic green birefringence under polarized light. Both effects are due to the interaction of the dye molecule with the regularly spaced peptide chains, in many ways analogous to the binding of iodine to amylase, which gives an intense purple colour. For protein aggregates to be properly described as amyloid, detection of the characteristic 'cross-β' structures in X-ray diffraction and typical morphology in EM micrographs are generally considered as requisites.

which are twisted around each other in a rope-like structure (for a recent review of amyloidoses, see Stefani, 2004).

The fact that amyloid fibres, albeit constructed from completely different proteins, are structurally very similar, seems to imply that their aggregation is a property of the polypeptide backbone which does not depend on the specific amino acid sequence. This implies that once they have been synthesized, polypeptide chains usually fold into their correct three-dimensional tertiary structure (**Figure 2.23**). However, native or misfolded monomers, despite the attention of well-intentioned chaperones, like heat shock protein Hsp, nonetheless progress down the primrose path of formation of distinct, misfolded monomers, and continue to the everlasting bonfire of inclusion body formation.

REFERENCES

Adams, J.M. and Cory, S. (1998) *Science*, **281**, 1322–1326.
Arai, M., Imai, H., Koumura, T., Yoshida, M. *et al.* (1999) *J. Biol. Chem.*, **274**, 4924–4933.
Baranano, D.E. and Snyder, S.H. (2001) *Proc. Natl. Acad. Sci., USA*, **98**, 10996–10002.
Barja, G. and Herrero, A.J. (1998) *J. Bioenerg. Biomembr.*, **30**, 235–243.
Beal, M.F. (2002) *Free Radic. Biol. Med.*, **32**, 797–803.
Berlett, B.S. and Stadtman, E.R. (1997) *J. Biol. Chem.*, **272**, 20313–20316.
Black, H.S. (2004) *Photochem Photobiol Sci.*, **3**, 753–758.
Boehning, D., Moon, C., Sharma, S., Hurt, K.J. *et al.* (2003) *Neuron*, **40**, 129–137.
Bowie, A. and O'Neill, L.A. (2000) *Biochem. Pharmacol.*, **59**, 13–23.
Boveris, A., Cadenas, E. and Stoppani, A.O.M. (1976) *Biochem. J.*, **156**, 435–444.
Cadenas, E. (2004) *Mol. Aspects Med.*, **25**, 17–26.
Chen, B. and Deen, W.M. (2001) *Chem. Res. Toxicol.*, **14**, 135–147.
Crapo, J.D., Oury, T., Rabouille, C., Slot, J.W. and Chang, L.Y. (1992) *Proc. Natl. Acad. Sci., USA*, **89**, 10405–10409.
Crichton, R.R. (2001) in *Inorganic Biochemistry of Iron Metabolism from Molecular Mechanisms to Clinical Consequences.* John Wiley and Sons, Chichester.
Crichton, R.R. and Pierre, J.L. (2001) *Biometals*, **14**, 99–112.
Dalle-Donne, I, Giustarini, D., Colombo, R., Rossi, R. and Milzani, A. (2003) *TRENDS Mol. Med.*, **9**, 169–176.
Dedon, P.C. and Tannenbaum, S.R. (2004) *Arch. Biochem. Biophys.*, **423**, 12–22.
Fenton, H.J.H. (1894) *Trans. Chem. Soc.*, **65**, 899–910.
Forman, H.J. and Torres, M. (2001) *Mol. Aspects Med.*, **22**, 189–216.
Foster, M.W., McMahon, T.J. and Stamler, J.S. (2003) *TRENDS Mol. Med.*, **9**, 160–168.
Genova, M.L., Ventura, B., Giuliani, G., Bovina, C. *et al.* (2001) *FEBS Lett.*, **505**, 364–368.
Gerasimov, O.V. and Lymar, S.V. (1999) *Inorg. Chem.*, **38**, 4317–4321.
Gong, X., Tang, X., Wiedmann, M., Wang, X. *et al.* (2003) *Neuron*, **38**, 33–46.
Greenacre, S.A. and Ischiropoulos, H. (2001) *Free Radic. Res.*, **34**, 541–581.
Grossmann, A. and Wendel, A. (1983) *Eur. J. Biochem.*, **135**, 549–552.
Guo, Q. (2003) *Sci. Aging Knowledge Environ.*, **50**, pe36.
Haber, F. and Weiss, J. (1934) *Proc. Roy. Soc. Ser. A*, **147**, 332–351.
Halfpenny, E. and Robinson, P.L. (1952a) *J. Chem. Soc.*, 928–938.
Halfpenny, E. and Robinson, P.L. (1952b) *J. Chem. Soc.*, 938–946.
Halliwell, B. (1989) *Brit. J. Exp. Path.*, **70**, 735–757.
Hanisch, U.K. (2002) *Glia*, **40**, 140–155.
Imai, H. and Nakagawa, Y. (2003) *Free Radic. Biol. Med.*, **34**, 145–169.
Kaltschmidt, B. and Kaltschmidt, C. (2000) *Exp. Brain Res.*, **130**, 100–104.

Karin, M. and Lin, A. (2002) *Nat. Immunol.*, **3**, 221–227.

Kreutzberg, G.W. (1996) *TRENDS Neurosci.*, **19**, 312–318.

Kushnareva, Y., Murphy, A.N. and Andreyev, A. (2002) *Biochem. J.*, **368**, 545–553.

Lewis, R.S., Tamir, S., Tannenbaum, S.R. and Deen, W.M. (1995) *J. Biol. Chem.*, **270**, 29350–29355.

Lindahl, T. (1993) *Nature*, **362**, 709–715.

Liou, W., Chang, L.Y., Geuze, H.J., Strous, G.J. *et al.* (1993) *Free Radic. Biol. Med.*, **14**, 201–207.

McCay, P.B. (1985) *Am. Rev. Nutr.*, **5**, 323–340.

McCullough, L., Wu, L., Haughey, N., Liang, X. *et al.* (2004) *J. Neurosci.*, **24**, 257–268.

McGeer, E.G. and McGeer, P.L. (1999) *Curr. Pharm. Des.*, **5**, 821–836.

Mark, L.P., Prost, R.W., Ulmer, J.L., Smith, M.M., *et al.* (2001) *Am. J. Neuroradiol.*, **22**, 1813–1824.

Nakamura, Y. (2002) *Biol. Pharm. Bull.*, **25**, 945–953.

Pfeiffer, P., Goedecke, W. and Obe, G. (2000) *Mutagenesis*, **15**, 289–302.

Pierre, J.L., Fontecave, M. and Crichton, R.R. (2002) *Biometals*, **15**, 341–346.

Pryor, W.A. and Squadrito, G.L. (1995) *Am. J. Physiol.*, **268**, L699–L722.

Riobo, N.A., Melani, M. Sanjuan, N., Fiszman, M.L. *et al.* (2002) *J. Biol. Chem.*, **277**, 42447–42455.

Schacter, E. (2000) *Drug Metab. Rev.*, **32**, 307–326.

Schelman, W.R., Andres, R.D., Sipe, K.J., Kang, E. *et al.* (2004) *Brain. Res. Mol. Brain. Res.*, **128**, 160–169

Schreck, R., Rieber, P. and Baeuerle, P.A. (1991) *EMBO J.*, **10**, 2247–2258.

Schroeter, H., Boyd, C.S., Ahmed, R., Spencer, J.P.E. *et al.* (2003) *Biochem. J.*, **372**, 359–369.

Shigeri, Y., Seal, R.P., Shimamoto, K. (2004) *Brain Res. Rev.*, **45**, 250–265.

Shiozaki, E.N. and Shi, Y. (2004) *TRENDS Biochem. Sci.*, **29**, 486–494.

Sies, H. and Arteel, G.E. (2000) *Free Radic. Biol. Med.*, **28**, 1451–1455.

Shigeri, Y., Seal, R.P., Shimamoto, K. (2004) *Brain Res. Rev.*, **45**, 250–265.

Slupphaug, G., Kavli, B. and Krokan, H.E. (2003) *Mutat. Res.*, **531**, 231–251.

Smith, D.S., Greer, P.L., Tsai, L-H. (2001) *Cell Growth Diff.* **12**, 277–283.

Stefani, M. (2004) *Biochim. Biophys. Acta*, **1739**, 5–25.

Stralin, P. and Marklund, S.L. (2001) *Am. J. Physiol. Heart Circ. Physiol.*, **281**, H1621–1629.

Thomas, J.P., Maiorino, M., Ursini, F. and Girotti, A.W. (1990) *J. Biol. Chem.*, **265**, 454–461.

Torres, M. and Forman, H.J. (2003) *Biofactors*, **17**, 287–296.

Turrens, J.F. (2003) *J. Physiol.*, **552**, 335–344.

Turrens, J.F., Freeman, B.A., Levitt, J.G. and Crapo, J.D. (1982) *Arch. Biochem. Biophys.*, **217**, 401–410.

Turrens, J.F., Alexandre, A. and Lehninger, A.L. (1985) *Arch. Biochem. Biophys.*, **237**, 408–414.

Uchida, K. (2000) *Free Radic. Biol. Med.*, **28**, 1685–1696.

Uchida, K. (2003) *Prog. Lipid Res.*, **42**, 318–343.

Voet, D. and Voet, J.G. (1995) *Biochemistry* 2nd *edn.* pp. 1360.

Voet, D. and Voet, J.G. (2004) *Biochemistry* 3rd *edn.* pp. 1591.

Vogt, T.M., Mayne, S.T., Graubard, B.I., Swanson, C.A. *et al.* (2002) *Am. J. Epidemiol.*, **155**, 1023–1032.

Wang, T., Zhang, X. and Li, J.J. (2002) *Internat. Immunopharm.*, **2**, 1509–1520.

Ward, R.J., Abiaka, C. and Peters, T.J. (1994) *J. Nephrol.*, **7**, 89–96.

Wood, R.D., Mitchell, M., Sgouros, J. and Lindahl, T. (2001) *Science*, **291**, 1284–1289.

Yoo, H.J., Chang, M.S. and Rho, H.M. (1999) *Mol. Gen. Genet.*, **262**, 310–313.

Zelko, I.N., Mariani, T.J. and Folz, R.J. (2002) *Free Radic. Biol. Med.*, **33**, 337–349.

3

Parkinson's Disease

Parkinson's disease (PD) was initially described as Shaking Palsy in 1817 by the English surgeon James Parkinson (Parkinson, 1817). The second most common form of motor system degeneration, it is characterized by a progressive loss of dopaminergic neurons in the substantia nigra pars compacta in the ventral midbrain. The aetiology of the disease is unknown. It is possibly multifactorial, with input from a variety of genetic, environmental and endotoxin factors, as well as iron, which increases in specific brain regions with aging. As was already mentioned in Chapters 1 and 2, oxidative stress together with abnormal protein turnover and degradation, are likely to be key factors in the development and progression of this disease.

With aging, >65y, there is a significantly higher incidence rate of Parkinson's disease, particularly in men where the relative risk found is 1.5x greater than women. Possible reasons for the increased Parkinson's risk in man are toxicant exposure, head trauma, neuroprotection by oestrogen, mitochondrial dysfunction or X-linkage of genetic risk factors. Animal studies suggest that oestrogen may protect the nigrostriatal dopaminergic pathway, by influencing the synthesis, release and metabolism of dopamine, but only in female rats. In addition, oestrogens can modulate dopamine receptor expression and function (Shulman 2002). After the menopause when PD symptoms may be exacerbated, hormone-replacement therapy may delay or alleviate the development of Parkinson's disease, as well as being of benefit in certain types of memory impairment (Shulman 2002).

Excessive dietary intake of iron, particularly in combination with manganese might be a risk factor for PD (Powers et al., 2003), although the tight control of iron intake at the intestinal mucosa (see Chapter 1), is likely to preclude such an occurrence. Genotyping of Parkinson's patients for the inheritance of mutations associated with genetic haemochromatosis, i.e. C282Y and the 282Tyr allele, indicated that the presence of the C282Y mutation did increase the risk of PD (Dekker et al., 2003). However, no iron status measurements were given for these patients, an important criterion, since the presence of the C282Y mutation is not necessarily associated with increased iron loading. The presence of the 282Tyr allele did offer some protection against the development of PD (Buchanan et al., 2002). A recent magnetic resonance study of the brains of 4 GH patients, did show that 3 patients had increased iron accumulation in the basal ganglia which was associated with neurological symptoms of Parkinson's disease (Costello et al., 2004).

Metal-based Neurodegeneration: From Molecular Mechanisms to Therapeutic Strategies R. R. Crichton and R. J. Ward
© 2006 John Wiley & Sons, Ltd

There is strong evidence implicating the abnormal processing of a number of cellular proteins (see 3.1.1 to 3.1.4) via the ubiquitin/26S proteosomal system in PD. Such proteins are present in the cytosol as insoluble, unfolded, ubiquitinated polypeptides. The characteristic inclusion bodies of PD, Lewy bodies (LB), present in affected neurons in the brains, are eosinophilic intracytoplasmic inclusions, with a core of granular and filamentous material surrounded by radiating filaments 10–15 nm in diameter. Wild type α-synuclein is found as a major component of Lewy bodies, suggestive that α-synuclein is involved in the pathophysiology of PD. A diverse group of other neurodegenerative proteinopathies (Lewy body disorders, multiple system atrophy and Hallervorden-Spatz disease) are also characterized by the presence of α-synuclein aggregates within specific neurons. Together with PD, these neurodegenerative diseases are termed synucleinopathies.

3.1 PROTEINS INVOLVED IN PARKINSON'S DISEASE

Synucleins are a family of small (between 123–143 amino acids), highly charged proteins, expressed predominantly in neural tissue and in some tumours (George, 2002). Three human synuclein proteins α, β and γ are known, and they are encoded by separate genes on three different chromosomes, 4q21.3-q22, 5q23 and 10q23.2-q23.3, respectively. The sequences of sixteen vertebrate synucleins are presented in **Figure 3.1**. They all consist of a highly conserved amino-terminal domain, including a variable number of 11-residue repeats and a less-conserved carboxy-terminal domain which has a preponderance of acidic residues. There is a deletion of 11 amino acids (residues 53-63) in all β-synucleins. The 11-mer repeats (which recur up to seven times) constitute a highly conserved α-helical lipid-binding motif, similar to that found in class-A_2 apolipoprotein.

The synucleins, in common with the microtubule-associated protein tau, as well as mutants of α-synuclein and tau, are associated with inherited forms of neurodegenerative disease, and have a very similar type of structure. They are classed as natively unfolded proteins with practically no organized secondary structure in solution. However, when they bind to phospholipid vesicles the lipid binding is accompanied by a large shift in protein secondary structure, from around 3% to over 70% α-helix (Perrin et al., 2000).

Bowman-Birk protease inhibitors are good examples of proteins which, while not natively unfolded, nonetheless have non-regular structures. They are small single-chain proteins of molecular mass around 7–9 kDa with seven disulfide links which stabilize a native fold comprising two tandem homologous domains (de la Sierra, 1999). The X-ray crystal structure (PDB code 1 pi2) of soybean Bowman-Birk inhibitor is shown in **Figure 3.2**. It has been suggested, on the basis of the similarity of their Raman optical activity (Syme et al., 2002) that the major conformational elements are similar and hence that the structures of the synucleins and tau may be envisaged as more open, hydrated, longer-chain (and non-globular) versions of the structure of the Bowman-Birk inhibitor.

Alpha- and β-synucleins are found primarily in brain tissue, predominantly in the neocortex, hippocampus, striatum, thalamus and cerebellum: immunoreactive proteins are enriched in presynaptic terminals. Gamma-synuclein is found primarily in the peripheral nervous system (in primary sensory neurons, sympathetic neurons and motor neurons) and in retina: its expression in breast tumours is a marker of tumour progression (George, 2002).

It has been proposed that α-synuclein may play an important biological role in the modulation of dopamine release, as a regulatory protein, which binds and inhibits tyrosine hydroxylase, the rate-limiting enzyme in dopamine biosynthesis (Perez and Hastings 2004).

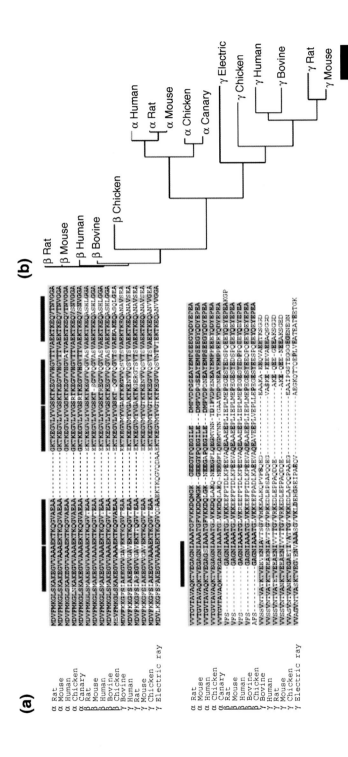

Figure 3.1: Amino acid sequence alignment and relationships of 16 known synuclein sequences (from George, 2002) The imperfect 11-residue repeats are identified. Reproduced with permission from Genome Biology, 3(1). Copyright (2001) BioMed Central Ltd.

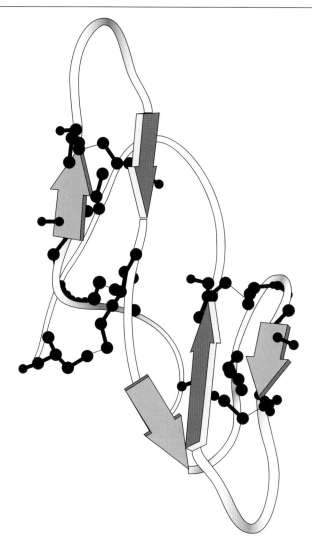

Figure 3.2: A MOLSCRIPT diagram of the X-ray crystal structure of soybean Bowman-Birk inhibitor. From Syme et al. 2002. Reproduced by permission of Blackwell Publishing Ltd.

Alpha-synuclein is localized within the cytosol, in close proximity to synaptic vesicles at presynaptic termini. It shares both physical and functional homology with 14-3-3 proteins, a family of ubiquitous cytoplasmic chaperones, which are, like α-synuclein, particularly abundant in brain. The 14-3-3 proteins bind to target proteins at sites containing phospho-serine residues. Regions of α-synuclein and 14-3-3 proteins share over 40% homology, α-synuclein binds to 14-3-3 proteins, and also binds to 14-3-3 target proteins, including protein kinase C and BAD (Ostrerova et al., 1999). BAD, as will be recalled from Chapter 2, is a pro-apoptotic member of the Bcl-2 family proteins, whose activation is involved in the initiation of the intrinsic pathway of apoptosis.

In idiopathic Parkinson's disease, aggregates of wild type α-synuclein, which are heavily ubiquinated, are found in Lewy bodies within dopaminergic neurons, axons and synapses of

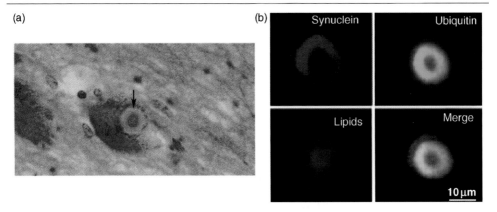

Figure 3.3: A Lewy body contains a mass of proteins, including synuclein, and is a characteristic feature of Parkinson's disease of neural tissue. (**a**) Midbrain Lewy body with easily recognized round shape with surrounding pallor (**b**) Lewy bodies stained with antibodies α-synuclein, ubiquitin and lipids. From Stewart, 2003. Reproduced with permission from the BMJ Publishing Group.

the substania nigra (**Figure 3.3**). The dopaminergic neurons seem to be particularly and selectively vulnerable to the toxic effects of α-synuclein (Eriksen et al., 2003). Over-production of wild type α-synuclein, as seen in the Iowan kindred (Singleton et al., 2003), exhibits a triplication of the α-synuclein gene, which results in autosomal dominant PD giving four copies of the gene rather than the usual two.

The presence of Lewy bodies in affected regions of PD brains indicates improper handling of this protein. Alpha-synuclein may be the actual building block of the fibrillary components of LBs, binding tubulin amongst a host of other ubiquitinated proteins, such as, transglutaminase (Junn et al., 2003), synphilin-1 and parkin (Chung et al., 2001), and acts as the focal point for the aggregations. Its polymerization is associated with concomitant changes in secondary structure which can range from the natively unfolded state in solution, to α-helical in the presence of lipid containing vesicles to anti-parallel β-pleated sheet structures or amyloid structure in fibrils. Such products will initiate disturbances in the cytosolic cellular compartment interacting with vesicles, dopamine transporters and intra-neuronal mitochondria, which may lead to cellular death.

The importance of α-synuclein in the development of PD can be exemplified in knock-out and knock-in mice for the gene. Mice lacking the gene have decreased striatal dopamine function, reduced locomotive responses to amphetamines and showed increased dopamine release with paired-pulse stimuli, but were resilient to the mitochondrial toxin MPTP, possibly due to altered synaptic function in dopaminergic neurons, thereby preventing MPTP from inhibiting Complex 1 (Dauer et al., 2002). Over-expression and gene triplication of α-synuclein in transgenic mice induces inclusions in brain regions which are typically affected by Lewy bodies and cause neurodegeneration (Trojanowski et al., 1998; Wirdefeldt et al., 2001; Singleton et al., 2003). Increased levels of α-synuclein in transfected human cultured foetal dopaminegic neurons resulted in apoptotic cell death. It was noteworthy that if dopamine synthesis was inhibited in these latter cells, apoptosis was prevented perhaps implicating a reaction between α-synuclein and endogenous levels of dopamine in the generation of ROS. In experiments in yeast, a specific protein-protein interaction between α-synuclein and cytochrome c oxidase, the terminal electron transporter of the mitochondrial respiratory system, was established, suggesting that α-synuclein aggregation might enhance mitochondrial dysfunction, (Elkon et al., 2002) (see mitochondrial dysfunction and PD, 3.4.).

A link between iron and α-synuclein has been identified *in vitro*. Iron enhances intracellular aggregation of α-synuclein (Ostrerova et al., 1999; Golts et al., 2002; Hasegawa et al., 2004) leading to the formation of advanced glycation end products (Uversky et al., 2001; Munch et al., 2000) while α-synuclein liberated hydroxy radicals when incubated with Fe^{2+} (Turnbull et al., 2001). Extracellular α-synuclein will generate ROS (Sung et al., 2001). Pretreatment of cells with cell-permeable iron chelators, transferrin-receptor antibodies or transfection with glutathione peroxidase inhibited intracellular oxidant generation, α-synuclein expression/aggregation as well as apoptosis (Kalivendi et al., 2004). Interestingly magnesium inhibited aggregation, by preventing conformational changes.

β-synuclein, while having similar properties to α-synuclein, is non-amyloidogenic and may be an inhibitor of α-synuclein aggregation (Hashimoto et al., 2001; 2004). In doubly transgenic mice expressing both human α- and β-synuclein, β-synuclein protected against motor defects, neurodegenerative alterations and neuronal accumulation of α-synuclein which was observed in the single transgenic mice model of α-synuclein (Hashimoto et al., 2001). More recent results (Hashimoto et al., 2004) indicate that the neuroprotective effects of β-synuclein may involve direct interactions with the serine-threonine kinase Akt (protein kinase B) and suggest that this signalling pathway might be a potential therapeutic target.

In contrast to the other two synucleins, γ-synuclein is most abundant in the peripheral nervous system and is distributed throughout the neuronal cytosol.

Parkin is located on chromosome 6, 6q25-27, and has a distinct domain structure (**Figure 3.4**) consisting of a ubiquitin-like (Ubl) domain at its amino terminus and two carboxy-terminal cysteine-rich RING[1] (really interesting new gene) fingers flanking an in-between RING (IBR) domain (Cookson, 2003a). Wild type parkin has been shown to have E3 ubiquitin-protein ligase activity, whereas autosomal recessive juvenile parkinsonian-related mutant parkin proteins do not have this activity (Imai et al., 2000: Shimura et al., 2000: Zhang, et al., 2000). Parkin is thus one of the large number of E3 ubiquitin-protein ligases whose cellular role is to add the polyubiquitin tail to targeted proteins for their degradations, through the binding of their Ubl to proteosomes, as described in Chapter 2 (**Figure 3.4**). The Ubl of parkin has a typical ubiquitin fold and binds to the Rpn10 subunit (Rnt6 and C3) of the 26S proteasome complex (Sakata et al., 2003), while the extreme C-terminal region interacts with at least one membrane protein, CASK (Fallon et al., 2002), and co-localizes with it in lipid rafts. This means that parkin is tethered to membranes where it can recruit proteasomes (**Figure 3.4**). Mutations affecting Ubl function have been identified in both human (R42P) and Drosophila (A46T) which cause neurodegeneration in humans and mitochondrial dysfunction in Drosophila.

Parkin can also recruit other proteins, such as the heat-shock chaperone Hsp70 (Imai et al., 2002), another E3 ubiquitin ligase, CHIP (Imai et al., 2002), and a component of modular E3 ligase systems, hsel10 (Staropoli et al, 2003). Putative substrates that may be ubiquinated by parkin are shown in **Table 3.1**, and include the O-glycosylated form of α-synuclein,

---

[1] A RING finger is a cysteine-rich zinc-binding motif, which is found in a wide variety of proteins. The domain mediates binding to other proteins, either via their RING domains or other motifs. In several proteins, RING domains are found in combination with other cysteine-rich binding motifs and some proteins, like parkin, contain two RING domains. Recent evidence suggests that RING finger proteins function in the ubiquitin pathway as E3 ligases.

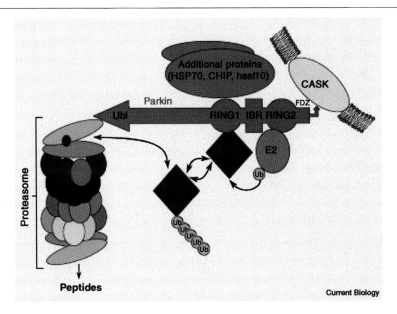

Figure 3.4: Parkin and its role in protein degradation. Parkin has a distinct domain structure, consisting of an amino-terminal ubiquitin-like (Ubl) domain and two carboxy-terminal RING domains separated by an in-between RING (IRB) domain. Two Ubl domains interact with the proteosome whilst the very carboxy-terminal region interacts with at least one membrane protein CASK. From Cookson, 2003a. Parkin can also recruit a number of accessory proteins such as HSP70, CHIP and components of other modular E3 ligases such as hsel10. Reprinted from Cookson, Copyright 2003a, with permission from Elsevier.

synphilin 1 and Pael-R (Cookson, 2003b). The substrates of parkin associate with the RING1 domain, whereas the E2 enzyme carrying the activated ubiquitin binds to the IBR and RING2 domains (**Figure 3.4**). Most of the mutations in parkin are loss-of-function mutations whereby parkin does not ubiquitinate and remove substrates which subsequently accumulate

Table 3.1: Reported substrates of Parkin. Reprinted from Imai and Takahashi, Copyright 2004, with permission from Elsevier

Protein	Physiological or pathological function	Immunopositivity detected in LBs
CDCrel-1	Septin family protein with unknown function	—
O-glycosylated α-synuclein	Isoform of α-synuclein with unknown function	N.D.
Pael receptor	Orphan G-protein coupled receptor	+
p38 subunit of the aminoacyl-tRNA synthetase	Role in protein biosynthesis	+
Synaptotagmin XI	Regulates exocytosis of neurotransmitters	+
Expanded polyglutamine (polyQ) proteins	Aberrant proteins responsible for polyQ diseases	N.D.
α/β-tubulins	Microtubule proteins	+
Synphilin-1	α-synuclein-binding protein	+
Cyclin E	Cell cycle regulation of mitotic cells; unknown function in neurons	N.D.
SEPT5_v2/CDCrel-2	SEPT5_v2 is highly homologous with CDCrel-1	N.D.

with toxic consequences. One of these is an endoplasmic reticulum-resident substrate, a putative G-protein-coupled receptor (Pael-R), which is abundantly expressed in dopaminergic neurons in the substantia nigra, and has the tendency to unfold, even under physiological conditions. Accumulation of insoluble Pael-R could lead to neuronal death as a result of unfolded protein stress: indeed, insoluble Pael-R accumulates in the brains of AR-JP patients, suggesting that accumulation of unfolded Pael-R could lead to selective death of dopaminergic neurons in AR-JP. Hsp70 and CHIP enhance the ability of parkin to inhibit cell death induced by Pael-R (Takahashi and Imai, 2003). Pael-R is selectively toxic to dopaminergic neurons in *Drosophila* which over-express it (Yang et al., 2003). Therefore an important role of parkin is to protect against the toxicity induced by mutant forms of α-synuclein and by Pael-R, by promoting their ubiquitination and proteasomal degradation.

Since the cysteine residues of parkin are integral to its E3 activity, their modification by reactive oxygen species (possibly catalysed by the increasing iron accumulation) may impair its function. Two recent reports indicate that S-nitrosylation may alter parkin's ability to ubiquitate target proteins, although they report opposite effects (Chung et al., 2004; Yao et al., 2004). Peroxide will induce mis-folded parkin which can be prevented if heat shock chaperones, Hsp70 and its co-chaperone Hsp40, are induced. The three carboxy-terminal amino acids of parkin are necessary for proper folding as well as function. Impairment of proteosomal activity by stable expression of parkin mutants leads to accumulation of oxidized proteins and lipids, thereby sensitizing the neurons to various forms of stress leading to neuronal death. Caspase 1 and 8 can directly cleave parkin leading to loss of ubiquitin ligase activity, causing accumulation of toxic parkin substrates and triggering dopaminergic cell death (Kahns et al., 2003). Lymphocytes from patients with AR-JP, homozygous for the Cys212Tyr parkin mutation, show increased sensitivity to dopamine, iron and hydrogen peroxide (Jimenez Del Rio et al., 2004).

Studies of parkin-deficient mice suggest that the function of parkin is to maintain synaptic function in dopaminergic neurons. A decrease in several subunits of mitochondrial complexes I and IV in the ventral midbrain were identified in parkin-deficient mice, while functional assays showed reduced respiratory capacity. Decreased levels of cytoprotective enzymes were also identified which resulted in increased protein and lipid peroxidation (Palacino et al., 2004). Such results reveal an essential role for parkin in the regulation of mitochondrial function. Over expression of parkin is beneficial to dopaminergic neurons protecting them from mutant forms of α-synuclein and from Pael-R. Parkin may also protect against aberrant accumulation of cyclin E (Staropoli et al., 2003), facilitate the clearance of proteins which have polyglutamine expansions (Tsai et al., 2003) (see Chapter 5), protect against ER stress, proteasomal inhibition, kainin acid excitotoxicity and ceramide-induced mitochondrial apoptosis (reviewed in Cookson, 2003b).

Synphilin-1, α-synuclein and parkin represent the major components of Lewy bodies. Synphilin-1 is an α-synuclein-binding protein that is ubiquitinated by parkin, and promotes the formation of cytosolic inclusions. It also interacts with the E3 ubiquitin-ligases SIAH-1 and SIAH-2 (Liani et al., 2004). SIAH proteins ubiquitinate synphilin-1 *in vivo*, and promote its degradation by the ubiquitin-proteasome system. An inability of the proteasome to degrade the synphilin-1/SIAH complex will lead to the formation of ubiquitinated cytosolic inclusions. The importance of this protein in Parkinson's disease awaits further clarification although SIAH immuno-reactivity has been shown in Lewy bodies.

Park 3 and **Park 4**, located respectively on chromosomes 2 and 4 have been identified by linkage analysis and may play an important role in Parkinson's disease but further clarification at the protein levels is required. **Park 5** is an ubiquitin carboxy-terminal hydrolase, otherwise known as UCH-L1, which is involved in regulation of the ubiquitin-proteasomal degradation pathway. Its most likely role is to regulate the degradation of free ubiquitin monomers by the lysosomal degradation pathway. It is expressed in neuronal, testicular and ovarian mammalian cells, and is associated and co-localizes with mono-ubiquitin, thereby prolonging the half-life of ubiquitin. Ubiquitin-targeted protein degradation is terminated by recycling of ubiquitin from the polyubiquitin tail followed by digestion of the target protein. Ubiquitin release is catalysed by UCH-L1 An inability to release ubiquitin from the polyubiquitin tail, as a result of reduced UCH-L1 activity, will lead to incomplete degradation of the target protein and accumulation of neurotoxic proteins, **Figure 3.5**. The protein level of UCH-L1 is down regulated in the brains

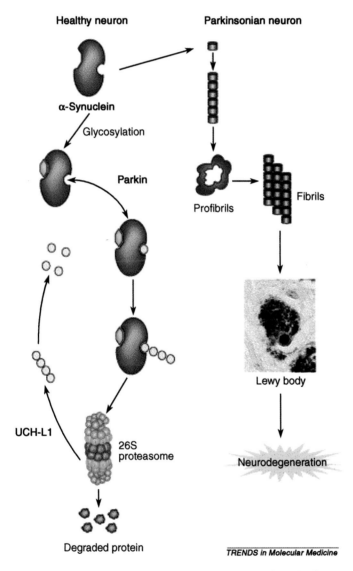

Figure 3.5: A putative model of the role of 3 proteins linked with Parkinson's disease. Reprinted from Barzilai and Melamed, Copyright 2003, with permission from Elsevier.

of idiopathic Parkinson's disease (Choi et al., 2004). Over-expression of this gene increases levels of ubiquitin in both cultured cells and mice and thereby ensures ubiquitin stability within neurons. A mutation in UCH L1 (Ile93Met) decreases the enzymatic activity of UCH L1 but its link with Parkinson's disease remains undefined. UCH L1 protein is a major target for oxidative damage, with carbonyl formation, methionine and cysteine oxidation.

Park 6 (also known as PINK1) appears to encode a putative protein kinase, which locates primarily to the mitochondria (Valente et al., 2002). The *PARK 6* gene provides a direct molecular link between PD and mitochondria, which had been suspected from indirect evidence. However, the targets for phosphorylation by Park 6 remain unknown.

Park 7 (also known as DJ-1) protein maps to the frontal cortex and substantia nigra in the human brain and is particularly prominent in astrocytes. Located on chromome 1, 1p36' its function may be to directly buffer cytosolic redox changes since an acidic isoform accumulates after oxidative stress, thereby reducing neuronal death (Bandopadhyay et al., 2004). In the presence of oxidative stress, wild type Park 7 translocates to the outer mitochondrial membrane where it is associated with neuroprotection (Canet-Aviles et al., 2004): the translocation is induced by oxidation of a key cysteine residue to cysteine-sulphinic acid in the active site of Park 7. Two mutations in the DJ-1 gene have recently been identified which cause early onset, autosomal recessive Parkinson's disease (Bandopadhyay et al., 2004). One mutation is a large deletion that is predicted to produce knock out of the gene while the other is a point mutation, L166P, which destabilizes the DJ-1 protein and promotes its degradation through the ubiquitin-proteasome system, thereby decreasing DJ-1 protein within the cell. Down-regulation of endogenous DJ-1 of the neuronal cell line enhanced cell death that was induced by oxidative stress, ER stress and proteasome inhibition.

Park 8-11 are all genes which have been identified associated with Mendelian forms of PD through genome-wide linkage analysis: the causative genes have not yet been reported (Healy et al., 2004).

NR4A2 which encodes a member of nuclear receptor super family, is essential for the differentiation of nigral dopaminergic neurons. Two mutations, (−291T del and −245T-G) were identified in one allele of 10 out of 107 individuals with familial PD but not in individuals with sporadic PD (n = 94) by comparison to 221 age-matched unaffected controls. Such mutations result in a marked decrease of NR4A2 mRNA levels in transfected cell lines and in lymphocytes of affected individuals. Such mutations may affect transcription of the gene encoding for tyrosine hydroxylase (Le et al., 2003).

3.2 METAL INVOLVEMENT IN PARKINSON'S DISEASE

An inevitable consequence of ageing is an elevation of brain iron in specific brain regions, e.g. in the putamen, motor cortex, prefrontal cortex, sensory cortex and thalamus (Hallgren and Sourander 1958); localized within H-ferritin (Connor et al., 1995; Zecca et al., 2001) H- and L-ferritin in substantia nigra. (Zecca et al., 2001; 2004), and neuromelanin (Zecca et al., 2004), with no apparent adverse effect, **Figure 3.6**. The concentrations of iron vary considerably between different brain regions; areas associated with motor function tend to have more iron than non-motor related regions.

The only differences in the brains of Parkinson's patients is that there is a specific elevation of iron in the substania nigra and the lateral globus pallidus, by approximately

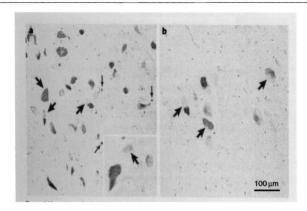

Figure 3.6: Iron deposits in the ageing brain. Iron histochemistry with modified Perls' staining of (**a**) human substantia nigra and (**b**) locus coeruleus, from a normal male subject aged 88 y. Neuromelanin in dopaminergic neurons of SN and noradrenaline neurons of LC are seen as brown granules and iron deposits stain blue. Reproduced with permission from Zecca et al. Copyright (2004) Nature Publishing Group.

2 fold in comparison to age-matched controls (Götz et al., 2004) – see **Figure 1.5**. The cause of such changes in brain iron content in specific brain region remains undefined, and may be caused by a number of factors which include changes in iron release mechanisms across the BBB; or the regulation of iron transport across the cellular membranes of specific brain regions (Moos, 2002). Evidence for the first hypothesis comes from *in vivo* studies of radiolabelled verapamil, a specific substrate for P-glycoprotein (which normally does not cross the blood-brain barrier), but showed increased penetration into the brains of Parkinson's patients in comparison with controls. Such excess iron accumulates in both Lewy bodies and within cytosolic compartments of dopaminergic neurons of the substantia nigra in PD patients, (Wolozin and Golts 2002). Changes in the activity of proteins involved in cellular iron homeostasis may contribute to the increasing cellular iron excesses. DMT1 facilitates the release of iron from the endosomes after internalization of the transferrin-transferrin receptor complex; an increased expression of DMT1 has been reported in the dopaminergic neurons of the substantia nigra of Parkinson's patients (Andrews, 1999), which could reflect an up-regulation of transferrin receptors on such neurons although this needs to be clarified *in vivo*. Neurons are thought to be devoid of ferritin, such that excess iron would be incorporated into neuromelanin which is abundant in dopaminergic neurons. Neurons can also take up iron from non-transferrin iron forms. However, as yet there have been no studies of protein content of DMT1 in the neurons of Parkinson's patients in comparison with controls.

It is remarkable that, in contrast to other iron storage diseases, where 10-20-fold increases in iron stores must be attained before clinical abnormalities occur, e.g. untreated genetic haemochromatosis, GH, and thalassaemia patients, THAL, it requires only a two-fold increase in the iron content of the substantia nigra of PD brains to produce extensive pathological consequences. Although haemosiderin is the predominant iron storage protein in GH and THAL (the result of lysosomal degradation of L-ferritin) it is of interest that in PD H-ferritin is the predominant ferritin present. However, it may be a less effective iron storage protein. This may explain why excess iron accumulates within neuromelanin contained in the dopaminergic neurons of SN and LGP. As these neurons degenerate, the iron-neuromelanin complex is released into the extraneuronal environment to stimulate microglial proliferation. Ferritin increases in the microglial cells which are in close proximity to the degenerating neurons of the SN of PD (reviewed in Götz et al., 2004).

Homozygous knock-out mice for H-ferritin die *in utero*, whereas heterogenous mice are viable (Ferreira et al., 2001) and show brain iron comparable to controls although H-ferritin content is half that of controls. However, transferrin, transferrin receptors, L-ferritin, DMT1 and ceruloplasmin are increased. Oxidative stress was increased in these mice, as shown by oxidatively modified proteins and reduced activities of cytoprotective enzyme, e.g. super-oxide dismutase (Thompson et al., 2003).

Cells which over-expressed human H-chain ferritin accumulated the protein at levels 14-16-fold over background, and showed an iron-deficient phenotype manifested by a 5-fold increase of IRP activity, 2-fold increases in both transferrin receptor, and iron-transferrin iron uptake, and approximately 50% reduction of the labile iron pool (Cozzi et al., 2000). Over-expression of the H-ferritin strongly reduced cell growth and increased resistance to H_2O_2 toxicity; these effects were reverted by prolonged incubation in iron-supplemented medium.

It is noteworthy that, despite the increasing brain iron content in PD, there is no reciprocal up-regulation of L-ferritin expression in response to the iron increase (Dexter et al., 1991; Connor et al., 1995 ; Faucheux et al., 2002). Neuromelanin, a granular dark brown pigment, is produced in catecholaminergic neurons of the SN and locus coeruleus and is possibly the product of reactions between oxidized catechols with a variety of nucleophiles, including thiols from glutathione and proteins (Zucca et al., 2004), **Figure 3.7a**. The function of neuromelanin in the pigmented neurons is unknown but it could play a protective role via attenuation of free radical damage by binding transition metals, particularly iron, **Figure 3.7b**. Whether the ability of the neurones to synthesize neuromelanin is impaired in PD patients is unknown; it is reported that the absolute concentration of nigral neuromelanin is less than 50% in PD with respect to age-matched controls. *In vitro* it has been shown that melanin can bind a significant amount of iron at two sites (Double et al., 2003) although the pigment appears to be only 50% saturated with iron in PD. Iron is bound to the catechol groups. EPR studies of the SN show that ferric iron is bound to neuromelanin as a high spin complex with an octahedral configuration (Zecca and Swartz, 1993; Zecca et al., 1996). Mossbauer spectroscopy (MS) shows that the ferric iron is bound in

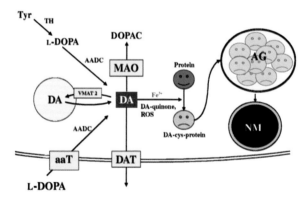

Figure 3.7a: Formation of neuromelanin from the oxidation of dopamine by monoamine oxidase and reactive oxygen species. From Zucca et al. 2004. Reproduced by permission of Blackwell Publishing Ltd.

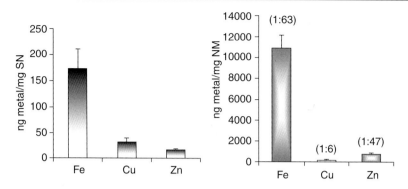

Figure 3.7b: Iron, copper and zinc content in neuromelanin in comparison with substantia nigra. From Zucca et al. 2004. Reproduced by permission of Blackwell Publishing Ltd.

ferritin-like oxyhydroxide clusters; the spectra obtained were comparable to that of ferritin (see Ward et al., 1994 for MS blocking temperatures of ferritin and haemosiderin). Degenerating neurons contain high amounts of iron and neuromelanin but no calbindin 28K, and are poorly protected against oxidative stress. In contrast, neurons that survive in PD are free of melanin, are calbindin 28K-positive, contain low amounts of iron and are better protected against oxidative stress.

Iron regulatory proteins, IRP-1 and IRP-2 act as iron sensors (see Chapter 1) and regulate ferritin synthesis. Studies have therefore been undertaken to ascertain whether changes in post-translational control of ferritin synthesis have occurred in SN of Parkinson's patients. Since changes in ubiquination appear to be an important facet of Parkinson's disease, there may also be changes in the degradation of IRP-2, which may be an explanation for the high cellular iron content within the substantia nigra and the lateral globus pallidus. No studies of IRP-2 binding activity have been reported, although studies of IRP-1 in the SN of Parkinson's patients showed no significant changes by comparison to age-matched controls (Faucheux et al., 2002). This may explain why ferritin mRNA translation is not up regulated despite the increased iron accumulation. However, recent evidence has suggested that IRP2 dominates post-transcriptional regulation of iron metabolism such that further studies are currently needed to clarify the roles played by IRP-1 and IRP-2 in controlling iron homeostasis (see Chapter 2).

No IRP-2 polymorphisms are reported in subjects with sporadic PD and normal controls which might have played an important role in the development of the disease. Genetically engineered mice which lack IRP-2 but have the normal complement of IRP-1, develop adult onset neurodegenerative disease associated with inappropriately high expression of ferritin in degenerating neurons, while mice that are homozygous for a targeted deletion of IRP-2 and heterozygous for a targeted deletion of IRP-1 developed severe neurodegeneration with severe axonopathy, with increase levels of ferric iron and ferritin expression as well as neuronal cell bodies degenerating in the substantia nigra.

The increase in SN iron content, detectable in 90% of individuals affected by the disease by ultrasound measurements, was also detectable in 45% of relatives of Parkinson's disease patients, indicating a degree of inheritance of this disorder (Ruprecht-Dorfler et al., 2003).

Some interest has been directed towards the increased expression of lactoferrin receptors on SN neurons and microvessels of PD patients which may be secondary to iron accumulation (Faucheux et al., 1999). The explanation for their up-regulation is unknown but may be related to lactoferrin's protective properties – it is released in response to inflammation and infection, removing iron from the circulation and allowing it to be sequestered within macrophages.

Melanotransferrin or melanoma tumor antigen p97 is a transferrin homologue with one iron binding site, which can exist either as a membrane-bound associated GPI anchored form or as a soluble form in the CSF or serum. It may be a marker for AD; the soluble form may cross the BBB and accumulate in mouse brain following intravenous infusion (Moroo et al., 2003). *In vitro* studies show that melanotransferrin can bind and internalize iron into cells from iron citrate but not from iron-loaded transferrin. While it may play an important role in Alzheimer's disease, no evidence for an involvement in Parkinson's disease has been reported.

3.3 RISK FACTORS FOR PARKINSON'S DISEASE

Inherited forms of PD have been identified. In an autosomal dominant familial form, α-synuclein, has two rare mis-sense mutations (Polymeropoulos et al., 1997) while in Japanese autosomal recessive juvenile PD, linkage studies revealed mutations in the parkin gene (Kitada et al., 1998). Since then, further mutations of parkin have been identified world-wide. In such PD patients, there is loss of dopaminergic neurons but the typical Parkinsonian symptoms occur without Lewy body formation (Mizuno et al., 1998). Since these early identifications of mutations in α-synuclein and parkin, over 20 other genes have been identified as being associated with PD (Healy et al., 2004).

There is little evidence for transferrin polymorphism despite one study of Borie et al. (2002), which suggested that the increase of iron could be due to G258S transferrin polymorphism, particularly in PD patients with onset of the disease over 60 years and negative family history. Similarly there is no evidence for ferritin mutations; in one study of 186 PD patients, two silent mutations were detected in L-ferritin and one sequence variation in H-ferritin but none in the controls (Felletschin et al., 2003). A recent study indicates that mitochondrial polymorphisms may significantly reduce the risk of Parkinson's disease (van der Walt et al., 2003).

Complex 1 inhibitors such as rotenone, benzylisoquinoline derivatives and acetogenins (found in tropical herbal teas or tropical fruits of the Annonaceae) reproduce the features of Parkinson's disease, possibly by influencing downstream signal transduction processes such as impairment of energy production (Lannuzel et al., 2003).

Enviromental toxins such as fertilizers, pesticides and herbicides have been proposed as causes of Parkinson's disease. MPTP (*N*-methyl-4-phenyl-1,2,3,6-tetrahydropyridone) produces clinical and neuropathologic findings similar to Parkinson's disease.

Manganese is an essential trace element at low concentrations, but at higher concentrations it is neurotoxic, accumulating particularly in the globus pallidus producing the typical clinical symptoms of PD, with rhythmic tremor and muscular rigidity. In addition there is an important psychiatric aspect associated with Mn intoxication, which is manifested by behavioural aggressivity. Chronic occupational metal exposure, particularly to Mn and Cu, has been shown to be a risk factor for Parkinsonism (Gorell et al., 1999). Studies in the rat have shown that Mn and Fe interact during transfer from the plasma to the brain and other organs, and that this transfer is synergistic rather than competitive in nature, suggesting that excessive intake of Fe plus Mn may accentuate the risk of tissue damage by one metal alone, particularly in the brain. Chronic Mn exposure in rats alters iron homeostasis apparently by causing a unidirectional influx of iron from the systemic circulation across the BBB (Zheng et al., 1999). Manganese intoxication in rhesus monkeys results in a Parkinsonian syndrome (in two of three animals), which did not respond to L-DOPA (Olanow et al., 1996). Focal mineral deposits, primarily consisting of iron and aluminium, were found in both the globus pallidus and the substantia nigra pars reticularis.

Zn and Mn influence the neurotransmitter concentrations in the synapic cleft, probably via action against neurotransmitter receptors and transporters as well as ion channels (Takeda, 2004). Zn may be an inhibitory neuromodulator of glutamate release in the hippocampus while manganese may induce functional and toxic effects in the synapse.

In vitro, manganese induced cell death in the dopaminergic cells, SH-SY5Y and CATH.a cells, increasing the expression of endoplasmic reticulum stress-associated genes including parkin (Higashi et al., 2004). However, no changes in proteasome activity was observed. Transient infection of these cells with the parkin gene inhibited cell death. When SK-N-MC neuroblastoma cells, which over-expressed α-synuclein, were exposed to various doses of MPTP, dopamine or Mn, only Mn induced a significantly decreased viability of these cells after 72h, which suggested that Mn may co-operate with α-synuclein in triggering cell death (Pifl et al., 2004).

Both the cytotoxicity and plastogenicity of levodopa and dopamine in cultured cells lines is enhanced by concomitant exposure to either Mn and Cu salts (Snyder and Friedman, 1998). Mn increased LPS-stimulated NO production from microglial cells, unlike other transition metals tested which included iron, cobalt, copper and zinc. Mn appeared to exert its effect at the level of transcription of the inducible NO synthase, but unlike other transition metals, Mn did not appear to be cytotoxic to microglial cells. It is suggested that Mn could induce sustained production of neurotoxic NO by activated microglial cells, which might be detrimental to surrounding neurons.

While our present dietary heterogeneity (at least in the developed world) makes it unlikely that we will encounter many cases of Mn deficiency, the increasing tendency for a vegetarian regime, may induce iron deficiency, which may simultaneously increase both iron and Mn intake at the intestinal level. Manganese may interfere with iron regulation by altering the binding of iron regulatory proteins; *in vitro* incubation of 1, 10, and 50 mM manganese with undifferentiated PC12 cells increased the labile iron pool, resulting in a decrease in IRP binding activity (Kwik-Uribe et al., 2003).

Post-mortem studies have demonstrated a substantial loss of nicotinic receptors in Parkinson's disease (Kelton et al., 2000). Epidemiological studies show that smoking is associated with a decreased incidence of Parkinson's disease (Ross and Petrovitch, 2001; Quik, 2004); a decreased PD risk in twin studies (Tanner, 2002) and a decrease in monoamine oxidase activity. Furthermore, nicotine treatment relieves some of the symptoms of the disease (Quik and Kulak, 2002). Intravenous administration of nicotine, followed by its chronic administration by transdermal patch for 2 weeks, to non-demented early to moderate PD patients, showed improvements in both cognitive performance and motor measures (Kelton et al., 2000). Nicotine has been shown in animal models to stimulate the release of dopamine in the striatum and to preserve nigral neurons and striatal dopamine levels in animals with lesioned nigristriatal pathways.

There are multiple nicotinic receptor populations in the brain with different functional properties, such that the identification of specific subunits involved in nigrostriatal dopami-nergic activity is essential. Nicotine stimulates striatal dopamine neurons via its nicotinic

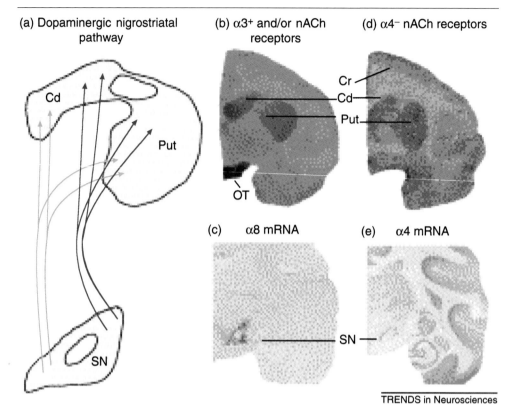

(a) Dopaminergic nigrostriatal pathway

(b) α3+ and/or nACh receptors

(d) α4− nACh receptors

(c) α8 mRNA

(e) α4 mRNA

TRENDS in Neurosciences

Figure 3.8: Autoradiographic distribution of nicotinic nACh receptor mRNA and receptor sites at the level of the substania nigra and striatum in monkey brains. Reprinted from Quik, Copyright 2001, with permission from Elsevier.

receptors, nACh, **Figure 3.8**. Neuronal nACh receptors are pentameric ligand-gated ion channels, composed of α and β subunits. Certain subunits are altered in brains of PD patients, namely α2–α6 are reduced, indicating that nicotine-evoked dopamine release is reduced, while α7 do not appear to be significantly altered. Other investigators have indicated a role for α4 subtypes in nicotine-mediated protection against nigrostriatal injury. Since nAch receptor is a Ca^{2+} ions channel, changes in the calcium fluxes will alter intracellular signalling cascades, as well as nitric oxide-cGMP pathway, caspases and apoptopic signaling. Immune modulators such as IL-1α, IL-1β IL-6 and TNFa, may be activated by nicotine exposure. This may lead to some neuroprotection through inhibition of apoptosis, **Figure 3.9**.

However, a crucial question which needs to be addressed for the use of nicotine supplementation as a therapeutic agent in PD is whether the function of nACh receptors in the degenerating nigrostriatal dopaminergic neurons in PD is affected by denervation (are the receptors still coupled to their effector mechanisms?), as this would have an impact on the subsequent actions of administered nicotine.

In one study where the protective effects of nicotine were studied *in vitro* and *in vivo* (Linert et al., 1999) a reduction in the formation of the neurotoxin 6-hydroxydopamine was assayed in cells (possibly as a result of reduced monoamine oxidase activity), while there was enhanced memory retention in nicotine-treated rats *in vivo* compared to controls. Another effect of nicotine is to preserve mitochondrial function in the rat central nervous

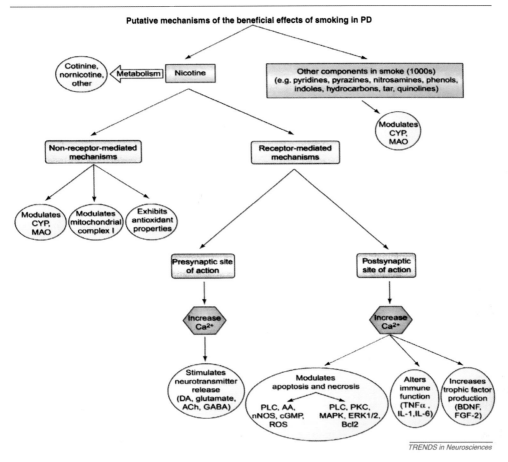

Figure 3.9: Potential mechanisms whereby smoking could result in an apparent beneficial effect in PD. Reprinted from Quik, Copyright 2004, with permission from Elsevier.

system by decreasing the respiratory control ratio and superoxide anion generation in brain mitochondria (Cormier et al., 2003). Other cytochromes such as CYP2E1 (also induced by chronic alcohol ingestion), CYP2B6 are stimulated by nicotine which could enhance the metabolism of toxic agents thereby reducing toxicity. Nicotine metabolites, e.g. cotinine, exhibit cytoprotective properties in cultured cells while another metabolite, nornicotine reduces β-amyloid aggregation.

Coffee and caffeine consumption have been shown in epidemiological studies to be inversely related to Parkinson's disease risk (Ross and Petrovitch, 2001). Caffeine is an adenosine A (2A) receptor antagonist which enhances locomotor activity in animal models of Parkinson's.

An increased consumption of alcohol may reduce the risk of Parkinson's disease. In one study 13,977 residents of a southern California community were studied from 1981 to 1998 and showed that alcohol consumption was inversely associated with risk of Parkinson's disease. In a Dutch study, from the Erasmus Medical Center in Rotterdam, The Netherlands, abstainers from alcohol appeared more likely to develop Parkinson's disease. However, as yet there has been no evidence that there is a genetic links between particular alcohol dehydrogenase (ADH) genotypes and the incidence of Parkinson's disease.

The neurobiology to explain why ethanol may reduce the incidence of PD remains unclear. In experimental animals, microdialysis experiments show that ethanol, both acute and chronic, will alter dopamine release in the nucleus accumbens, where the dopaminergic pathways originates from the ventral tegmental area, VTA. Whether such 'priming' of the dopaminergic neurons elicits some long-term benefit remains to be clarified.

The neurons of the VTA possess nAChRs, such that their activation by nicotine will cause a release of dopamine in the nucleus accumbens. Therefore low doses of alcohol possibly combined with nicotine will result in an additive dopamine release in the nucleus accumbens (Tizabi et al., 2002).

3.4 MITOCHONDRIAL DYSFUNCTION

There is considerable evidence that strongly suggests mitochondrial dysfunction as a major causative factor in PD. However, the molecular mechanisms responsible remain poorly understood.

Mitochondria play a major role in cellular metabolism, not only as ATP producers through oxidative phosphorylation but also as regulators of intracellular calcium homeostasis and endogenous producers of reactive oxygen species. Increasing mitochondrial calcium overload as a result of excitotoxicity is associated with the generation of ROS and may induce the release of pro-apoptotic mitochondrial proteins, culminating in the demise of the cell by apoptosis and/or necrosis (Rego and Oliveira, 2003). Protein mis-folding and aggregation *in vivo* can be suppressed and promoted by several factors such as molecular chaperones, protein degradation systems and free radicals, many of which are under the control of normal mitochondrial function. Mitochondrial defects can lead to aggregation of α-synuclein. Furthermore translocation of misfolded proteins to the mitochondrial membrane may play an important role in triggering or perpetuating neurodegeneration by causing changes in membrane permeability and cytochome c release.

A defect in mitochondrial oxidative phosphorylation, resulting in a reduction in the activity of NADH CoQ reductase (complex 1), occurs in the striatum of patients with Parkinson's disease (Ebadi et al., 2001). The reduction in the activity of complex 1 is found specifically in the SN and not in other parts of the brain. Such specificity of mitochondrial impairment may play a major role in the degeneration of nigrostriatal dopaminergic neurons.

Current evidence suggests that complex 1 inhibition may be the central cause of sporadic PD. Both *in vivo* and *in vitro* iron accumulation in mitochondria will adversely alter complex 1 (Ward and Crichton, unpublished observations). In addition, derangement in complex I causes α-synuclein aggregation contributing to the demise of dopamine neurons. Aggregates of α-synuclein may enhance such dysfunction by specific protein-protein interaction of α-synuclein with cytochrome c oxidase, the terminal complex of the mitochondrial electron transport chain (Elkon et al., 2002), while dopamine-oxidized metabolites may interact with complex I of the chain. Other mitochondrial complexes II and IV are also implicated. Nitric oxide production, either from mitochondrial NOS or from inducible NOS within the cell cytosol inhibits components of the mitochondrial respiratory chain, complexes I, II and IV (particularly when GSH is reduced), causing a cellular energy-deficient state if damage is severe. However, the activation of iNOS in iron-loaded cells will be modulated by the effects of NF-IL6. Dlaska and Weiss (1999) identified a regulatory region on iNOS between -153 to -142 bp upstream of the transcriptional start site of the iNOS promoter that was sensitive to regulation by iron perturbation.

Substantial amounts of parkin are present on the mitochondrial outer membrane which has led to suggestions that this protein may have an important role in maintaining mitochondrial function, possibly protecting the cell from oxidative stress. Indeed, over-expression of parkin has been shown to attenuate C2-ceramide-mediated mitochondrial swelling.

The mitochondrial dysfunctional seen in manganese neurotoxicity might be related to the accumulation of reactive oxygen species. Mitochondrial Mn superoxide dismutase (MnSOD) is found to be low or absent in tumour cells and may act as a tumour suppressor. It is induced by inflammatory cytokines, such as TNF, presumably to protect host cells. In a rat model, iron-rich diets were found to decrease MnSOD activity, although a recent study reported that in rat epithelial cell cultures, iron supplementation increased MnSOD protein levels and activity, but did not compromise the ability of inflammatory mediators like TNF to further increase the enzyme activity (Kuratko, 1999).

3.5 ROLE OF DOPAMINE IN PARKINSON'S DISEASE

In the normal healthy brain, dopamine is produced in the substantia nigra and transmitted to the putamen and caudate nucleus with the net result of an inhibitory effect on movement.

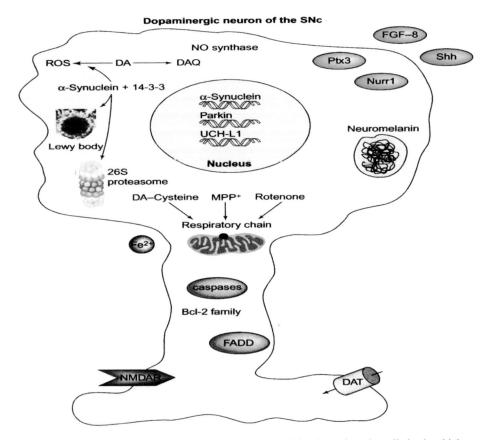

Figure 3.10: Factors that have been shown to be involved in dopaminergic cell death which may be involved in Parkinson's disease. Reprinted from Barzilai and Melamed, Copyright 2003, with permission from Elsevier.

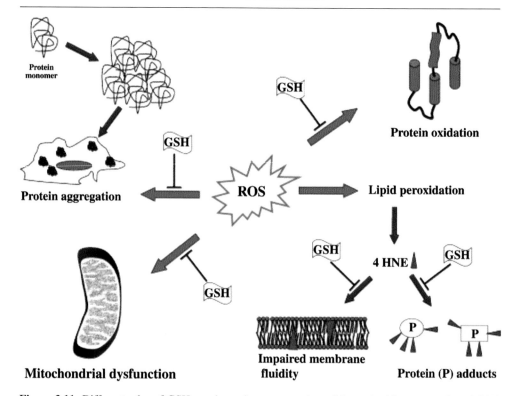

Figure 3.11: Different roles of GSH: a schematic representation of the antioxidant properties of GSH as relevant to SN dopaminergic neuronal cells in PD. Reprinted from Bharath et al., Copyright 2002, with permission from Elsevier.

Acetyl choline, synthesized throughout the basal ganglia will have an excitatory effect on movement such that degeneration of the dopaminergic neurons in the substantia nigra pars compacta, particularly in the subpopulation of melaninized neurones, as observed in Parkinson's brain, will result in an imbalance between acetyl choline and dopamine. The predominance of cholinergic activity produces the characteristic symptoms of rigidity, tremor and bradykinesia.

During a normal life span of 70–80 years, the number of dopamine neurons decreases by around 3–5% every decade. However, by the time that Parkinson's disease is identified, approximately 60–80% of the dopamine-containing neurons have been lost. An increasingly popular hypothesis is that the continued degeneration of dopaminergic neurones in Parkinson's disease may be the consequences of aberrant oxidation of dopamine, **Figure 3.10**. Cumulative evidence supports an 'oxidative stress hypothesis' for initiation of nigral dopamine neuron loss, **Figure 3.11** with depletion of glutathione, **Figure 3.12**. The nigral dopaminergic neuronal cells die by a process of apoptosis. Cellular metabolism of dopamine generates H_2O_2 which is reduced to hydroxyl radicals in the presence of iron (Kim et al., 2002) thereby propagating neuronal damage, **Figure 3.13**.

A multitude of malfunctions occur in Parkinson's disease as a result of the initial alteration in the handling of specific proteins and their degradation by the proteosomal apparatus. As yet, as discussed in Chapter 11, therapeutic strategies are directed only at the pathogenesis of the disease. As our knowledge of the primary and secondary

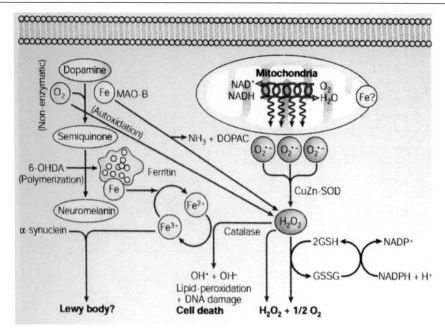

Figure 3.12: Oxidative stress of PD. Iron induces oxidative stress in PD. From Zecca et al., 2004. Reproduced by permission of the National Academy of Sciences.

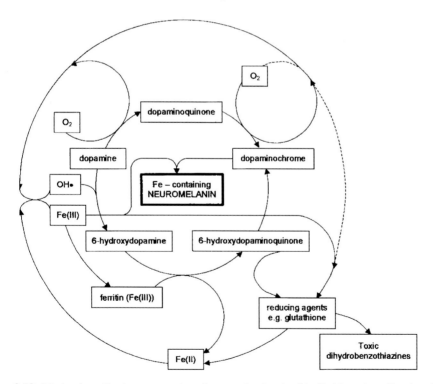

Figure 3.13: Mechanisms for the propagation of cytotoxins involved in Parkinsonism. Reprinted from Linert and Jamieson, Copyright 2000, with permission from Elsevier.

structures of such proteins increases, combined with a better understanding of the ubiquitination and proteasome processes within the cell, further advances will be possible.

REFERENCES

Andrews, N.C. (1999) *Int. J. Biochem. Cell Biol.*, **31**, 991–994.
Bandopadhyay, R., Kingsbury, A.E., Cookson, M.R., Reid, A.R. *et al.* (2004) *Brain*, **127**, 420–430.
Barzilai, A. and Melamed, E. (2003) *TRENDS Mol. Med.*, **9**, 126–132.
Bharath, S., Hsu, M., Kaur, D., Rajagopalan, S. and Andersen, J.K. (2002) *Biochem. Pharmacol.*, **64**, 1037–1048.
Borie, C., Gasparini, F., Verpillat, P., Bonnet, A.M. *et al.* (2002) *J. Neurol.*, **249**, 801–804.
Buchanan, D.D., Silburn, P.A., Chalk, J.B., Le Couteur, D.G. and Mellick, G.D. (2002) *Neurosci. Lett.*, **327**, 91–94.
Canet-Aviles, R.M., Wilson, M.A., Miller, D.W., Ahmad, R. *et al.* (2004) *Proc. Natl. Acad. Sci. USA*, **101**, 9103–9108.
Choi, J., Levey, A.I., Weintraub, S.T., Rees, H.D. *et al.* (2004) *J. Biol. Chem.*, **279**, 13256–13264.
Chung, K.K., Zhang, Y., Lim, K.L., Tanaka, Y. *et al.* (2001) *Nat. Med.*, **7**, 1144–1150.
Chung, K.K., Thomas, B., Li, X., Pletnikova, O. *et al.* (2004) *Science*, **304**, 1328–1331.
Connor, J.R., Snyder, B.S., Arosio, P., Loeffler, D.A. *et al.* (1995) *J. Neurochem.*, **65**, 717–724.
Cookson, M.R. (2003a) *Curr. Biol.*, **13**, R522–R524.
Cookson, M.R. (2003b) *Neuromolecular Med.*, **3**, 1–13.
Cormier, A., Morin, C., Zini, R., Tillement, J.P. *et al.* (2003) *Neuropharmacology*, **44**, 642–652.
Costello, D.J., Walsh, S.L., Harrington, H.J. and Walsh, C.H. (2004) *J. Neurol. Neurosurg. Psychiatry*, **75**, 631–633.
Cozzi, A., Corsi, B., Levi, S., Santambrogio, P. *et al.* (2000) *J. Biol. Chem.*, **275**, 25122–25129.
Dauer, W., Kholodilov, N., Vila, M., Trilat, A.C., *et al.* (2002) *Proc. Natl. Acad. Sci., USA*, **99**, 14524–14529.
Dekker, M.C., Giesbergen, P.C., Njajou, O.T., van Swieten, J.C. *et al.* (2003) *Neurosci. Lett.*, **348**, 117–119.
De la Sierra, I.L., Quillien, L., Flecker, P., Gueguen, J. *et al.* (1999) *J. Mol. Biol.*, **285**, 1195–1207.
Dexter, D.T., Carayon, A., Javoy-Agid, F., Agid, Y. *et al.* (1991) *Brain*, **114**, 1953–1975.
Dlaska, M. and Weiss, G. (1999) *J. Immunol.*, **162**, 6171–6177.
Double, K.L., Gerlach, M., Schunemann, V., Trautwein, A.X. *et al.* (2003) *Biochem. Pharmacol.*, **66**, 489–494.
Ebadi, M., Govitrapong, P., Sharma, S., Muralikrishnan, D. *et al.* (2001) *Biol. Signals Recept.*, **10**, 224–253.
Eriksen, J.L., Dawson, T.M., Dickson, D.W. and Petrucelli, L. (2003) *Neuron*, **4**, 453–456.
Elkon, H., Don, J., Melamed, E., Ziv, I., *et al.* (2002) *J. Mol. Neurosci.*, **18**, 229–238.
Fallon, L., Moreau, F., Croft, B.G., Labib, N. *et al.* (2002) *J. Biol. Chem.*, **277**, 486–491.
Faucheux, B.A., Bonnet, A.M., Agid, Y. and Hirsch, E.C. (1999) *Lancet*, **353**, 981–982.
Faucheux, B.A., Martin, M.E., Beaumont, C., Hunot, S. *et al.* (2002) *J. Neurochem.*, **83**, 320–330.
Felletschin, B., Bauer, P., Walter, U., Behnke, S. *et al.* (2003) *Neurosci. Lett.*, **352**, 53–56.
Ferreira, C., Santambrogio, P., Martin, M.E., Andrieu, V. *et al.* (2001) *Blood*, **98**, 525–532.
George, J.M. (2002) *Genome Biol. Rev.*, **3**, 3002.1–3002.6.
Golts, N., Snyder, H., Frasier, M., Theisler, C., *et al.* (2002) *J. Biol. Chem.*, **277**, 16116–16123.
Gorell, J.M., Johnson, C.C., Rybicki, B.A., Peterson, E.L. *et al.* (1999) *Neurotoxicology*, **20**, 239–247.
Götz, M.E., Double, K., Gerlach, M., Youdim, M.B. *et al.* (2004) *Ann. N.Y. Acad. Sci.*, **1012**, 193–208
Hallgren, B. and Sourander, P. (1958) *J. Neurochem.*, **3**, 41–51.
Hasegawa, T., Matsuzaki, M., Takeda, A., Kikuchi, A., *et al.* (2004) *Brain Res.*, **1013**, 51–9.

Hashimoto, M., Rockenstein, E., Mante, M., Mallory, M. and Masliah, E. (2001) *Neuron*, **32**, 213–223.

Hashimoto, M., Bar-On, P., Ho, G., Takenouchi, T., *et al.* (2004) *J. Biol. Chem.*, **279**, 23622–23629.

Healy, D.G., Abou-Sleiman, P.M. and Wood, N.W. (2004) *Lancet, Neurol.*, **3**, 652–662.

Higashi, Y., Asanuma, M., Miyazaki, I., Hattori, N. *et al.* (2004) *J. Neurochem.*, **89**, 1490–1497.

Imai, Y., Soda, M. and Takahashi, R. (2000) *J. Biol. Chem.*, **275**, 35661–35664.

Imai, Y., Soda, M., Hatakeyama, S., Akagi, T. *et al.* (2002) *Mol. Cell*, **10**, 55–67.

Imai, Y. and Takahashi, R. (2004) *Curr. Opin. Neurobiol.*, **14**, 384–389.

Jimenez Del Rio, M., Moreno, S., Garcia-Ospina, G., Buritica, O. *et al.* (2004) *Mov. Disord.*, **19**, 324–330.

Junn, E., Ronchetti, R.D., Quezado, M.M., Kim, S.Y. and Mouradian, M.M. (2003) *Proc. Natl. Acad. Sci., USA*, **100**, 2047–2052.

Kahns, S., Kalai, M., Jakobsen, L.D., Clark, B.F. *et al.* (2003) *J. Biol. Chem.*, **278**, 23376–23380.

Kalivendi, S.V., Cunningham, S., Kotamraju, S., Joseph J. *et al.* (2004) *J. Biol. Chem.*, **279**, 15240–15247.

Kelton, M.C., Kahn, H.J., Conrath, C.L. and Newhouse, P.A. (2000) *Brain Cogn.*, **43**, 274–282.

Kim, J.R., Kwon, K.S., Yoon, H.W., Lee, S.R. *et al.* (2002) *Arch. Biochem. Biophys.*, **397**, 414–423.

Kitada, T., Asakawa, S., Hattori, N., Matsumine, H. *et al.* (1998) *Nature*, **392**, 605–608.

Kuratko, C.N. (1999) *Toxicol. Lett.*, **104**, 151–158.

Kwik-Uribe, C.L., Reaney, S., Zhu, Z. and Smith, D. (2003) *Brain Res.*, **973**, 1–15.

Lannuzel, A., Michel, P.P., Hoglinger, G.U., Champy, P. *et al.* (2003) *Neuroscience*, **121**, 287–296.

Le, W.D., Jankovic, J., Jiang, H., Appel, S.H. *et al.* (2003) *Nat. Genet.*, **33**, 214.

Lianni, E., Eyal, A., Avraham, E., Shemer, R. *et al.* (2004) *Proc. Natl. Acad. Sci. USA*, **101**, 5500–5505.

Linert, W., Bridge, M.H., Huber, M., Bjugstad, K.B. *et al.* (1999) *Biochem. Biophys. Acta.*, **1454**, 143–152.

Linert, W. and Jamieson, G.N. (2000) *J. Inorg. Biochem.*, **79**, 319–326.

Mizuno, Y., Hattori, N. and Matsumine, H., (1998) *J. Neurochem*, **71**, 893–902.

Moos, T. (2002) *Dan. Med. Bull.*, **49**, 279–301.

Moroo, I., Ujiie, M., Walker, B.L., Tiong, J.W. *et al.* (2003) *Microcirculation*, **10**, 457–462.

Munch, G., Luth, H.J., Wong, A., Arendt, T. *et al.* (2000) *J. Chem. Neuroanat.*, **20**, 253–257.

Olanow, C.W., Good, P.F., Shinotoh, H., Hewitt, K.A. *et al.* (1996) *Neurology*, **46**, 492–498.

Ostrerova, N., Petrucelli, L., Farrer, M., Mehta, N. *et al.* (1999) *J. Neurosci.*, **19**, 5782–5791.

Palacino, J.J., Sagi, D., Goldberg, M.S., Krauss, S. *et al.* (2004) *J. Biol. Chem.*, **279**, 18614–186122.

Parkinson, J. (1817) *An essay on the shaking palsy.*

Perez, R.G. and Hastings, T.G. (2004) *J. Neurochem*, **89**, 1318–1324.

Perrin, R.J., Woods, W.S., Clayton, D.F. and George, J.M. (2000) *J. Biol. Chem.*, **275**, 34393–34398.

Pifl, C., Khorchide, M., Kattinger, A., Reither, H. *et al.* (2004) *Neurosci. Lett.*, **354**, 34–37.

Polymeropoulos, M.H., Lavedan, C., Leroy, E., Ide, S.E. *et al.* (1997) *Science*, **276**, 2045–2047.

Powers, K.M., Smith-Weller, T., Franklin, G.M., Longstreth, W.T. *et al.* (2003) *Neurology*, **60**, 1761–1766.

Quik, M. and Kulak, J.M. (2002) *Neurotoxicology*, **23**, 581–594.

Quik, M. (2004) *Trends Neurosci.*, **27**, 561–569.

Rego, A.C. and Oliveira, C.R. (2003) *Neurochem. Res*, **28**, 1563–1574.

Ross, G.W. and Petrovitch, H. (2001) *Drugs Aging*, **18**, 797–806.

Ruprecht-Dorfler, P., Berg, D., Tucha, O., Benz, P. *et al.* (2003) *Neuroimage*, **18**, 416–422.

Sakata, E., Yamaguchi, Y., Kurimoto, E., Kikuchi, J. *et al.* (2003) *EMBO Rep.*, **4**, 301–306.

Shimura, H., Hattori, N., Kubo, S., Mizuno, Y., *et al.* (2000) *Nat. Genet.*, **25**, 302–305.

Shulman, L.M. (2002) *Parkinsonism Relat. Disord.*, **8**, 289–295.

Singleton, A.B., Farrer, M., Johnson, J., Singleton, A. *et al.* (2003) *Science*, **302**, 841.

Snyder, R.D. and Friedman, M.B. (1998) *Mutat. Res.*, **405**, 1–8.

Staropoli, J.F., McDermott, C., Martinat, C., Schulman, B. *et al.* (2003) *Neuron*, **3**, 735–749.

Stewart, J.T. (2003) *Postgrad. Med.*, **113**, 71–75.

Sung, J.Y., Kim, J., Paik, S.R., Park, J.H. *et al.* (2001) *J. Biol. Chem.*, **276**, 27441–27448.

Syme C.D., Blanch E.W., Holt C., Jakes R. *et al.* (2002) *Eur. J. Biochem.*, **269**, 148–156.

Takahashi, R. and Imai, Y. (2003) *J. Neurol.*, **250**, Suppl 3, 25–29.

Takeda, A. (2004) *Yakugaku. Zasshi.*, **124**, 577–585.

Tanner, C.M. (2002) *Neurology*, **58**, 581–588.

Tizabi, Y., Copeland, R.L. Jr, Louis, V.A. and Taylor, R.E. (2002) *Alc. Clin. Exp. Res.*, **26**, 394–399.

Thompson, K., Menzies, S., Muckenthaler, M., Torti, F.M. *et al.* (2003) *J. Neurosci. Res.*, **71**, 46–63.

Trojanowski, J.Q., Goedert, M., Iwatsubo, T. and Lee, V.M. (1998) *Cell Death Differ.*, **5**, 832–837.

Tsai, Y.C., Fishman, P.S., Thakor, N.V. and Oyler, G.A. (2003) *J. Biol. Chem.*, **278**, 22044–22055.

Turnbull, S., Tabner, B.J., El-Agnaf, O.M., Moore, S. *et al.* (2001) *Free Radic. Biol. Med.*, **30**, 1163–1170.

Uversky, V.N., Li, J. and Fink, A.L. (2001) *J. Biol. Chem.*, **276**, 44284–44296.

Valente, E.M., Brancati, F., Caputo, V., Graham, E.A. *et al.* (2002) *Neurol. Sci.*, **23**, S117–118.

Van der Walt, J.M., Nicodemus, K.K., Martin, E.R., Scott, W.K. *et al.* (2003) *Am. J. Hum. Genet.*, **72**, 804–811.

Ward, R.J., Ramsey, M., Dickson, D.P., Hunt, C., Douglas, T. *et al.* (1994) *Eur. J. Biochem.*, **225**, 187–194.

Wirdefeldt, K., Bagdanovic, N., Westerberg, L., Payami, H. *et al.* (2001) *Brain Res. Mol. Brain Res.*, **92**, 58–65.

Wolozin, B. and Golts, N. (2002) *Neuroscientist*, **8**, 22–32.

Yang, Y., Nishimura, I., Imai, Y., Takahashi, R. and Lu, B. (2003) *Neuron*, **37**, 911–924.

Yao, D., Gu, Z., Nakamura, T., Shi, Z.Q. *et al.* (2004) *Proc. Natl. Acad. Sci. USA*, **101**, 10810–10814.

Zecca, L., Gallorini, M., Schunemann, V., Trautwein, A.X. *et al.* (2001) *J. Neurochem.*, **76**, 1766–1773.

Zecca, L., Stroppolo, A., Gatti, A., Tampelline, D. *et al.* (2004) *Proc. Natl. Acad. Sci. USA*, **101**, 9843–9848.

Zecca, L., Shima, T., Stroppolo, A., Goj, C. *et al.* (1996) *Neurosci.*, **73**, 407–415.

Zecca, L., Gallorini, M., Schunemann, V., Trautwein, A.X. *et al.* (2001) *J Neurochem*.

Zecca, L. and Swartz, H.M. (1993) *J. Neural. Transm. Park. Dement. Sect.*, **5**, 203–213.

Zhang, Y., Gao, J., Chung, K.K., Huang, H. *et al.* (2000) *Proc. Natl. Acad. Sci. USA.*, **97**, 13354–13359.

Zheng, W., Zhao, Q., Slavkovich, V., Aschner, M. *et al.* (1999) *Brain Res.*, **833**, 125–132.

Zucca, F.A., Giaveri, G., Gallorini, M., Albertini, A. *et al.* (2004) *Pigment Cell Res.*, **17**, 610–617.

4

Alzheimer's Disease

Alzheimer's disease, AD, is one of the most common neurodegenerative maladies in Western societies. Clinical symptoms occur between the ages of 60–70 y. This disease, for which no effective treatment is currently available, initially presents with symptoms of memory loss, after which a progressive decline of both cognitive and motor function occurs. Both genetic and environmental factors are implicated in its development.

Estimates of prevalence vary but 1–5% of the population over 65 may be affected by the disease. Initially there is short term memory loss followed by widespread cognitive impairment and emotional dysfunction due to widespread neuronal loss in the hippocampus and selected cortical and subcortical areas. High systolic blood pressure, which often occurs with aging, has also been associated with higher relative risk of AD.

Females are more susceptible than males, which may be attributable to the higher constitutive activity of the synaptic zinc transporter ZnT3. Studies showed that female mice exhibited age-dependent hyperactivity of the ZnT3 transporter which was associated with increased Aβ deposition (Lee et al., 2002).

Rats fed on a diet where the energy intake is 70% of normal, have vastly improved life spans, retain the physiology of a young animal and possibly show increased resistance to neurodegeneration. With obesity becoming an ever-increasing problem in modern society, measures to reduce corporal weight might have significant effects in reducing neurodegeneration.

The amyloidosis which occurs in AD involves abnormal protein processing; a structural transition of a polypeptide chain from a natively folded protein to one with an improperly folded conformation which leads to inefficient protein degradation. Truncated proteins are formed, and the resulting peptides tend to aggregate. There is considerable evidence that defective homeostasis of redox-active metals, i.e. iron and copper, together with oxidative stress, contribute to the neuropathology of AD. The characteristic histology of AD is the deposition of both the amyloid peptide, Aβ, as neurotic plaques, **Figure 4.1a**, and of the protein tau, as neurofribrillary tangles, **Figure 4.1b**, predominantly in the cerebral cortex and hippocampus.

Metal-based Neurodegeneration: From Molecular Mechanisms to Therapeutic Strategies   R. R. Crichton and R. J. Ward
© 2006 John Wiley & Sons, Ltd

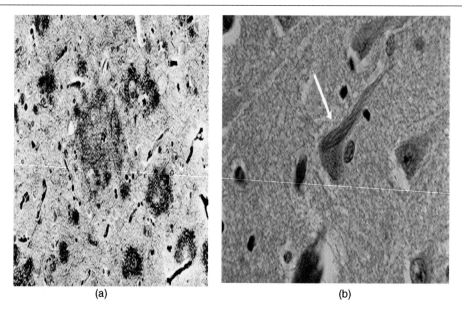

(a)   (b)

Figure 4.1: (**a**) Characteristic histo-pathological findings of Alzheimer's disease are senile plaques – a collection of degenerative presynaptic endings with astrocytes and microglia. Plaques are stained with silver stain, and are of varying size. (**b**) Neurofibrillary tangles of Alzheimer's diseasae. The tangles are present as long pink filaments in the cytoplasm. Each is composed of cytoskelatal intermediate filaments.

4.1 PROTEINS INVOLVED IN ALZHEIMER'S DISEASE

Amyloid precursor protein (APP), a type I membrane protein, resembles a cell surface receptor and is physiologically processed by site-specific proteolysis. APP is cleaved by α-secretase (within the Aβ domain between Lys^{687} and Leu^{688}) to yield APPsα and the C-terminal fragment containing p3. The production of the amyloid peptide, Aβ, is thus precluded. The presence of increasing amounts of iron may alter α-secretase activity; one hypothesis suggested that iron might be required as a co-factor or be an allosteric modifier of α-secretase activity. Iron may also decrease α-secretase cleavage rates (Rogers et al., 2002). The membrane-anchored α-carboxy terminal fragment, α-CTF, is then cleaved by γ-secretase within the membrane, releasing p3 peptide and the APP intracellular domain (AICD), **Figure 4.2** (Wilquet and De Strooper, 2004). AICD may function in nuclear signalling; it can fuse to the DNA binding domain of the Gal4 transcription factor to induce the expression of an upstream activating sequence (UAS)-dependent reporter in combination with the adaptor protein Fe65 and the histone acetyl-transferase Tip60. The fate of p3 is unknown.

Aβ can exist in three biochemical fraction in the brain: membrane-associated, aggregated and soluble; in healthy individuals, most of the Aβ will be membrane-associated, with small amounts of the soluble monomers detectable in CSF and blood. Aβ possibly exists as an α-helical conformation when it is part of the transmembrane protein, APP, with the hydrophobic C terminus embedded in the membrane lipid (**Figure 4.3a**). *In vitro* studies of Aβ (in organic solvent/aqueous mixtures) show that it assumes helical conformations which are characterized by two helical segments interrupted by a central tract, (the kink region).

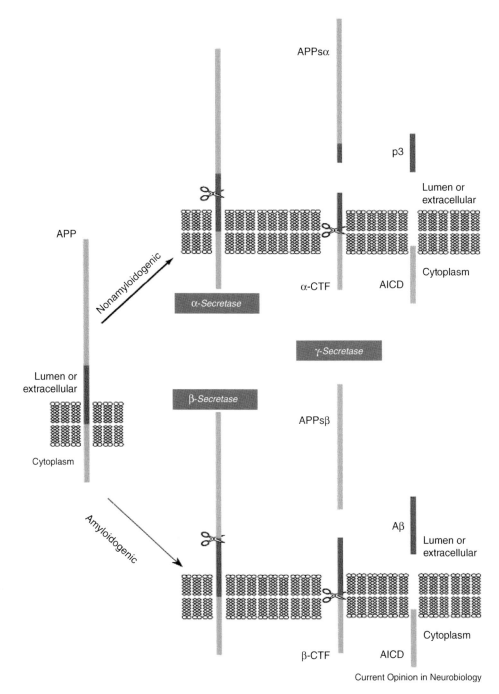

Figure 4.2: Proteolytic processing of amyloid precursor protein (APP) by the secretases. APP is a type 1 transmembrane glycoprotein. The majority of APP is processed in the non-amyloidogenic pathway (thick arrow); APP is first cleaved by α-secretase within the amyloid-β protein (Aβ) domain leading to APPsα secretion and precluding Aβ generation. Membrane-anchored α-carboxy terminal fragment (CTF) is then cleaved by γ-secretase within the membrane releasing the p3 peptide and the APP intracellular domain (AICD). Alternatively amyloidgenesis takes place when APP is first cleaved by β-secreatase, producing APPsβ. Aβ and AICD are generated upon cleavage by γ-secretase of the β-CTF fragment retained in the membrane. Reprinted from Wilquet and De Strooper, Copyright 2004, with permission from Elsevier.

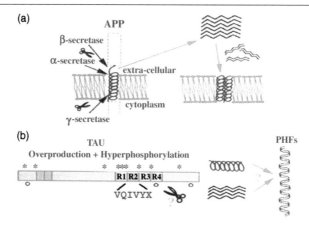

Figure 4.3: Hypothetical mechanisms of conformational transitions for Aβ peptides (**a**) and tau (**b**). (**a**) The peptides are proteolytically cleaved from APP, precipitate as B structures in equilibrium with oligomers which may eventually redissolve into the membrane. (**b**) A schematic picture of the architecture of tau. The four repeats are indicated as R1-R4. The sites identified as calpain and caspase-3 cleavage are indicated with stars and open circles respectively. From Temussi et al., 2003. Reproduced by permission of the Nature Publishing Groups and the Journal of Biological Chemistry.

In amyloidogenesis, the APP is cleaved sequentially by the proteolytic enzymes β-secretase (aspartyl protease, BACE or Asp-20) and then by γ-secretase. Beta-secretase has a C-terminal transmembrane domain and two active site motifs located in the luminal domain. Beta secretase cleaves APP between Met[671] and Asp[672] and yields APPβs and C99 fragments. The enzyme γ-secretase, a multi-subunit complex (containing presenilins 1 and 2 (PS1 and PS2)) will then cleave APPβs to produce β-amyloid peptide, Aβ (Aβ$_{42}$ and Aβ$_{40}$) and AICD. Some recent studies indicate that there may be other factors involved in the action of PSs on the intramembranous proteolysis of APP (Sisodia et al., 2001). Mutations in PS1 or PS2 genes will increase the production of the toxic Aβ$_{42}$.

In individuals with AD, the aggregated and soluble fractions of Aβ are markedly increased (McLean et al., 1999); the two β-amyloid peptides, Aβ$_{42}$ and Aβ$_{40}$, migrate from the cell to form aggregates, fibrils and eventually neuritic plaques. The structure of Aβ$_{40}$ consists of two helices spanning residues 15–23 and 31–35, which are separated by a disordered region. The Aβ$_{42}$ peptide adopts a regular type I β-turn, yielding a well defined tertiary structure (Crescenzi et al., 2002), **Figure 4.4**, which shows similarities with the fusion domain of the haemagglutinin of the influenza virus.

Aβ accumulation and aggregation is considered to be the initiating factor in AD pathogenesis although it is known that such deposition occurs over many years, if not

▶

Figure 4.4: (**a**) Bundle of the best 10 structures of Aβ$_{42}$ after AMBER minimization, superimposed for: A, backbone atoms of residue 8–38 (RMSD = 0.86 Å); B, backbone atoms of residues 8–25 (RMSD = 0.38 Å); C, backbone atoms of residues 26–27 (RMSD = 0.048 Å); D, backbone atoms of residues 23–38 (RMSD = 0.59 Å) (from Crescenzi et al., 2002). (**b**) Stereo view of the lowest energy structure colored according to the electrostatic potential. (**c**) Comparison of the shapes of the lowest energy structure of influenza haemagglutinin (A) and of the 1–35 region of the Aβ$_{(1-42)}$. From Crescenzi et al., 2002. Reproduced by permission of Blackwell Publishing Ltd.

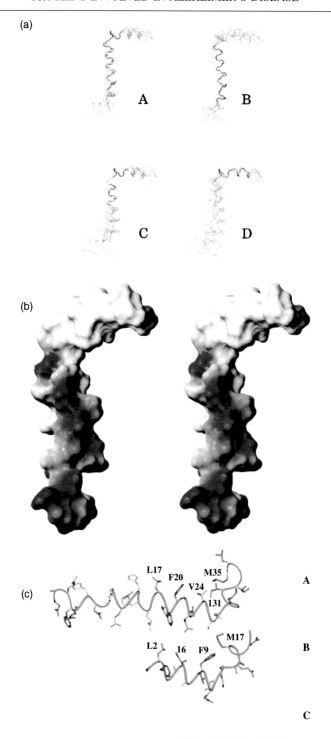

(a)

A   B

C   D

(b)

(c)

L17 F20   M35   A
         V24
              I31

L2   16 F9   M17   B

C

AB-(1-42) DAEFRHDSGYEVHHQKLVFFAEDVGSNKGAIIGLMVGGVVIA

HA_fd   GLFGAIAGFIENGWEGMIDG

decades, prior to the clinical cognitive impairment. Aβ may be oxidized within the membrane, perhaps as a result of the increased Cu and Fe levels in the brain (Bush, 2003), from where it is ultimately liberated in a soluble form, to precipitate in the amyloid plaques. Aβ peptides will increase calcium influx through voltage-gated calcium channels (N and L types) by reducing magnesium blockade of NMDA receptors, as well as forming cation-selective ion channels after Aβ peptide incorporation into the cellular membrane, thereby increasing excitotoxicity. Aβ peptides may interfere with long-term hippocampal potentiation and cause synaptic dysfunction in Alzheimer's disease (Walsh et al., 2002).

The balance between the α- and β- secretase processing of APP is partially regulated by subcellular transport. Alpha secretase typically cleaves the protein during the transport route to and at the cell surface. Beta secretase apparently meets APP at the cell surface and both are internalized together into early endosomes. Therefore the bulk of β-secretase cleavage of APP occurs in the endosomes which is related to the acid pH optimum for β-secretase. Cleavage of APP may also be regulated by ligands although no such functionally active ligands have yet been identified. F-spondin will bind to the central APP domain (CAPPD) and inhibit the initial α-and β- cleavage of APP, thereby regulating cleavage. This may indicate a potential pharmaceutical target to inhibit APP cleavage by synthesizing new molecules which bind to this CAPPD motif (Ho and Sudhof, 2004). Trafficking and processing of APP can also be regulated by many adaptor proteins, e.g. members of the XII and the Fe65 families, which can bind to the APP cytosolic tail. Fe65 is involved in gene transcription regulation and appears to promote Aβ secretion (Wilquet and De Strooper 2004).

It is unknown whether Aβ, which is continuously secreted under normal physiological conditions, may have a physiological role, possibly functioning as an antioxidant. There is an inverse relationship between Aβ content and *in vivo* oxidative damage, suggesting that Aβ might be a modulator of ROS generation. (Perry et al., 2002; Zhu et al.,2004). The precipitation of Aβ into plaques, associated with increased levels of metal ions, may be an efficient means of presentation to phagocytic cells for its removal from the cell, **Figure 4.5**. Other physiological functions assigned to Aβ are as a superoxide scavenger (SOD activity), a cholesterol binding molecule, and an acute phase reactant (reviewed in Obrenovich et al.,

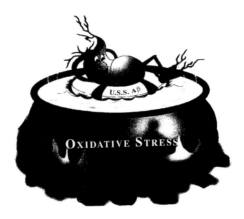

Figure 4.5: Amyloid Aβ life preservers afford protection to neurons adrift in a caldron of oxidative stress. Reprinted from Obrenovich et al., Copyright 2002, with permission from Elsevier.

2002). Many forms of stress, including head injury and trauma, may be regulated via β-amyloid. It has also recently been suggested (Atamna and Frey, 2004) that β-amyloid interacts directly with haem thereby provoking functional haem deficiency, notably in mitochondria.

Tau is a natively unfolded protein, containing neither α-helix nor β-sheet, which regulates microtubule function in the axon. It shows an even distribution of hydrophobic fragments along its sequence with up to four repeats of approx 30 residues in its central region, **Figure 4.3b**. Peptides from tau are more soluble than Aβ. Short synthetic peptides spanning tau repeat sequences are able to aggregate as β-structures. A peptide from the C-terminus (residues 423-441) forms a regular helix in an organic solvent/aqueous mixture, with a helical stabilizing C-capping motif (Esposito et al., 2000).

Tau proteins are highly hydrophilic microtubule-associated proteins, **Figure 4.3b**. There are six isoforms of tau, ranging between 352 and 441 amino acids in length, which are produced as a result of alternative mRNA splicing from a single gene on chromosome 17 (Lee et al., 2001), and are differentially expressed in neurons. In the normal brain, the functions of tau include stabilization of axonal microtubules, modulation of signal transduction and regulation of vesicle transport (reviewed by Friedhoff et al., 2000). Tau protein monomers can polymerize to form fibrils known as paired helical filaments (aggregated hyperphosphorylated tau protein), which become the building blocks for the neurofibrillary tangles, neuropil threads and dystrophic neuritis that accumulate in AD. Such tau hyperphosphorylation may be associated with an increase in kinase activity or a decrease in phosphatase activity. PS1 mutations also modulate neurofilament-H protein phosphorylation (Avila, 2000), which in turn can modulate tau phosphorylation, leading to disruption of neurofilament-microtubule binding. This will disrupt axonal transport of APP and other proteins increasing accumulation and subsequent degradation of APP.

Neurofibrillary tau lesions are not restricted to AD; they are also the defining feature of other neurodegenerative diseases collectively referred to as tauopathies and include frontotemporal dementias including Pick's disease, progressive supranuclear palsey and corticobasal degeneration. When such protein aggregates occur, their normal cellular function is lost and neurotoxicity occurs.

NFTs contain redox active iron. Accumulation of tau in neurofibrillary tangles is associated with the induction of haem oxygenase 1, a potent antioxidant which plays an important role in metabolizing haem released from damaged mitochondria. Although this will reduce oxidative damage (Perry et al., 2002), Fe^{2+} will be released which may participate in Fenton chemistry to produce hydroxyl radicals. Tau within the neurofibrillary tangles is oxidatively damaged.

4.2 METAL INVOLVEMENT IN ALZHEIMER'S DISEASE

High levels of Zn, Cu and Fe are constitutively found in the neocortical regions which are most prone to AD pathology. Enriched amounts of copper, iron and zinc are also present in the insoluble amyloid plaques in post-mortem AD brain (Huang et al., 2004). Alternatively is has been suggested that the formation of the β-sheet configuration of Aβ may actually be a protective mechanism. It may be that the increased synthesis of APP and Aβ is an attempt by the brain cells to detoxify the elevated levels of redox active metals, copper and iron; other studies suggest that zinc and copper are inhibitory and prevent β-sheet formation (Yoshiike et al., 2001).

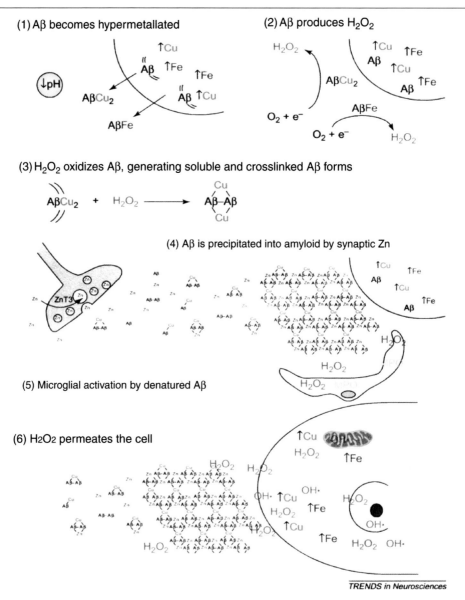

(1) Aβ becomes hypermetallated

(2) Aβ produces H_2O_2

(3) H_2O_2 oxidizes Aβ, generating soluble and crosslinked Aβ forms

(4) Aβ is precipitated into amyloid by synaptic Zn

(5) Microglial activation by denatured Aβ

(6) H2O2 permeates the cell

TRENDS in Neurosciences

Figure 4.6: Hypothetical model for the metallobiology of Aβ in Alzheimer's disease. (from Bush, 2003). The proposed sequence of events: 1. Concentration of iron and copper increase in the cortex with aging. There is an overproduction of APP and Aβ in an attempt to suppress cellular metal-ion levels. 2. Hypermetallation of Aβ occurs which may facilitate H_2O_2 production. 3. Hypermetallated Aβ reacts with H_2O_2 to generate oxidized and cross-linked forms which are liberated from the membrane. 4. Soluble Aβ is released from the membrane and is precipitated by zinc which is released from the synaptic vesicles. Oxidized Aβ are the major components of the plaque deposits. 5. Oxidized Aβ initiate microglia activation. 6. H_2O_2 crosses cellular membranes to react with Cu and Fe, and generate hydroxyl radicals which oxidize a variety of proteins and lipids. Reprinted from Bush, Copyright 2003, with permission from Elsevier.

Membrane-bound Aβ may be damaged by metal-induced reactive oxygen species prior to their liberation from the membrane, and consequently precipitated by zinc which is released from synaptic vesicles, **Figure 4.6**. *In vitro*, zinc rapidly accelerates Aβ aggregation, the zinc being associated with the N-terminal region of Aβ which has an autonomous zinc binding domain. Zinc induces conformational change of the 1-16 N-terminal region of AP3 (Zirah et al., 2004). In adult rat brain, pools of zinc are detectable within glutamatergic synaptic vesicles in the neocortex which represents 30% of total brain zinc, **Figure 4.7**. Zinc is released during synaptic transmission, possibly in conjunction with glutamate, and induces cerebral Aβ deposition in a transgenic mouse model for AD. The transporter ZnT3 carries zinc into vesicles such that its genetic ablation will inhibit Aβ deposition in Tg2576 mice (Lee et al., 2002).

Iron may modulate APP processing, by virtue of the presence of a putative iron response element in APP mRNA (based on sequence homology). The IRE was mapped within the

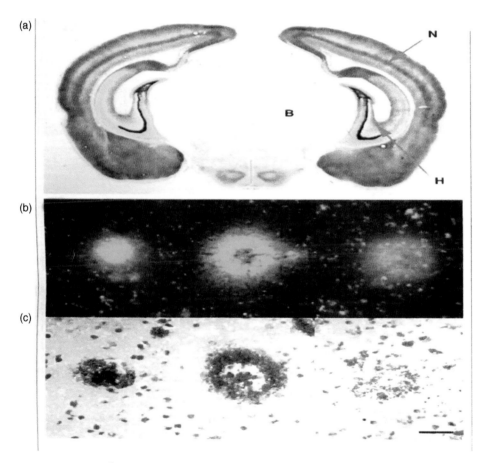

Figure 4.7: Brain Zn^{2+} localization in normal necortex and in an amyloid plaque from AD brain. (**a**) Timm's stain for pools of dissociable ionic Zn^{2+} or low affinity-bound Zn^{2+} in adult rat brain. The stain detects Zn^{2+} within the glutamatergic synaptic vesicles in the neocortex. (**b**) Basal ganglia H hippocamous N neocortex. (**c**) Zinc staining of amyloid plaques in AD. The plaques are attained with TSQ fluorescent stain for zinc, top panel and Anti-Aβ antibody. Reprinted from Bush, Copyright 2003, with permission from Elsevier.

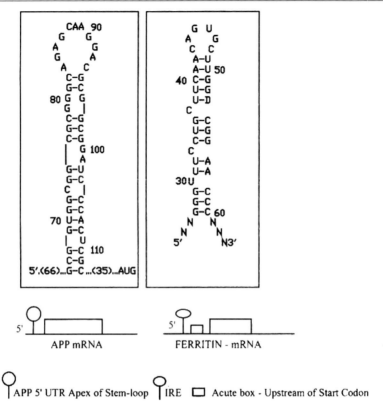

Figure 4.8: Evidence for an iron-responsive element in the 5′-UTR of APP mRNA. APP 5′-UTR sequences were computer-folded to generate the predicted RNA stem. From Rogers et al., 2002. Reproduced by permission of the Journal of Biological Chemistry.

5′-untranslated regions (5′-UTR) of the APP transcript (+51 to +94) from the 5′cap site, **Figure 4.8**. The APP mRNA IRE is located immediately upstream of an interleukin-1 responsive acute box domain (+101 to +146). In response to intracellular iron chelation, translation of APP was selectively down regulated (Rogers et al., 2002) thereby causing a striking decrease in the production of APP_{sol}. Iron influx reversed this inhibition, by a pathway similar to iron control of the translation of the ferritin-L mRNAs by iron responsive elements in its 5′UTRs (Venti et al., 2004). In addition, increase in cytokine production, namely IL-1, increased IRP binding to the APP 5′-UTR, thereby decreasing APP production. When the APP cRNA probe is mutated in the core IRE domain, IRP binding is abolished. In addition, binding of the IRP to the IRE might interfere with APP translation and transloca-tion across the endoplasmic reticulum membrane. This interference could be significant since α-secretase activity has been shown to require membrane-bound APP. The role played by IRP-2 in Alzheimer's disease remains undefined but may be more important than was previously thought.

Aβ has a very effective binding domain for copper in its N-terminal domain and can bind copper in nmol amounts, **Figure 4.9**. It is unclear whether APP and Aβ, when associated with copper, are in fact neuronal metallochaperones. Knock-out and knock-in mice for APP show that in the former, cerebral cortex copper levels are increased, whereas in the latter reduced copper levels were assayed. Copper was also influential in APP processing in the

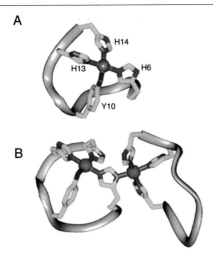

Figure 4.9: Binding domain for copper in APP. (A) the initial coordination site of Cu^{2+} on Aβ in solution (His[6], His[13], His[14], and Tyr[10]) as determined by NMR and EPR spectroscopy. (B) a proposed model explaining the aggregation, cooperative binding, and redox properties of metal-bound Aβ peptides. The imidaole ring of His[6] is shown forming a bridge between copper atoms to form a dimeric species; this residue is used as an example, and other histidine residues could form similar bridges and therefore lead to aggregation. From Curtain et al., 2001. Reproduced by permission of the Journal of Biological Chemistry.

cell, copper will reduce levels of Aβ and cause an increase in the secretion of the APP ectodomain.

No review on Alzheimer's disease would be complete without some comments of the role of aluminium in the aetiology and pathogenesis of Alzheimer's disease. In early studies, cognitive impairment was reported in men exposed to high aluminium concentrations during the course of their work, Hereby was the early evidence for the link between aluminium and neurotoxicity! From one point of view, it is possible to obtain considerable evidence for an association between aluminium and Alzheimer's disease. For example, epidemiological studies show that the rates of Alzheimer's disease were marginally increased, 1.5x, in areas with high aluminium levels in the water supply; *in vitro* biochemical studies show that aluminium will induce toxicity, by acting as a pro-oxidant and promoting Aβ oxidation in the presence of iron, accelerating β-pleated sheets formation of Aβ as well as antagonizing IRE binding of IRPs in cell cultures (Yamanaka et al., 1999). *In vivo* cognitive impairment occurs in rats after administration of high doses of aluminium. On the other hand, we have consistently questioned whether aluminium would even be able to traverse cellular membranes, since its ability to use iron transporters, e.g. DMT1 at the apical membrane of enterocytes and in the endosomal membrane during the transferrin to cell cycle described in Chapter 1, will be constrained by its inability to change its valency state. Furthermore, one of the earliest electron probe microanalysis studies, which identified increased content of both aluminium and silicon in about half of the tangles and plaques in the brains of Alzheimer's disease, post mortem (Wisniewski and Wen, 1992) may have been flawed as the aluminium was from an extrinsic source. Later pathological studies were unable to assay aluminium in such brain sections.

Elevated ferritin iron is possibly a risk factor for AD. It is reported that the iron cores of AD ferritin may show significant differences in their mineral composition to that of physiological ferritin, neither ferrihydrite nor hematite were present, the core mineralization product being identified as wustite and magnetite (Quintana et al., 2004). Such results have implications not only for the disease progression but also for possible early diagnosis.

The glycoprotein, lactoferrin, specifically binds iron, and removes it from the circulation in situations of infection and inflammation. Analysis of iron binding protein distribution in the brain of AD patients post mortem, showed that lactoferrin accumulates within a subpopulation of neurofibrillary tangles, senile plaques as well as tau in the hippocampus and inferior temporal cortex. Such accumulation of lactotransferrin may lead to cytotoxic effect and neuronal death (Leveugle et al., 1994).

4.3 GENETIC AND RISK FACTORS

Mutations in the genes encoding for APP (Chromosome 21) (the most common being a valine to isoleucine substitution at codon 717), PS-1 (Chromosome 14) (single amino acid mis-sense substitution, located in the transmembrane domains of the protein) or PS2 (Chromosome 1) are linked to early onset of familial AD, via autosomal dominant inheritance, **Figure 4.10**. In addition, three different dominant early-onset AD mutations have been identified as single base substitutions in the stem of the APP-IRE.

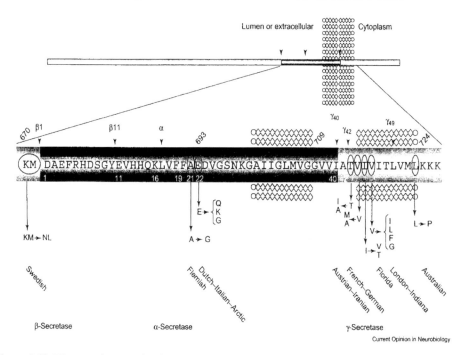

Figure 4.10: The mutations causing familial Alzheimer's disease in APP surround the cleavage sites of the three secretases. Reprinted from Wilquet and De Strooper, Copyright 2004, with permission from Elsevier.

Familial British dementia, FBD, is a rare autosomal dominant neurodegenerative disease (chromosome 13), which shows neuropathological similarities to Alzheimer's disease, such as parenchymal amyloid plaques and neurofibillary degeneration. The underlying genetic lesion is a T-A transversion at the termination codon of the BRI membrane protein (Vidal et al., 1999), which creates an arginine codon. A novel protein, termed BRI-L is created, that is extended by 11 amino acids at the carboxy-terminus. Both BRI and its mutant counterpart are constitutively processed by furin which results in the secretion of carboxyl-terminal peptide derivatives that correspond to ABri (Kim et al., 2000). BRI-L is the precursor of the ABri peptide, a component of amyloid deposits in FBD brain. Elevated levels of peptides are generated from the mutant BRI precursor, suggesting that subtle conformational alterations at the carboxy-terminus may influence furin-mediated processing. Electron microscopic studies reveal that synthetic ABri peptides assemble into insoluble β-pleated fibrils. Enhanced furin-mediated processing of mutant BRI generates amyloidogenic peptides that initiate the pathogenesis of FBD. Familial Danish dementia, FDD, is associated with a different mutation in the BRI_2 gene to that of FBD, but with similar neurodegenerative changes.

Cholesterol plays a role in Aβ metabolism and may directly influence Aβ production by altering the activities of the secretase enzymes. Apolipoprotein E (ApoE) has three genotypes, ε2, ε3 and ε4, with ε3 being the most common coding sequence variant. In sporadic and late-onset AD, the frequency of Apoε4 gene is higher, and may increase the risk of developing Alzheimer's disease by promoting the formation of Aβ. *In vitro* studies showed that Apoε4 induces higher Aβ aggregation in the presence of zinc and copper than either Apoε2 or Apoε3 (Moir et al., 1999). *In vitro*, ApoE administration to multiple neural and non-neural cell lines reduced $A\beta_{40}$ by 60–80% and AB_{42} to a lesser extent, 20–30%. ApoE treatment resulted in the accumulation of APP-C terminal fragments which is consistent with diminished γ-secretase processing of APP. Cholesterol-lowering drugs may have an impact on AD disease. Retrospective studies of β-hydroxy-β-methylglutaryl-Coenzyme A (HMG-CoA) reductase inhibitors (statins) show a large reduction in the risk of AD development (by lowering Aβ levels) in comparison to individuals with elevated cholesterol.

The α-$_2$ macroglobulin gene plays an important role in the fate of protein degradation by proteases. Alpha$_2$ macroglobulin traps the proteases and delivers them to a specific receptor protein (low density lipoprotein receptor related protein) – in fact the same receptor protein that acts as a receptor for ApoE to deliver blood fats. There may be some genetic link between Alzheimer's disease and two different variants of α-$_2$ macroglobulin gene; both of these variants are at higher frequencies in Alzheimer's patients than the general population.

4.4 MITOCHONDRIAL FUNCTION IN ALZHEIMER'S DISEASE

Cerebral metabolism is altered in AD, with activities of specific mitochondrial enzyme complexes reduced, e.g. cytochrome oxidase, pyruvate dehydrogenase complex and the α-ketoglutarate dehyrogenase complex. As a consequence of these alterations there may be an increase in ROS production. Defective ATP production combined with increased oxygen radicals may induce mitochondrial-dependent cell death. It is currently unknown whether there is increased deposition of iron in mitochondria of AD brains.

4.5 OXIDATIVE STRESS

Recent evidence indicates that oxidative stress occurs during the early stages of Alzheimer's disease. *In vitro* there is concomitant production of ROS, e.g. hydrogen peroxide and hydroxyl radicals, after metal-induced aggregation into tinctorial Aβ (Huang et al., 2004). However, the production of hydrogen peroxide should diminish APP production, the translation of APP being selectively down regulated. $A\beta_{42}$ induces the release of pro-inflammatory cytokines that trigger the inflammatory cascades which occur before the development of the neurofibrillary tangles and senile plaques. The altered mitochondrial function, together with increased levels of the redox transition metals, iron and copper, will increase ROS and RNS levels as well as calcium fluxes **Figure 4.11**. Apoptotic cell death

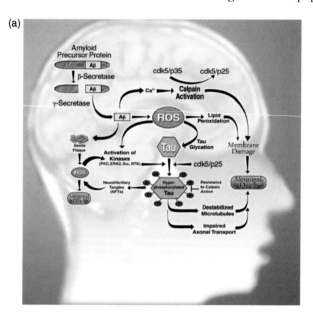

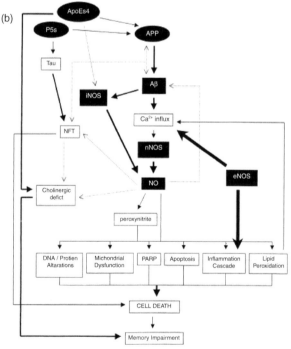

Figure 4.11: (a) Oxidative stress and Alzheimer's disease. From Calbiochem Biologics 2000. **(b)** Nitric oxide neurotoxicity and neuroprotectivity in relation to Alzheimer's disease. Reprinted from Law et al., Copyright 2001, with permission from Elsevier.

will occur as a result of this milieu of cellular function. A variety of oxidative markers are elevated in susceptible neurons, such as reactive carbonyls (Smith et al., 1996), protein adducts, the consequences of lipid peroxidation products, such as hydroxynonenal (Montine et al., 1996), and the modification of nucleic acid bases like 8-hydroxyl-2deoxyguanosine and 8-hydroxyguanosine (reviewed by Zhu et al., 2004).

Stress-activated protein kinase pathways, SAPK, are activated by oxidative stress and propagate stress signals from the membrane to the nucleus. JNK/SAPK and p38/SAPK2 are the two major SAPKs, **Figure 4.12**. The entire JNK/SAPK pathway is altered in AD. JNK2 and JNK3 are related to neurofibrillary pathology while JNK1 is related to Hirano bodies in cases of AD. JNK is redistributed from the nucleus to the cytoplasm in a manner that correlates with the progression of the disease, and may play a role in the phosphorylation and modulation of tau protein. JNK/SAPK activation precedes amyloid deposition, which may suggest that oxidative stress, rather than Aβ is the initial activator of this pathway. It is also suggested that JNK/SAPK is activated by Aβ which may involve oxidative stress but this awaits clarification. Interestingly it was found that JNK/SAPK is strongly activated in AβPP mice (amyloid β protein precursor), and is associated with extensive iron accumulation and oxidative damage, which suggests that this pathway is important in Aβ toxicity (Zhu et al., 2004). The activation of the JNK/SAPK pathway can also modulate the induction of several antioxidant enzymes, haem oxygenase 1 and SOD-1.

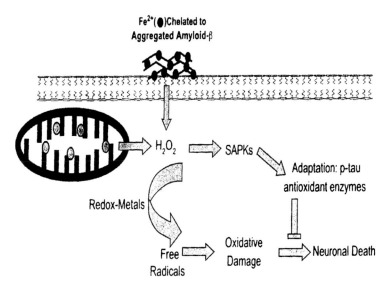

Figure 4.12: Schematic illustration of oxidative stress signalling in AD. Reprinted from Zhu et al., Copyright 2004, with permission from Elsevier.

One molecular mediator that could link the pathological hallmarks of AD, plaques, tangles and neuronal death, is the proline-directed serine-threonine protein kinase cyclin-dependent kinase 5 (cdk5). Cdk5 phosphorylation of its numerous substrates has a pivotal role in the normal development of the central nervous system. Deregulation of this kinase is neurotoxic and might contribute to the pathogenesis of AD. Neurotoxic insults such as $A\beta_{42}$ elevate intracellular calcium levels in neurons and activate the cysteine-protease calpain. When calpain is activated, it cleaves p35 into an N-terminal p10 fragment and a C-teminal p25 fragment, **Figure 4.13**. The truncated p25 activator contains all the necessary elements to bind to and activate cdk5. The introduction of p25 in primary neurons causes the

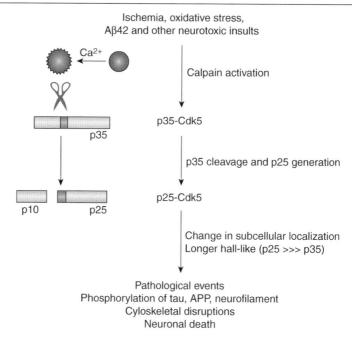

Ischemia, oxidative stress,
Aβ42 and other neurotoxic insults

Ca²⁺

Calpain activation

p35

p35-Cdk5

p35 cleavage and p25 generation

p10   p25

p25-Cdk5

Change in subcellular localization
Longer hall-like (p25 >>> p35)

Pathological events
Phosphorylation of tau, APP, neurofilament
Cyloskeletal disruptions
Neuronal death

Figure 4.13: The deregulation of cyclin-dependent kinase 5 (cdk5) activity. Reprinted from Cruz and Tsai, Copyright 2004, with permission from Elsevier.

deregulation of cdk5 and leads to tau hyperphosphorylation, cytoskeletal disruptions and neuronal cell death. (reviewed in Cruz and Tsai, 2004). Amyloid, Aβ, will increase the converson of p35 to p25, indicating an important role for the aberrant activation of Cdk5 by p25.

In addition, iron induces an imbalance in the function of p25-cdk5 system of the hippocampal neurons resulting in a marked decrease in tau phosphorylation at typical Alzheimer's epitopes, possibly reducing p25-cdk5 complex activator as a result of depletion of the activator p25, possibly mediated by calcium (Egana et al., 2003). The loss of phosphorylated tau epitopes correlated with an increase in 4-hydroxy-nonenal adducts revealing damage by oxidative stress.

Cytokine-mediated inflammatory processes play an important role in AD. Cytokines mediate cellular mechanisms sub-serving cognition (cholinergic and dopaminergic pathways) and can modulate neuronal and glial cell function to facilitate neuronal regeneration or degeneration (Wilson et al., 2002). Peripheral administration of cytokines can penetrate the BBB either directly or indirectly and can produce adverse cognitive effects in humans. Interestingly it is suggested that complex cognition systems such as those which underlie religious beliefs can modulate the effects of stress on the immune system.

Cyclooxygenases are members of a haem enzyme family that catalyse the rate limiting reaction to produce prostaglandins, see Chapter 2. COX-1 is constitutively expressed while COX-2 is the inducible form that is up-regulated by cytokines and mitogens. COX-2 may play an important role in AD, its expression is linked to the progression and severity of AD in affected regions of the brain (Ho et al., 2001). COX-2 over-expression in primary neurons potentiates Aβ neurotoxicity *in vitro* (Xiang et al., 2002). Aβ is a strongly active peptide that may react with COX-2 in the presence of hydrogen peroxide to form an Aβ-COX-2 cross linking (Nagano et al., 2004), the tyrosine of Aβ co-ordinating with the metal active site of COX-2. NSAI may inhibit the formation of COX-2-Aβ cross-linking by decreasing tyrosyl radicals in COX-2, such that Aβ clearance could be enhanced. Alternatively there may be a direct interaction between Aβ and NSAIs. A COX-3 isoform has also been identified, which may also play ancillary roles in membrane-based COX signalling (Cui et al. 2004).

4.6 ROLE OF ACETYL CHOLINE IN ALZHEIMER'S DISEASE

AD is initially and primarily associated with the degeneration and alteration in the metabolism of acetyl choline. AD patients present with a loss of many cholinergic neurons, especially those located in the nucleus basalis of Meynert. In addition there is a decrease of choline acetyl transferase activity. This would indicate that the cognitive deficit is caused by the loss of cholinergic input. It is noteworthy that in subjects with mild cognitive impairment, despite the presence of Aβ plaques and NFTs in the neocortex and allocortex, there were relatively normal levels of choline acetyl transferase. This would indicate that the cholinergic system is preserved during the early stages of the disease (Lopez and DeKosky, 2003). Both Aβ and pro-inflammatory cytokines may exert degenerating actions on cholinergic cells. Light and electron microscopical investigations of the cerebral cortex of aged Tg2576 mice (see Chapter 11) in addition to showing pathology of activated microglia, astroglia proliferation etc. also showed degeneration of ChAT- reactive fibres in the region of Aβ plaques and activated glial cells by immunostaining (Luth et al., 2003). *In vitro* studies of nerve growth factor showed its importance as an essential component for cholinergic neurons; cholinergic neurons rapidly degenerate when incubated without NGF, while a number of neurons could be rescued when reincubated with the growth factor (Humpel and Weis, 2002). This may indicate that NGF may be a promising candidate for the treatment of AD.

REFERENCES

Atamna, H. and Frey II, W.H. (2004) *Proc. Natl. Acad. Sci. USA*, **101**, 11153–11158.
Avila, J. (2000) *FEBS Lett.*, **476**, 89–92.
Bush, A.I. (2003) *Trends Neurosci.*, **26**, 207–214.
Calbiochem Biologics 2000, http://www.emdbiosciences.com/html/CBC/biologics.htm, viewed . . . 2005.
Crescenzi, O., Tomaselli, S., Guerrini, R., Salvadori, S. *et al.* (2002) *Eur. J. Biochem.*, **269**, 5642–5648.
Cui, J.G., Kuroda, H., Chandrasekharan, N.V., Pelaez, R.P., *et al.* (2004) *Neurochem. Res.*, **29**, 1731–1737.
Cruz, J.C. and Tsai, L.H. (2004) *Curr. Opin. Neurobiol.*, **14**, 390–394.
Curtain, C.C., Ali, F., Volitakis, I., Cherny, R.A. *et al.* (2001) *J. Biol. Chem.*, **276**, 20466–20473.
Egana, J.T., Zambrano, C., Nunez, M.T., Gonzalez-Billault, C. *et al.* (2003) *Biometals,* **16**, 215–223.
Esposito, L., Viglino, P., Novak, M., Cattaneo, A. (2000) *Pept. Sci.*, **6**, 550–559.
Friedhoff, P., von Bergen, M., Mandelkow, E.M., Mandelkow, E. (2000) *Biochim. Biophys. Acta.*, **1502**, 122–132.
Ho, A., and Sudhof, T.C. (2004) *Proc. Natl. Acad. Sci. USA*, **101**, 2548–2553.
Ho, L., Purohit, D., Haroutunian, V., Luterman, J. D. *et al.* (2001) *Arch. Neurol.*, **58**, 487–492.
Huang, X., Moir, R.D., Tanzi, R.E., Bush, A.I. and Rogers, J.T. (2004) *Ann. N. Y. Acad. Sci.*, **1012**, 153–163.
Humpel, C. and Weis, C. (2002) *J. Neural. Transm. Suppl.*, **62**, 253–263.

Kim, S-H., Wang, R., Gordon, D.J., Bass, J. *et al.* (2000) *Ann. N. Y. Acad. Aci.*, **920**, 93–99.

Law, A., Gauthier, S. and Quirion, R. (2001) *Brain Res. Rev.*, **35**, 73–96.

Lee, J-Y., Cole, T.B., Palmiter, R.D., Suh, S.W. and Koh, J.Y. (2002) *Proc. Natl. Acad. Sci. USA*, **99**, 7705–7710.

Lee, V.M., Goedert, M. and Trojanowski, J.Q. (2001) *Annu. Rev. Neurosci.*, **24**, 1121–1159.

Lee V.M-Y., Giasson, B.I. and Trojanowski, J.Q. (2004) *Trends Neurosci.*, **27**, 129–134.

Leveugle, B., Spik, G., Perl, D.P., Bouras, C. *et al.* (1994) *Brain Res.*, **650**, 20–31.

Lopez, O.L. and DeKosky, S.T. (2003) *Rev. Neurol.*, **37**, 155–163.

Luth, H.J., Apelt, J., Ihunwo, A.O., Arendt, T. and Schliebs, R. (2003) *Brain Res.*, **977**, 16–22.

McLean, C.A., Cherny, R.A., Fraser, F.W., Fuller, S.J. *et al.* (1999) *Ann. Neurol.*, **46**, 860–866.

Moir, R.D., Atwood, C.S., Romano, D.M., Laurans, *et al.* (1999) *Biochemistry*, **38**, 4595–4603.

Montine, T.J., Amarnath, V., Martin, M.E., Strittmatter, W.J. *et al.* (1996) *Am. J. Pathol.*, **148**, 89–93.

Nagano, S., Huang, X., Moir, R.D., Payton, S.M. *et al.* (2004) *J. Biol. Chem.*, **279**, 14673–14678.

Obrenovich, M.E., Joseph, J.A., Atwood, C.S., Perry, G. and Smith, M.A. (2002) *Neurobiol. Aging*, **23**, 1097–1099.

Perry, G., Nunomura, A., Raina, A.K. and Smith, M.A. (2000) *Lancet*, **355**, 757.

Perry, G., Nunomura, A., Hirai, K., Zhu, X. *et al.* (2002) *Free Radic. Biol. Med.*, **33**, 1475–1479.

Pietrzik, C.U., Yoon, I.S., Jarger, S., Busse, T. *et al.* (2004) *J. Neurosci.*, **24**, 4259–4265.

Quintana, C., Cowley, J.M. and Marhic, C. (2004) *J. Struct. Biol.*, **147**, 166–178.

Rogers, J.T., Randall, J.D., Cahill, C.M., Eder, P.S. *et al.* (2002) *J. Biol. Chem.*, **277**, 45518–45528.

Rottkamp, C.A., Raina, A.K., Zhu, X., Gaier, E. *et al.* (2001) *Free Radic. Biol. Med.*, **30**, 447–450.

Roses, A.D. (1997) *Neurobiol. Dis.*, **4**, 170.

Sisodia, S.S., Annaert, W., Kim, S.H. and De Strooper, B. (2001) *Trends Neurosci.*, **24**, S2–6.

Smith, C.D., Perry, G., Richey, P.L., Sayre, L.M. *et al.* (1996) *Nature*, **382**, 120–121.

Temussi, P.A., Masino, L.A. and Pastore, A. (2003) *EMBO J.*, **22**, 355–361.

Venti, A., Giodano, T., Eder, P., Bush, A.L. *et al.* (2004) *Ann. N. Y. Acad. Sci.*, **1035**, 34–48.

Vidal, R., Frangione, B., Rostagno, A., Mead, S. *et al.* (1999) *Nature*, **399**, 776–778.

Walsh, D.M., Klyubin, I., Fadeeva, J.V., Cullen, W.K. *et al.* (2002) *Nature*, **416**, 483–484.

Wilson, C.J., Finch, C.E., Cohen, H.J. (2002) *J. Am. Geriatr. Soc.*, **50**, 2041–2056.

Wisniewski, H.M. and Wen, G.Y. (1992) *Ciba Found. Symp.*, **169**, 142–154.

Wilquet, V. and De Strooper, B. (2004) *Curr. Opin. Neurobiol.*, **14**, 582–588.

Xiang, Z., Ho, L., Valdellon, J., Borchelt, D. *et al.* (2002) *Neurobiol. Aging*, **23**, 327–334.

Yamanaka, K., Minato, N. and Iwai, K. (1999) *FEBS Lett.*, **462**, 216–220.

Yoshiike, Y., Tanemura, K., Murayama, O., Akagi, T. *et al.* (2001) *J. Biol. Chem.*, **276**, 32293–32299.

Zhu, X., Raina, A.K., Lee, H-G., Casadesus, G. *et al.* (2004) *Brain Res.*, **1000**, 32–39.

Zirah, S., Stefanescu, R., Manea, M., Tianm, X. *et al.* (2004) *Biochem. Biophys. Res. Commun.*, **321**, 324–328.

5

Huntington's Disease and Polyglutamine Expansion Neurodegenerative Diseases

5.1 INTRODUCTION – AN OVERVIEW OF TRINUCLEOTIDE EXPANSION DISEASES

In 1968, Dr. William Kennedy and colleagues (Kennedy et al., 1968) defined a clinical disorder now known as spinobulbar muscular atrophy (SBMA), or Kennedy's disease, which was mapped and identified as an expanded trinucleotide repeat in the androgen receptor gene on the X chromosome in 1991 (La Spada et al., 1991). This turned out to be the first in a series of neurodegenerative diseases which are all characterized by the repeated expansion of a trinucleotide sequence either in a coding or in a non-coding region of the corresponding gene (for reviews see Masino and Pastore, 2001; Cummings and Zoghbi, 2000; Zoghbi, 2000). In patients with Kennedy's disease the causative mutation is the expansion of a CAG[1] trinucleotide repeat in the first exon of the androgen receptor to two to three times its normal length. As with other repeat expansion diseases, this repeat is unstable, and it shifts in length as it is passed from one generation to the next: the longer it gets, the earlier the onset, and the more severe the manifestations of the disease (La Spada et al., 1992). With the repeat expansion, there is an extended polyglutamine tract near the N-terminus of the protein.

At least fifteen human genetic diseases involving triplet expansion have been identified. They are grouped into two sub-families depending on whether the expansion occurs in a coding or a non-coding region of the gene. In this chapter we consider the first class, which includes Huntington's disease as well as a number of spinocerebral ataxias[2], all of which are characterized by an extended segment of poly-glutamines (polyQ); they are listed in **Table 5.1** (Poletti, 2004). The second class, considered in Chapter 6, includes Friedreich's

---

[1] CAG is the trinucleotide sequence which codes for the amino acid glutamine (in the one letter amino acid alphabet, Q).
[2] Ataxias are disorders associated with total or partial inability to coordinate voluntary bodily movements, particularly muscular movements.

Metal-based Neurodegeneration: From Molecular Mechanisms to Therapeutic Strategies   R. R. Crichton and R. J. Ward
© 2006 John Wiley & Sons, Ltd

Table 5.1: Polyglutamine expansions and neurodegenerative diseases (reprinted from *Brain Research Bulletin*, Vol 56, Masino and Pastore, A structural approach to trinucleotide expansion diseases, pp 183–189, Copyright 2001, with permission from Elsevier)

Disease	Protein	Nres
Coding triplets		
Huntington's disease (HD)	Huntingtin	3144
Spinobulbar muscular atrophy (Kennedy disease or SBMA)	Androgen receptor	919
Dentatorubral-pallidoluysian atrophy (Haw-River syndrome or DRPLA)	Atrophin-1	1182
Spinocerebellar ataxia 1 (SCA1)	Ataxin-1	816
Spinocerebellar ataxia 2 (SCA2)	Ataxin-2	1312
Spinocerebellar ataxia 3 (Machado-Joseph or SCA3)	Ataxin-3	360
Spinocerebellar ataxia 6 (SCA6)	α-VDCCS*	2505
Spinocerebellar ataxia 7 (SCA7)	Ataxin-7	892
Non-coding triplets		
Fragile X syndrome	FMR1	632
Fragile XE syndrome	FMR2	1301
Friedreich's ataxia	Frataxin	210
Myotonic dystrophy	MD protein kinase	639
Spinocerebellar ataxia 8 (SCA 8)	KLHL1	748
Spinocerebellar ataxia 12 (SCA 12)	PP2A-PR55βS[†]	443

ataxia and the fragile X syndrome, in which the triplet expansion occurs either in an intron or in the untranslated region of the gene.

5.2 POLYQ DISEASES

Nine neurological disorders have been found to result from an expansion of CAG repeats coding for a polyQ tract in the corresponding proteins (Cummings and Zoghbi, 2000; Masino and Pastore, 2001). With the exception of Kennedy's disease (SBMA), which is X-linked, all of the others show an autosomal dominant pattern of inheritance. The proteins involved have no obvious sequence homology, apart from the polyQ tract, they all appear to be widely or ubiquitously expressed, yet their functions remain for the most part unknown. Each disease is characterized by a distinct pathology involving a specific subset of neuronal cells, but they do have some common features. All are progressive neuronal dysfunctions, with a typical midlife onset and a duration of between 10 to 20 years (Zoghbi and Orr, 2000) and the threshold for most of the diseases appears to be a glutamine repeat of between 35 to 40 residues (Paulson, 1999). In the case of Huntington's disease, individuals with 35 CAG repeats or fewer do not develop the disease; those with 36-39 repeats have an increased risk of developing the disease; repeats of 40 or greater will always lead to the disease within a normal lifespan (Myers et al., 1998). The age of onset, as well as the severity of the symptoms are in all cases a function of the length of the glutamine stretches. This is illustrated in **Figure 5.1** for Huntington's disease, where the relationship between the CAG repeat number and the age of onset is represented. Another common feature of most of the diseases is the presence of neuronal intranuclear aggregates, or inclusions, which contain the

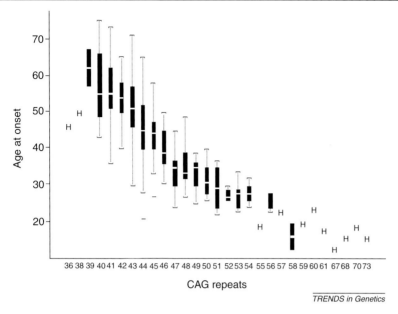

Figure 5.1: Relationship between CAG repeat number on HD disease chromosome and age of onset of disease (reprinted from *Trends in Genetics*, Vol 18, Rubinsztein, Lessons from animal modes of Huntington's disease, pp 202–209, Copyright 2002, with permission from Elsevier).

protein with the polyQ repeat; in several cases these inclusions are formed by insoluble amyloid-like fibrils (McGowan et al., 2000; Scherzinger et al., 1999), reminiscent of the presence of inclusions containing aggregated forms of the protein involved in the disease in other neurological diseases such as Alzheimer's disease, Parkinson's disease, prion disease and amyotrophic lateral sclerosis (Kaytor and Warren, 1999; Paulson, 1999). This aggregation process, which we discuss below, seems to involve misfolding of the protein involved in the disease. The disease protein is found in aggregated deposits, often within intracellular inclusion bodies, which also contain chaperones (components of the normal folding process) and elements of the cytosolic protein degradation pathway, ubiquitin and components of the proteosomal apparatus (Cummings and Zoghbi, 2000).

5.3 STRUCTURAL MODELS OF POLYQ PROTEIN AGGREGATION

While the aggregation of polyQ-containing proteins with the cell may involve interactions with other cellular components, there are quite strong *in vitro* arguments which indicate that aggregation is driven by the protein itself. Using preformed aggregates of simple polyQ peptides with 20 or 42Q residues, flanked at each end by a single lysine residue to confer solubility (Yang et al., 2002), it was shown in cultured mammalian cells that simple polyQ aggregates localized to the cytoplasm have little impact on cell viability. However, aggregates of polyQ peptides containing a nuclear localization signal effectively localize to the nucleus, and lead to dramatic cell death (Yang et al., 2002). Nuclear localization of an aggregate of the short Q_{20} polyQ peptide was just as toxic as that of the longer polyQ peptide, supporting the idea that the influence of the polyQ repeat length on age of onset and severity of the disease is at the level of aggregation efficiency. It was also demonstrated that the rate of formation of amyloid fibrils increases dramatically as the polyQ repeat expands in polyQ-containing huntingtin, from the normal to mutant range, again supporting the central role for the aggregation process in the pathogenesis (Scherzinger et al., 1999).

It is evident that the mechanism of the pathogenesis of polyQ diseases results from a toxic gain of function which depends only on the expanded polyQ sequence. It follows that, if we could determine what is the molecular event which causes the altered properties of the longer polyQ inserts compared to the shorter, non-pathogenic polyQ repeats, we would be better placed to devise effective therapeutic strategies. Some of the suggestions are presented in **Figure 5.2**. They include, most probably, the formation of large β-pleated sheet aggregates, originating either from random coil conformations or from β-hairpins (Perutz, 1996; Sharma et al., 1999): there is also the suggestion that they might form an unusual right-handed µ-helix, which, when inserted into membranes, could act as an ion channel (Monoi et al., 2000). This latter hypothesis was not borne out experimentally when N-terminal huntingtin fragment containing more than 100 CAG repeats were expressed in Xenopus oocytes or CHO cells without inducing any change in ion channel activity (Norremolle et al., 2003).

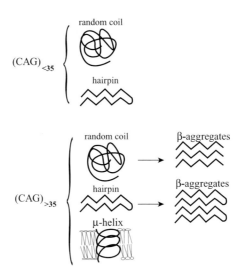

Figure 5.2: Summary of possible models for the aggregation of polyQ proteins (reprinted from *Brain Research Bulletin*, Vol 56, Masino and Pastore, A structural approach to trinucleotide expansion disease, pp 183–189, Copyright 2001, with permission from Elsevier).

Based on studies with synthetic polyQ peptides, a model of polyQ aggregate structure has been proposed (Thakur and Wetzel, 2002) which includes an alternating beta-strand/beta-turn structure, with seven glutamine residues per beta-strand. This model of a compact beta sheet structure is supported by studies using the huntingtin exon-1 N-terminal fragment in both mammalian cell cultures and in cultured primary cortical neurons (Poirier et al., 2005).

However, there does seem to be a consensus that initiation of aggregation requires a critical concentration of polyQ-containing aggregation precursor (**Figure 5.3**), associated with a lag time, which may account for the late onset of the disease (Chen et al., 2002). This is confirmed by the findings that the rate of formation of amyloid fibrils increases

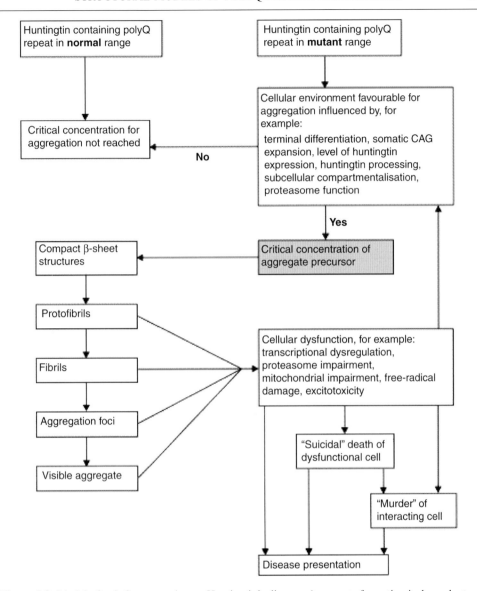

Figure 5.3: Model of polyQ aggregation on Huntingtin's disease. Aggregate formation is dependent on critical concentration of the aggregate precursor. Each aggregation state might act to make aggregation more likely. Disease occurs as a consequence of both cellular dysfunction and death (reprinted with permission from Elsevier (*The Lancet*, 2003, Vol 361, pp 1642–1644).

dramatically as the polyQ repeat expands from the normal to the mutant range, again supporting a central role for the aggregation process in the pathogenesis of the disease (Chen et al., 2002). The observation that polyQ repeats in the non-pathogenic range can also form fibrillar aggregates, which are as toxic as those containing expanded repeats provided they are targeted to the nucleus (Yang et al., 2002) suggests that it is the likelihood of aggregate formation that determines whether disease will occur. It also raises the interesting question of what causes the nuclear relocation of proteins with extended polyQ repeats. One

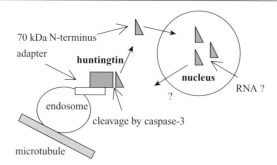

Figure 5.4: Model of relocation of huntingtin to the nucleus. At steady state, most of the huntingtin is in the cytoplasm associated with the surface of endosomes, perhaps through association with an adapter protein. Limited amounts of huntingtin are cleaved by caspase-3 and enter the nucleus, where they concentrate in RNAase-sensitive foci. The process is dramatically exaggerated upon caspase activation (reprinted from Tao and Tartakoff, Nuclear relocation of normal Huntington, *Traffic*, Vol 2, pp 385–394, Copyright 2001, with permission of Blackwell Publishing Ltd).

suggestion in the case of huntingtin is that the protein, which is normally located anchored to endosomes, has a potential caspase-3 cleavage site which, if cleaved, would release a 70kD N-terminal fragment (**Figure 5.4**). Since polyQ tracts stimulate caspase activation, mutant huntingtin would be transferred to the nucleus as the 70kD fragment containing the polyQ tract (Tao and Tartakoff, 2001).

It has also been demonstrated that other proteins, such as Creb binding protein (CRP, discussed in Chapter 10) containing polyQ could be recruited into aggregates of the huntingtin protein (Huang et al., 1998; Kazantzev et al., 1999).

5.4 MECHANISMS OF CELL DEATH IN POLYQ DISEASES

The processes by which proteins with polyglutamine expansions, and their associated protein aggregates, cause neuronal damage and cell death remain uncertain. Several hypotheses have been advanced (reviewed in Lipinski and Yuan, 2004).

A first possibility is that expanded polyQ aggregates might induce neuronal cell death by directly activating components of apoptotic pathways. Expression of expanded polyQ tracts in primary rat neurons led to recruitment of caspase-8 to the polyQ aggregates and its activation (Sanchez et al., 1999). The affinity of Hip-1, a putative huntingtin (Htt)-binding protein, for Htt is reduced in the presence of expanded polyQ. This results in increased cellular levels of Hip-1, which forms heterodimers with another protein, Hippi, which, like Hip-1, has pseudo death-effector domains (DED) (Hackam et al., 2000). Hip-1/Hippi complexes are able to bind and activate caspase-8, thus inducing apoptosis (Gervais et al., 2002). Neuroprotective effects of peptide caspase inhibitors in transgenic models of Huntington's disease suggest that, in addition to caspase-8, both caspase-1 and caspase-3 may also be involved in the mediation of neurodegeneration induced by mutant huntingtin (Chen et al., 2000).

A second mechanism involves the already alluded to critical role of the nuclear accumulation of expanded polyQ aggregates. Nuclear localization and aggregation of the affected proteins is a common feature of many of the polyQ triplet-repeat disorders (Ross, 1997; Orr, 2001) and seems to be key to trigger pathogenesis. This is particularly well illustrated by spinobulbar muscular atrophy (SBMA), in which the polyQ expansion is localized to the androgen receptor. Upon binding of androgens, like testosterone, the cytoplasmic androgen receptor undergoes a conformational change, translocates to the nucleus, where it binds DNA and mediates transcription of androgen-responsive genes. This explains why SBMA is restricted to males (Brooks and Fischbeck, 1995), but does not explain the mechanism of nuclear translocation.

Yet another explanation, consistent with the requirement for nuclear localization of polyQ proteins could be interference with transcription and in particular, its regulation. Expanded polyQ stretches in disease-causing genes have been shown to interact with short Q stretches present in many transcription factors (reviewed in Lipinski and Yuan, 2004). Interference with transcription might explain some of the cell-type specificity of polyQ expansion diseases. For example, in a mouse model of SCA-7, ataxin-7 with an expanded polyQ interacted with and suppressed the activity of the cone-rod homeobox protein (La Spada et al., 2001). Inactivation of this tissue-specific transcription factor could contribute to the cone-rod dystrophy observed in both SCA-7 mice and patients. Mutant ataxin-1 binds and inhibits a cerebellum-specific protein, PQBP-1 and RNA polymerase II, leading to decreased levels of RNA polymerase II, which could contribute to the specific death of cerebellar neurons in SCA-1 (Okazawa et al., 2002). Another possibility is that some polyQ proteins interfere with transcription through alteration of their normal function as transcriptional regulators. Both ataxin-3 (mutated in SCA-3) and atrophin-1 have been suggested to function as co-repressors. The former acts by a dual mechanism involving direct inhibition of transcription, as well as interference with histone acetylation (Li et al., 2002), while the latter functions as a transcriptional corepressor in multiple developmental processes in *Drosophila* (Zhang et al., 2002). Some of the effects could be explained by the progressive sequestration of transcription factors: as the polyQ-rich proteins aggregate they would titrate their normal binding partners away from the promoters that they regulate (Lipinski and Yuan, 2004).

Down-regulation of pro-survival pathways has also been proposed. Wild type huntingtin enhances the expression of brain-derived neurotrophic factor, necessary for survival of striatal neurons, which are the first to be affected by HD, whereas expanded polyQ huntingtin causes transcriptional down-regulation of this same factor (Zuccato et al., 2001). Treatment with insulin-like growth factor 1 can abolish the toxicity induced by cellular expression of mutant huntingtin, and the effect was at least partially dependent on direct phosphorylation of huntingtin by Akt (Humbert et al., 2002). Akt protein was altered in the brains of HD patients. Akt was also shown to phosphorylate polyQ-rich ataxin-1 in a cell-based model of SCA-1 (Chen et al., 2003).

Finally, it has been suggested that, since motor neurons rely on axonal transport of macromolecules to ensure their distribution along their long axons, interference with this process might also be involved in polyQ expansion diseases. For example, aggregates of androgen receptor with elongated polyQ tracts alter axonal trafficking and mitochondrial distribution in motor neurons (Piccioni et al., 2002). So, at least in SBMA, polyQ aggregates could cause the death of motor neurons by physically interfering with the process of axonal transport of macromolecules and organelles.

The cause of neuronal damage by expanded polyQ proteins most probably occurs by several pathways, some of which may be more pronounced in specific diseases, such as axonal transport in SBMA and activation of caspase-8 together with interference with transcriptional regulation in HD.

5.5 HUNTINGTON'S DISEASE

HD has a frequency of 4 in 10^5 among European populations (less than 1 in 10^6 in Japanese and African populations), and is the most common of the polyQ diseases. It causes movement disorders, cognitive deterioration and psychiatric disturbances. Symptoms begin appearing insidiously, typically between the ages of 35 to 50: the disease is progressive and fatal some 15–20 years after onset. Motor disturbances include choreiform[3] involuntary movements of proximal and distal muscles and progressive impairment of voluntary movements. In patients with juvenile onset HD the symptoms include bradykinesia (slowness of voluntary movements and of speech), rigidity and dystonia (intense irregular muscle spasms); the involuntary movements of the children often take the form of tremor, and they often suffer from epileptic seizures (Vonsattel and Di Figlia, 1998). HD is characterized by a remarkable specificity of neuronal loss. The most sensitive region (**Figure 5.5**) is the striatum, with loss of GABAergic medium spiny projection neurons. The caudate nucleus and the putamen are also particularly affected; in advanced cases there is also loss of neurons in the thalamus, substantia nigra and the subthalamic nucleus.

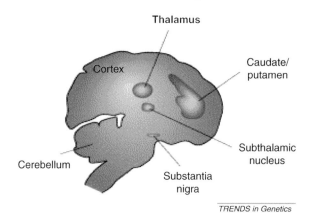

TRENDS in Genetics

Figure 5.5: Cartoon of a sagittal section of human brain showing major sites of axonal loss in HD (reprinted from *Trends in Genetics*, Vol 18, Rubinsztein, Lessons from animal modes of Huntington's disease, pp 202–209, Copyright 2002, with permission from Elsevier).

Alterations in brain iron metabolism have been reported, resulting in increased iron accumulation in Huntington's disease (Qian and Wang, 1998; Moos and Morgan, 2004). This was particularly the case in basal ganglia from patients with HD compared to normal controls (Bartzokis et al., 1999). In studies in embryonic stem cells, huntingtin was found to be iron-regulated, essential for the function of normal nuclear and perinuclear organelles and to be involved in the regulation of iron homeostasis (Hilditch-Maguire et al., 2000).

The gene for huntingtin (Htt) consists of 67 exons, extending over 180kb of DNA and codes for a polypeptide of 3144 residues, making it one of the longest proteins known (MacDonald et al., 1993). Encoded on chromosome 4, it has the CAG trinucleotide repeat within exon 1; huntingtin (Htt) has an interesting multi-domain structure (**Figure 5.6**). The polyQ domain, close to the N-terminus, is much larger in wild type human Htt than in other species. Adjacent to this, there is a glutamine/proline (Q/P)-rich region (a) and ten HEAT

---

[3] Choreiform movements are purposeless, involuntary movements such as flexing and extending of fingers, raising and lowering of shoulders or grimacing.

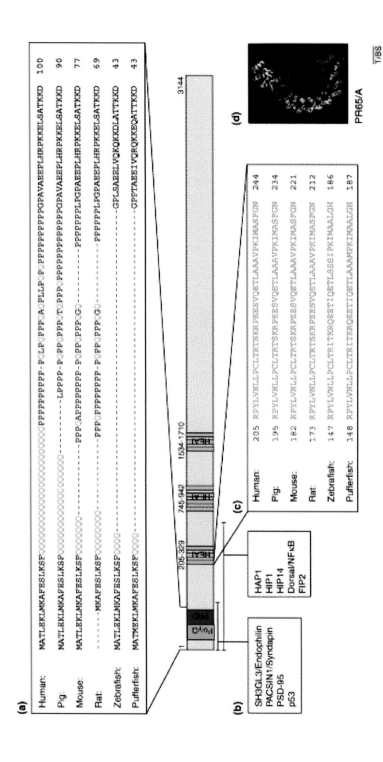

Figure 5.6: Huntingtin domain structure and sequence comparison between species. Huntingtin contains a glutamine/proline(Q/P)-rich region at the N-terminus (**a**) and ten highly conserved HEAT repeats, also clustered in the amino terminal region (**c**). Reprinted from *Trends in Biochemical Sciences*, Vol 28, Harjes and Wanker, The hunt for Huntingtin function: interaction partners tell many different stories, pp 524–533, Copyright 2003, with permission from Elsevier.

(for Htt, elongation factor 3, regulatory A subunit of protein phosphatase 2a and Tor1) repeats, clustered in three domains in the N-terminal half of the protein. Partners which might interact with either the Q/P-rich domain or the first cluster of HEAT domains are indicated in (b). Amino acid sequence comparison shows that, unlike the Q/P-rich domains, the HEAT domains are highly conserved between species (c).

Htt is expressed ubiquitously with highest levels in neurons of the central nervous system: intracellularly it is present in nuclei, cell bodies, dendrites and nerve terminals. The normal function of Htt in neurons remains elusive. Potential Htt-binding partners have been identified; some of them are indicated in **Figure 5.6b** for the Q/P-rich region and the first cluster of HEAT repeats. Evidence has been presented which suggests that htt plays a role in clathrin-mediated endocytosis, in neuronal transport processes and in postsynaptic signaling (reviewed in Harjes and Wanker, 2003). It protects neuronal cells from apoptotic stress, suggesting that it has a function in cell survival (Cattaneo et al., 2001), and it has been shown to interact with transcription factors, including some which contain a normal polyQ stretch (the TATA-binding protein, TBP, and the cAMP-responsive element-binding protein, CBP), indicating that it also plays a role in transcriptional regulation (Néri, 2001). That Htt appears to be involved in so many different cellular processes, which take place in distinct cellular compartments, suggests that Htt is a prime example of a protein which does not have a single unified function, but rather is a multifaceted and multifunctional protein.

A model for HD cellular pathogenesis (Ross, 2002) is presented in **Figure 5.7**. Huntingtin is normally predominantly cytoplasmic. It may cycle to the nucleus and have a normal role in the regulation of gene transcription, but this is uncertain. The mutation causes a conformational change and likely leads to partial unfolding or abnormal folding of the protein, which can be corrected by molecular chaperones. Proteolytic cleavage of mutant huntingtin takes place. The N terminus with the expanded repeat can assume a β-pleated sheet structure. Toxicity in the cytoplasm may be caused by mutant full-length protein or by cleaved protein, and the toxic species may be soluble monomers or oligomers or, possibly,

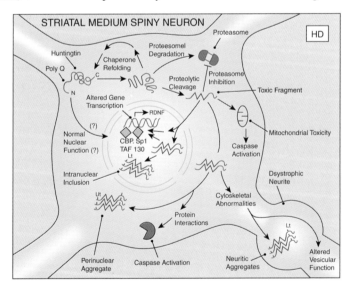

Figure 5.7: Model of HD cellular pathogenesis. Reprinted from *Neuron*, Vol 35, Ross, Polyglutamine pathogenisis: emergence of unifying mechanisms for Huntington's disease and related disorders, pp 819–822, Copyright 2002, with permission from Elsevier.

insoluble aggregates. Toxicity may involve inhibition of the proteasome or activation of caspases directly or be mediated through mitochondrial effects. Cytoplasmic aggregates accumulate in perinuclear or neuritic regions and are ubiquitinated. The mutant protein translocates to the nucleus, where it forms intranuclear inclusions. Nuclear toxicity is believed to be caused by interference with gene transcription.

5.6 OTHER POLYQ DISEASE PROTEINS

Spinal and bulbar muscular atrophy (SBMA), the neurodegenerative disease discovered by Kennedy et al. (1968), involves the death of motor neurons in the spinal cord and in the bulbar region of the brainstem and affects only men. This is one of the few polyQ diseases for which we know the function of the affected protein – it is the androgen receptor, a member of the nuclear receptor family of transcription factors, and is responsible for the biological actions of androgenic steroids in target tissues. In the absence of androgens, the receptor is confined to the cytosol in a complex with accessory heat-shock proteins (**Figure 5.8**). Upon binding of androgen, the receptor dissociates from the accessory proteins, dimerizes and translocates to the nucleus where it interacts with androgen responsive elements on androgen responsive genes, and activates transcription. The three-

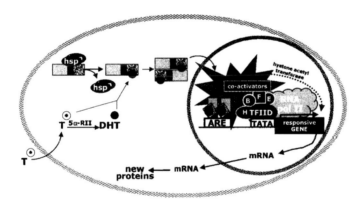

Figure 5.8: Mechanism of action of the androgen receptor. Testosterone (T) or its reduction product, dihydrotestosterone (DHT) bind to the androgen receptor, inducing the dissociation of the heat-shock proteins (hsp); the receptor dimerizes through an interaction between the N- and C-terminus, and translocates to the nucleus; there, the androgen receptor dimers bind androgen responsive elements (ARE) located in the promoter region of androgen responsive genes; a number of co-activators are recruited which interact with the general transcription factors of the TFII family and the activated androgen receptor dimers allow RNA polymerase II (RNA pol II) to transcribe the gene (reprinted from *Frontiers in Neuroendocrinology*, Vol 25, Poletti, the polyglutamine tract of androgen receptor: from function to dysfunction in motor neurons, pp 1–26, Copyright 2004, with permission from Elsevier).

dimensional structure of the ligand binding domain of the human androgen receptor (Matias et al., 2000), located in the C-terminal region of the protein, is illustrated in **Figure 5.9**. The fact that the dimerization of the androgen receptor occurs through an inter-molecular NH_2-COOH-terminal interaction involving the ligand binding domain of one molecule and the NH_2-terminal portion of another, and that this interaction is modified by the polyQ length of

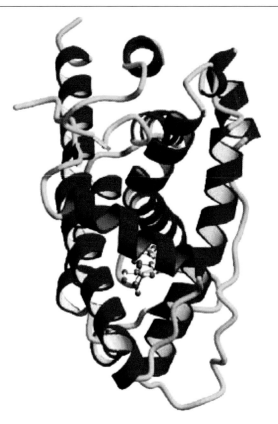

Figure 5.9: Diagram of the three-dimensional structure of the ligand binding domain of the human androgen receptor with a synthetic androgenic steroid bound (from Matias et al., 2000, reproduced by permission of The American Society for Biochemistry and Molecular Biology).

the androgen receptor monomers, may explain the loss of transcriptional activity as a function of the length of the polyQ tract.

A model for SBMA cellular pathogenesis (Ross, 2002) is presented in **Figure 5.10**. Upon binding of ligand (agonist or antagonist), the androgen receptor (AR) dimerizes, dissociates from the associated heat-shock proteins (not shown), which exposes its nuclear localization signal (NLS), resulting in nuclear translocation. Agonist binding results in association with androgen response elements (ARE), leading to the recruitment of coactivators and activation of gene transcription in the nucleus. Antagonist binding results in nuclear translocation without gene transcription. Upon binding of either agonist or antagonist, the mutant receptor translocates to the nucleus. After proteolytic cleavage (either in the nucleus or the cytoplasm), the polyglutamine stretch assumes an altered conformation, leading to aggregation and the formation of intranuclear inclusions. The mutation may confer a gain of a novel toxic property on the AR, such as abnormal interactions with CBP, leading to loss of neuronal survival signaling.

Spinocerebellar ataxias types 1, 2, 3 and 7 are all associated with polyQ expansions in proteins known as ataxins, for which the physiological role was unknown when the genes were first identified. Some individuals have been found with histidine interruptions in an expanded polyglutamine repeat in ataxin-1, the *SCA1* gene product. Although the repeat length was well within the disease range for SCA1, the individuals were found to be phenotypically normal (Quan et al. 1995; Calabresi et al. 2001), and the protein had a

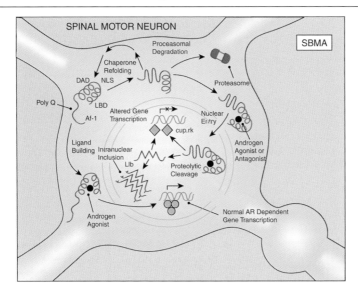

Figure 5.10: A model for SBMA cellular pathogenesis. Reprinted from *Neuron*, Vol 35, Ross, Polyglutamine pathogenisis, emergence of unifying mechanisms for Huntington's disease and related disorders, pp 819–822, Copyright 2002, with permission from Elsevier.

strikingly less propensity to aggregation (Sen et al., 2003). Subsequently, the application of structure-based multiple sequence alignments of homologous proteins (often referred to as integrative bioinformatics) has led to propositions for the latter three ataxins.

Ataxin-2, coded by chromosome 12q, and located principally in the Golgi apparatus, has 1312 amino acid residues, and is a highly basic protein apart from one acidic region consisting of residues 254–475 containing 46 acidic residues. This region is predicted to contain two globular Lsm domains (Like Sm), one of which is typical of RNA-binding Sm and Sm-like proteins. Generally Lsm domain proteins are involved in a variety of RNA processing events, and **Figure 5.11** presents a 3D model of the Lsm domain of ataxin 2

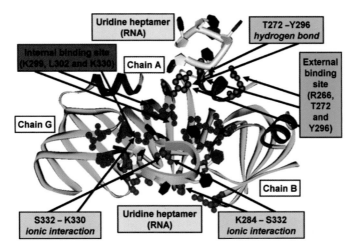

Figure 5.11: 3D model of the Lsm domain of ataxin-2 (reprinted from Albrecht et al., Structural and functional analysis of ataxin-2 and ataxin-3, *FEBS Journal*, Vol 271, pp 3155–3170, 2004, with permission from Blackwell Publishing Ltd), based on the crystal structure of Sm1 from *P. abyssi* as template.

(Albrecht et al., 2004), based on the crystal structure of Sm1 from *P. abyssi* bound to uridine heptamers (Thore et al., 2003). The physiological function of ataxin-2 in RNA processing remains to be established, but it has been observed to interact with a protein which has an RNA-binding homologue in *C. elegans* involved in the regulation of the tissue-specific splicing of RNA.

Ataxin-3 is the protein mutated in Machado Joseph Disease (SCA3), and found in both the nucleus and the cytoplasm of cells. Its longest splice variant, coded on chromosome 14, possesses 376 amino acids (including 22 in the polyQ stretch, which is contained unusually in exon 10, close to the C-terminus), belongs to a novel class of cysteine-proteases (Scheel et al., 2003), binds polyubiquitinated proteins and has ubiquitin protease activity (Burnett et al., 2003). Ataxin-3 has a globular N-terminal domain, named Josephin, comprising residues 1-170 and a more flexible C-terminal region, which includes several ubiquitin-interacting motifs and the polyQ region. The Josephin domain contains highly conserved amino acid residues similar to those found in a deubiquitinating cysteine protease (Scheel et al., 2003), and mutating the catalytic cysteine of ataxin-3 inhibits its ability to cleave ubiquitin from ubiquitinated protein substrates (Burnett et al., 2003). A 3D model of the deubiquitinating domain of ataxin-3 is presented in **Figure 5.12**, based on the structure of YUH1, a ubiquitin-specific protease from yeast, bound to the ubiquitin-like inhibitor Ubal (Albrecht et al., 2004). A recent report suggests that the Josephin domain of ataxin-3 has an intrinsic tendency to aggregate and to form temperature-induced fibrils similar to those described for expanded ataxin-3 (Masino et al., 2004).

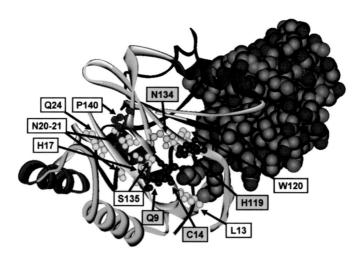

Figure 5.12: 3D model of the deubiquitinating Josephin domain of ataxin-3 using the structure of yeast YUH1 bound to the ubiquitin-like inhibitor Ubal (in CPK view mode) as template (reprinted from Albrecht et al., Structural and functional analysis of ataxin-2 and ataxin-3, *FEBS Journal*, Vol 271, pp 3135–3170, 2004, with permission from Blackwell Publishing Ltd).

For ataxin-7, the prediction from integrative bioinformatics is that it is a component of a multicomponent complex which is involved in histone acetylation (Scheel et al., 2003).

Ataxin-1 has been shown to bind to chromosomes and to interact with transcriptional corepressors and with histone deacetylase (Tsai et al., 2004). A region of ataxin-1, the AXH domain, has significant sequence homology to the transcription factor HBP1, and has been

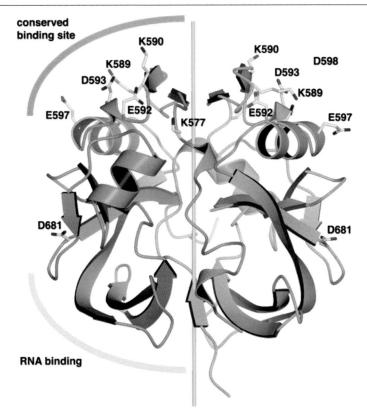

Figure 5.13: The putative RNA binding site of the AXH domain of ataxin-1 (from Chen et al., 2004 reproduced with permission of The American Society for Biochemistry and Molecular Biology).

implicated in RNA binding and in dimer formation. The crystal structure of the AXH domain of ataxin-1 has been determined (Chen et al., 2004). The AXH domain is dimeric and contains a structural motif found in many oligonucleotide-binding proteins. The putative RNA-binding site is represented in **Figure 5.13**. A cluster of well conserved charged surface residues has also been identified, which may constitute a second binding site for an as yet unidentified partner.

REFERENCES

Albrecht, M., Golatta, M., Wüllner, U. and Lengauer, T. (2004) *Eur. J. Biochem.*, **271**, 3155–3170.
Bartzokis, G., Cummings, J., Perlman, S., Hance, D.B. and Mintz, J. (1999) *Arch. Neurol.*, **56**, 569–574.
Bates, G. (2003) *Lancet*, **361**, 1642–1644.
Brooks, B.P. and Fischbeck, K.H. (1995) *Trends Neurosci.*, **18**, 459–461.
Burnett, B., Li, F. and Pittman, R.N. (2003) *Hum. Mol. Genet.*, **12**, 3195–3205.
Calabresi, V., Guida, S., Servadio, A., Fontali, M. and Jodice, C., (2001) *Brain Res. Bull.*, **56**, 337–342.
Cattaneo, E., Rigamonti, D., Goffredo, D. and Zuccato, C. (2001) *Trends Neurosci.*, **24**, 182–188.
Chen, M., Ona, V.O., Li, M., Ferrante, R.J. *et al.* (2000) *Nat. Med.*, **6**, 797–801.
Chen, S., Ferrone, F.A. and Wetzel, R. (2002) *Proc. Natl. Acad. Sci., USA*, **99**, 11884–11889.
Chen, H.K., Fernandez-Funez, P., Acevedo, S.F., Lam, Y.C. *et al.* (2003) *Cell*, **113**, 457–468.

Chen, Y.W., Allen, M.D., Veprintsev, D.B., Lowe, J. and Bycroft, M. (2004) *J. Biol. Chem.*, **279**, 3758–3765.

Cummings, C.J. and Zohgbi, H.Y. (2000) *Hum. Mol. Genet.*, **9**, 909–916.

Gervais, F.G., Singaraja, R., Xanthoudakis, S., Gutekunst, C.A. *et al.* (2002) *Nat. Cell Biol.*, **4**, 95–105.

Hackam, A.S., Yassa, A.S., Singaraja, R., Metzler, M. *et al.* (2000) *J. Biol. Chem.*, **275**, 41299–41308.

Harjes, P. and Wanker, E.E. (2003) *TRENDS Biochem. Sci.*, **28**, 425–433.

Hilditch-Maguire, P., Trettel, F., Passani, L.A., Auerbach, A. *et al.* (2000) *Hum. Mol. Genet.*, **9**, 2789–2797.

Huang, C.C., Faber, P.W., Persichetti, F., Mittal, V. *et al.* (1998) *Somat. Cell Mol. Genet.*, **24**, 217–233.

Humbert, S., Bryson, E.A., Cordelieres, F.P., Connors, N.C. *et al.* (2002) *Dev. Cell*, **2**, 831–837.

Kaytor, M.D. and Warren, S.T. (1999) *J. Biol. Chem.*, **274**, 37507–37510.

Kazantsev, A., Preisinger, E., Dranovsky, A., Goldhaber, D. and Housman, D. (1999) *Proc. Natl. Acad. Sci., USA*, **96**, 11404–11409.

Kennedy, W.R., Aleter, M. and Sung, J.H. (1968) *Neurology*, **18**, 671–680.

La Spada, A., Wilson, E.M., Lubahn, D.B., Harding, A.E. and Fischbeck, K.H. (1991) *Nature*, **352**, 77–79.

La Spada, A., Roling, D., Harding, A.E., Warner, C.L. *et al.* (1992) *Nat. Genet.*, **2**, 301–304.

La Spada, A.R., Fu, Y.H., Sopher, B.L., Libby, R.T. *et al.* (2001) *Neuron*, **31**, 913–927.

Li, F., Macfarlan, T., Pittman, R.N. and Chakravarti, D. (2002) *J. Biol. Chem.*, **277**, 45004–45012.

Lipinski, M.M. and Yuan, Y. (2004) *Current Opin. Pharmacol.*, **4**, 85–90.

MacDonald, M.E., Ambrose, C.M., Duyao, M.P., Myers, R.H., *et al.* (1993) *Cell*, **72**, 971–983.

Masino, L. and Pastore, A. (2001) *Brain Res. Bull.*, **56**, 183–189.

Masino, L., Nicastro, G., Menon, R.P., Dal Piaz, F. *et al.* (2004) *J. Mol. Biol.*, **344**, 1021–1035.

Matias, P.M., Donner, R., Coelho, M, Thomaz, C. *et al.* (2000) *J. Biol. Chem.*, **275**, 26164–26171.

McGowan, D.P., van Roon-Mom, W., Holloway, H., Bates, G.P. *et al.* (2000) *Neuroscience*, **100**, 677–688.

Monoi, H., Futaki, S., Kugiyama, S., Minakata, H. and Yoshihara, K. (2000) *Biophys. J.*, **78**, 2892–2899.

Moos, T. and Morgan, E.H. (2004) *Ann. N.Y. Acad. Sci.*, **1012**, 14–26.

Myers, R.H., Marans, K.S. and MacDonald, M.E. (1998) In *Genetic instabilities and hereditary neurodegenerative diseases*. ed. Wells, R.D. and Warren, S.T., Academic Press, San Diego, 301–323.

Néri, C. (2001) *TRENDS Mol. Med.*, **7**, 283–284.

Norremolle, A., Grunnet, M., Hasholt, L. and Sorensen, S.A. (2003) *J. Neurosci. Res.*, **71**, 132–137.

Okazawa, H., Rich, T., Chang, A., Lin, X. *et al.* (2002) *Neuron*, **34**, 701–713.

Orr, H.T. (2001) *Neuron*, **31**, 875–876.

Paulson, H.L. (1999) *Am. J. Hum. Genet.*, **64**, 339–345.

Perutz, M.F. (1996) *Curr Opin. Struct. Biol.*, **6**, 848–858.

Piccioni, F., Pinton, P., Simeoni, S., Pozzi, P. *et al.* (2002) *FASEB J.*, **16**, 1418–1420.

Poirier, M.A., Jiang, H. and Ross, C.A. (2005) *Hum. Mol. Genet.*, **14**, 765–774.

Poletti, A. (2004) *Front. Neuroendocrinol.*, **25**, 1–26.

Qian, Z.M. and Wang, Q. (1998) *Brain Res. Brain Res. Rev.*, **27**, 257–267.

Quan, F., Janas, J., and Popovich, B.W. (1995) *Hum. Mol. Genet.*, **4**, 2411–2413.

Ross, C.A. (1997) *Neuron*, **19**, 1147–1150.

Ross, C.A. (2002) *Neuron*, **35**, 819–822.

Rubinsztein, D.C. (2002) *TRENDS Genet.*, **18**, 202–209.

Sanchez, I., Xu, C.J., Juo, P., Kakizaka, *et al.* (1999) *Neuron*, **22**, 623–633.

Scheel, H., Tomiuk, S. and Hofmann, K. (2003) *Hum. Mol. Genet.*, **12**, 2845–2852.

Scherzinger, E., Sittler, A., Schweiger, K., Heiser, V. *et al.* (1999) *Proc. Natl. Acad. Sci., USA*, **96**, 4604–4609.

Sen, S., Dash, D., Pasha, S. and Brahmakari, S.K. (2003) *Protein Sci.*, **12**, 953–962.

Sharma, D., Sharma, S., Pasha, S. and Brahmachari, S.K. (1999) *FEBS Lett.*, **456**, 181–185.

Tao, T. and Tartakoff, A.M. (2001) *Traffic*, **2**, 385–394.

Thakur, A.K. and Wetzel, R. (2002) *Proc. Natl. Acad. Sci., USA*, **99**, 17014–17019.

Thore, S., Mayer, C., Sauter, C., Weeks, S. and Suck, D. (2003) *J. Biol. Chem.*, **278**, 1239–1247.

Tsai, C.C., Kao, H.Y., Mitzutani, A., Banayo, E. *et al.* (2004) *Proc. Natl. Acad. Sci., USA*, **101**, 4047–4052.

Vonsattel, J.P. and Di Figlia, M. (1998) *J. Neuropathol. Exp. Neurol.*, **57**, 369–384.

Yang, W., Dunlap, J.R., Andrews, R.B. and Weizel, R. (2002) *Hum. Mol. Genet.*, **11**, 29095–2917.

Zhang, S., Xu, L., Lee, J. and Xu, T. (2002) *Cell*, **108**, 45–56.

Zoghbi, H.Y. and Orr, H.T. (2000) *Annu. Rev. Neurosci.*, **23**, 217–247.

Zuccato, C., Ciammola, A., Rigamonti, D., Leavitt, B.R. *et al.* (2001) *Science*, **293**, 493–498.

6

Friedreich's Ataxia and Diseases Associated with Expansion of Non-Coding Triplets

6.1 INCIDENCE AND PATHOPHYSIOLOGY OF FRIEDREICH'S ATAXIA

Friedreich's ataxia is the most common hereditary ataxia and is the most prevalent cerebellar ataxia among children and adults in Europe. It was first described in 1863 by Nikolaus Friedreich (Friedreich, 1863), chief of the medical clinic in Heidelberg, where he occupied the chair of pathology and therapy from 1858 till 1882. His clinical observations described the essential characteristics of the disease as an adolescent-onset ataxia, particularly associated with clumsiness in walking, accompanied by sensory loss, lateral curvature of the spine, foot deformity and heart disease (Pandolfo, 1999). Detailed neuropathological examination showed cerebrospinal degeneration. However, many patients with cerebellar ataxia were diagnosed with Friedreich's ataxia, until it was recognized that recessive inheritance is a major diagnostic criterion for Friedreich's ataxia (Harding, 1981). Since the discovery of the gene responsible for the disease, and the application of molecular genetic methods, the molecular diagnosis of atypical cases of Friedreich's ataxia has become possible, and the clinical spectrum of the disease has been broadened, with documentation of age of onset as late as 62 years (previously thought to be typically before 25 years of age). Extraneurological involvement is not always clinically obvious, but increased heart wall thickness is observed in all patients and 70% of patients develop a life-threatening hypertrophic cardiomyopathy (Harding, 1981). Loss of ambulation occurs on average 15.5 ± 7.4 years after the onset of the disease (Delatcycki et al., 2000) and cardiomyopathy is the most common cause of death.

The prevalence of Friedreich's ataxia is estimated at 1–2 per 40,000 among the Caucasian population in Europe, with a frequency of heterozygous carriers of around 1% (Dürr, 2002). The disease is absent in Japan, and relatively rare among Asians and black Africans, and genetic analysis suggests that Friedreich's ataxia may be a condition that is restricted to the white population (Cossée et al., 1999; Dürr, 2002).

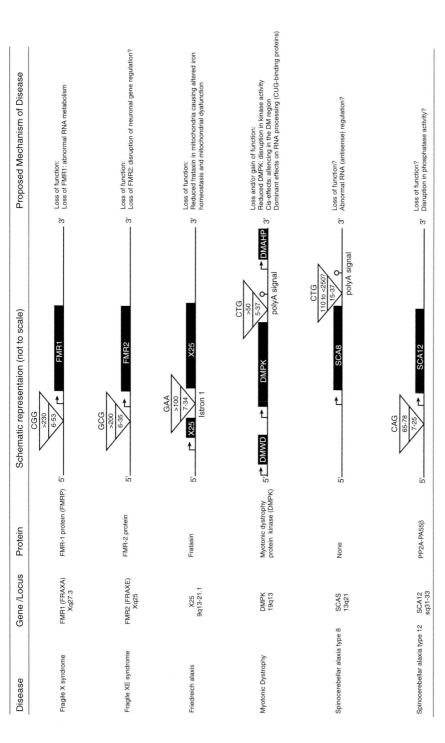

Figure 6.1: Diseases caused by expansion of non-coding trinucleotide repeats. From Cummings and Zoghbi, Fourteen and counting: unraveling trinucleotide repeat diseases, *Human Molecular Genetics*, 2001, 9(6), pp 909–916, by permission of Oxford University Press.

6.2 MOLECULAR BASIS OF THE DISEASE – TRIPLET REPEAT EXPANSIONS

Friedreich's ataxia (FRDA) is yet another of the fifteen neurological diseases in man which are known to be caused by the anomalous expansion of unstable trinucleotide repeats. However, unlike Huntington's disease, the trinucleotide expansion occurs in a non-coding region of the gene (**Figure 6.1**). The FRDA gene was mapped to chromosome 9 (Chamberlain et al., 1988), and finely mapped to a region small **enough to allow** a direct search for the candidate gene. Screening patients for a mutation in one of the candidate genes led to the identification of an expanded trinucleotide repeat (GAA) within the first intron of this gene (Campuzano et al., 1996). The FRDA gene was thus identified on chromosome 9q13 (Campuzano et al., 1996), and the encoded protein was named frataxin. The FRDA gene is composed of seven exons spread throughout 95kilobases of DNA (**Figure 6.2**), and encodes for the 210-residue frataxin protein. Frataxin protein levels are severely decreased in FRDA patients, and 96% of FRDA patients are homozygous for the GAA expansion in intron 1, while the remaining 4% are compound heterozygous for a GAA expansion and a point mutation within the coding part of the gene (**Figure 6.2**) (Campuzano

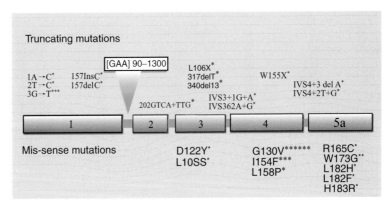

Figure 6.2: Frataxin mutations. The commonest mutation is the GAA expansion in the first intron of the frataxin gene (98% of cases). Boxes represent exons and bars represent introns of the frataxin gene. Asterisks indicate the number of families reported for each of the other mutations. Reprinted with permission from Elsevier (*The Lancet Neurology*, 2002, Vol 1, pp 370–374).

et al., 1996; Cossée et al., 1999). As we saw in Chapter 5, many neurological disorders, like Huntington's disease, are due to CAG expansions within coding regions of genes, resulting in polyglutamine expansions in the corresponding protein. FRDA is unique among trinucleotide repeat neurological disorders because it is autosomal recessive, the repeat is intronic, and it is the only one known with a GAA expansion. In FRDA patients, the first intron of the frataxin gene contains between 90 to 1700 GAA units. Most normal alleles carry six to nine GAA repeats, and never more than 34 repeats (Campuzano et al., 1996; Dürr et al., 1996; Epplen et al., 1997). The expansion of this GAA trinucleotide repeat severely decreases the expression of the frataxin protein. This decrease is due to reduction in the quantity of frataxin mRNA produced. It has been shown that the amount of frataxin mRNA depends on the length and orientation of the expansion and is due to disruption of transcription rather than to post-transcriptional splicing (Bidichandani et al., 1998; Ohshima et al., 1998; Grabcyk and Usdin, 2000). It has been suggested that the GAA-rich sequence is 'sticky' DNA, which forms a triple-helical structure, and impedes the transcription of the gene by RNA polymerase (Sakamoto et al., 1999). Although a number of point mutations in the frataxin gene have been observed (**Figure 6.2**), sometimes in individuals with a GAA expansion on one allele and the point mutation on the other, no patients have been found who have two point mutations and no triplet expansion. This may be because carriers of point mutations are rare in the population, or because double point mutations are lethal – embryonic lethality is observed in transgenic mice that lack frataxin (Cossée et al., 2000). If, as we will see in what follows, frataxin plays an important role in delivering iron for haem and iron-sulphur cluster synthesis in the mitochondria, it becomes clear why the total absence of the protein would prove to be fatal.

The screening of patients with ataxia for mutations in the frataxin gene has greatly broadened the clinical spectrum of FRDA. Applying the clinical criteria established by Harding (1981), only a few patients with this phenotype do not carry the GAA expansion in the frataxin gene. In contrast, many patients who do not fulfil these criteria, turn out to have confirmed FRDA. For a recent account of clinical knowledge of the disease see Dürr (2002).

Frataxin has been considered to be a mitochondrial protein conserved throughout evolution (Campuzano et al., 1996; Priller et al., 1997). Initially it was found that strains of yeast deficient in YFH1, the yeast frataxin homologue, accumulated iron in the mitochondrial matrix, presumably at the expense of cytosol iron (Babcock et al., 1997; Foury and Cazzalini, 1997). Current thinking on the pathogenesis of FRDA includes abnormal iron accumulation in mitochondria, hypersensitivity to oxidative stress, deficiency of Fe-S enzymes and respiratory chain electron transporters, free radical accumulation and cell degeneration (Bradley et al., 2001).

Frataxin is expressed ubiquitously with the highest concentrations found in heart, spinal cord and dorsal root ganglia (Koutnikova et al., 1997). The tissue-specific pathology of FRDA may reflect that tissues which are not affected by the disease, like liver, muscle, thymus and brown fat none the less express frataxin at significant levels. and are rich in mitochondria (Koutnikova et al., 1997). In contrast, affected tissues typically contain non- or slowly- dividing cells (e.g. CNS, heart and pancreas) whereas liver and skeletal muscle contain cells which can be replaced when they die (Delatycki et al., 2000; Puccio et al., 2001). Further, neurons and heart muscle depend exclusively on aerobic metabolism, and are therefore more vulnerable to mitochondrial defects and mitochondrial free radical damage.

6.3 MOLECULAR BASIS OF THE DISEASE – FRATAXIN AND ITS ROLE IN IRON METABOLISM

The discovery of frataxin as the product of the FRDA gene did not immediately indicate what its precise function might be. One of the first clues came from searches of DNA and protein databases, which found the presence of sequence homology to the CyaY proteins in the genomes of purple bacteria (Gibson et al., 1996), the closest relatives of the mitochondrial genome, but not in other bacteria, inferring a mitochondrial location for frataxin. The mitochondrial localization of frataxin was then experimentally confirmed (Campuzano et al., 1997). The N-terminal sequence, which directs the eukaryotic protein to the mitochondria and is cleaved upon entry into the mitochondria to yield the mature protein, is absent from the prokaryotic frataxin homologues. The frataxin family of proteins is widely distributed, ranging from mammals, through nematode worms, plants and yeast to Gram-negative bacteria, and they all have extensive sequence homology (**Figure 6.3**). The N-terminal

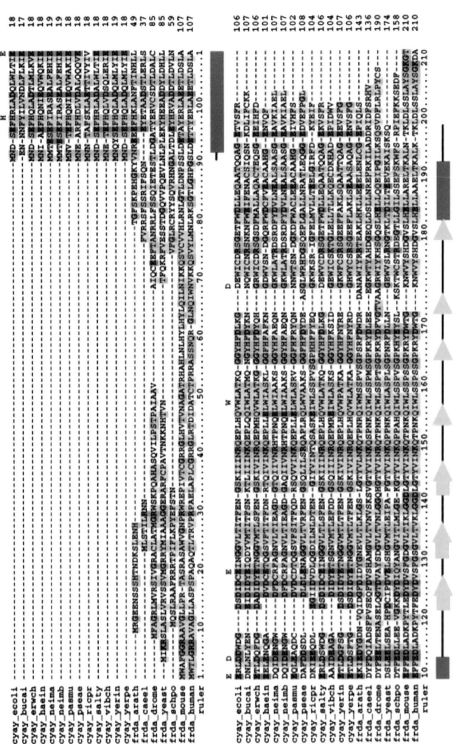

Figure 6.3: Alignment of the amino acid sequences of a number of eukaryotic frataxins (frda) and their prokaryotic orthologues (cyay). The numbering refers to human frataxin. The boxes and arrows indicate the positions of α-helices and β-strands respectively. From Adinolfi et al., A structural approach to understanding the import diversity of phylogenetically different frataxins. *Human Molecular Genetics*, 2002, 11(16), pp 1865–1877, by permission of Oxford University Press.

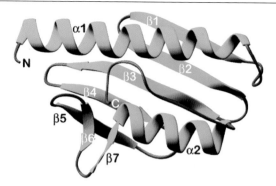

Figure 6.4: Structure of frataxin. Ribbon diagram showing the fold of frataxin, a compact αβ sandwich with α-helices in turquoise and β-strands in green. Strands β1–β5 form a large flat antiparallel β-sheet, which interacts with the two helices α1 and α2. The two helices are almost parallel to one another and to the plane of the large β-sheet. A second smaller β-sheet is formed by the C-terminus of β5 and strands β6 and β7. From Dhe-Paganon et al., 2000, reprinted with permission of The American Society for Biochemistry and Molecular Biology.

extensions which target eukaryotic frataxins to the mitochondria have no homology, whereas the C-terminal domain is highly conserved, with around 60% homology. The three-dimensional structure of the evolutionarily conserved C-terminal domain of human frataxin and of the *E. coli* CyaY protein have been determined (Dhe-Paganon et al., 2000; Cho et al., 2000; Musco et al., 2000). In agreement with their sequence homology, they have a very similar three-dimensional fold. This consists of a stable seven-stranded antiparallel β-sheet packed against a pair of parallel α-helices (**Figure 6.4**). This similarity of structure suggests that frataxin has similar functions in all species. This is underlined by studies which show that human frataxin can complement yeasts which are deficient in the protein YFH1, the yeast equivalent of frataxin (Cavadini et al., 2000). One striking feature of human frataxin is the clustering of 12 negatively charged residues on one surface of the molecule (**Figure 6.5**), which all point in the same general direction to form a large contiguous ionic patch on the protein surface. This is reminiscent of the clusters of acidic residues required for oxidation of Fe(II) to Fe(III) within the channels leading to the central iron core and for ferrihydrite nucleation at the inner surface of the iron storage protein ferritin. Because iron accumulates in the mitochondria of cells that lack frataxin, this led to the reasonable

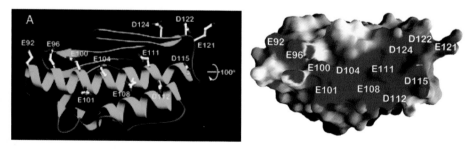

Figure 6.5: The anionic patch on the surface of the human frataxin molecule. In the ribbon diagram on the left, the side chains of the twelve Glu and Asp are represented. On the right hand side, the electrostatic potential of the molecular surface is represented with negative potential in red and positive in blue. From Dhe-Paganon et al., 2000, reprinted with permission of The American Society for Biochemistry and Molecular Biology.

conclusion that frataxin was involved in some way in mitochondrial iron homeostasis (Pandolfo, 1999).

There has been considerable debate on the role of frataxin in iron metabolism, with three hypotheses being advanced. The first was that frataxin was involved in iron transport out of the mitochondria, which would explain the accumulation of iron (Babcock et al., 1997) in frataxin deficiency. The second was that frataxin plays a role in mitochondrial iron storage, based on results obtained *in vitro* which showed that addition of Fe^{2+} to purified yeast YFH1 results in the assembly of a 48 subunit YFH1 multimer which can sequester an iron core containing up to 3000 atoms of iron (Adamec et al., 2000). More recent studies indicate that similar iron cores can be formed by human frataxin and that the iron cores have similar structures to the iron core of ferritin (Nichol et al., 2003). Other studies indicate that human frataxin has little or no tendency to bind iron (Dhe-Paganon, 2000; Musco et al., 2000; Adinolfi et al., 2002), and that the aggregation phenomena leading to multimer formation are not observed at physiological salt concentrations (Adinolfi et al., 2002). However, more recent studies indicate that human frataxin binds 6-7 iron atoms with a K_d of around $10 \, \mu M$ (Yoon and Cowan, 2003).

The third, and most promising hypothesis, is that frataxin is required for iron-sulphur cluster biosynthesis. The phylogenetic distribution of frataxin already indicated a role in iron-sulphur cluster assembly (Huynen et al., 2001) which was supported by the finding of reduced levels of iron-sulphur proteins in FRDA patients as well as in yeast and mouse frataxin-deficient models (Rötig et al., 1997; Foury, 1999; Bradley et al., 2000; Puccio et al., 2001). Many important proteins within the mitochondrial electron transport chain, as well as some key enzymes in metabolic pathways contain iron-sulphur clusters (**Figure 6.5**), and it has become clear that these metal centres are synthesized within the mitochondria itself, before being incorporated into proteins. Frataxin appears to play an important role in this process in yeast. It is necessary for assembly of the iron-sulphur cluster into yeast ferredoxin (Lutz et al., 2001) and it interacts both *in vivo* (Ramazzotti et al., 2004) and *in vitro* (Mühlenhoff et al., 2002; Gerber et al., 2003) with the iron-sulphur cluster scaffold protein Isu1. Isu1, together with the cysteine desulphurase Nfs1, constitutes the central Fe/S assembly complex. It seems reasonable to assume that frataxin supplies iron to this complex for Fe/S cluster assembly, as has been shown by *in vitro* experiments (Gerber et al., 2003; Yoon and Cowan, 2003).

Yeast cells which lack frataxin show low content of cytochromes, and it has been suggested from genetic studies (Lesuisse et al., 2003) and from *in vitro* studies with iron-containing frataxin and ferrochelatase, the enzyme which inserts iron into protoporphyrin IX (Park et al., 2003; Yoon and Cowan, 2004), that frataxin may also be the donor of iron for haem synthesis. This, however, remains to be established.

6.4 OTHER DISEASES ASSOCIATED WITH EXPANSION OF NON-CODING TRIPLETS

Altogether six neurological diseases are associated with the anomalous expansion of unstable trinucleotide repeats either in untranslated regions or in introns (**Figure 6.1**; Cummings and Zoghbi, 2000; Zoghbi and Orr, 2000). Unlike the polyQ family (Chapter 5), which all result from the same CAG trinucleotide repeat within a codon, different triplet expansions are observed in this family (CGG, GCC, GAA, CTG, and CAG). In **Figure 6.1**; the position of the expansion is shown and the upper and lower repeat sizes represent the disease and normal allele sizes, respectively. All of the proteins encoded by these genes are either absent, or, as in the case of FRDA, expressed with low efficiency.

In fragile X syndrome, the expansion is in the 5′-untranslated region of the gene, resulting in hypermethylation of the expanded repeats, transcriptional silencing and loss of the FMRP gene product. The expansion of a $(GCC)_n$ repeat in the promoter region of fragile XE patients also leads to hypermethylation, with the same consequences for FMR2 protein production as for FMRP. In myotonic dystrophy, the expanded CTG trinucleotide repeat is in the 3′-untranslated region of the protein kinase gene, DMPK, and a much larger CTG repeat is found in the same region of the gene involved in spinocerebral ataxia, type 8. Finally, in the rare disease SCA 12, the non-coding CAG repeat is in the 5′-untranslated region of the gene for a brain-specific regulatory subunit of protein phosphatase 2A.

We will not discuss all of the other five proteins, but rather focus on the FMRP protein, associated with fragile X syndrome (for a review see Masino and Pastore, 2001). This syndrome, an X-chromosome-linked dominant disorder is the most frequent cause of inherited mental retardation in humans (Hagerman, 1991), and is characterized by mental retardation of variable severity, autistic behaviour, enlarged testicles in adult males, a characteristic facial deformity and hyperextensible joints. The gene responsible, FMR1, is located at the Xq27.3 locus and is not expressed in fragile X syndrome (Pieretti et al., 1991), due to expansion of CGG trinucleotide repeats located in the 5′-untranslated region of the gene. This results in the absence of FMRP, a 630 residue protein (Verkerk et al., 1991). FRMP is an RNA-binding protein which can shuttle in and out of the nucleus (Jin et al., 2000). It is made up of four structurally distinct domains (**Figure 6.6**), a 200-residue N-terminal domain which forms a compact α-β fold, two so-called K-homology (KH) domains and a C-terminal region which contains an RGG box (Adinolfi et al., 1999; Siomi et al., 1993). The KH and RGG motifs are typical components of RNA binding proteins: FMRP associates with mRNAs within actively translating ribosomes (Corbin et al., 1997; Feng et al., 1997a,b), and it has recently been found to possess all of the properties of a potent RNA chaperone, suggestive of a role in the regulation of translation (Gabus et al., 2004).

As with frataxin, a number of protein partners have been identified which are presumed to bind to FMRP (reviewed in Masino and Pastore, 2001), although the way in which they affect its as yet undefined role of RNA binding protein remains to be established.

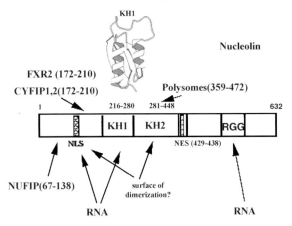

Figure 6.6: The domain architecture of FMRP. Reprinted from *Brain Research Bulletin*, Vol 56, Masino and Pastore, A structural approach to trinucleotide expansion diseases, pp 183–189, Copyright 2001, with permission from Elsevier.

REFERENCES

Adamec, J., Rusnak, F., Owen, W.G., Naylor, S. *et al.* (2000) *Am. J. Hum. Genet.*, **67**, 549–562.

Adinolfi, S., Bagni, C., Musco, G., Gibson, T. *et al.* (1999) *RNA*, **5**, 1248–1258.

Adinolfi, S., Trifluoggi, M., Politou, A.S., Martin, S. and Pastore, A. (2002) *Hum. Mol. Genet.*, **11**, 1865–1877.

Babcock, M., de Silva, D., Oaks, R., *et al.* (1997) *Science*, **276**, 1709–1712.

Bidichandani, S.I., Ashizawa, T. and Patel, P.I. (1998) *Am. J. Hum. Genet.*, **62**, 111–121.

Bradley, J.L., Blake, J.C., Chamberlain, S., Thomas, P.K. *et al.* (2000) *Hum. Mol. Genet.*, **9**, 275–282.

Campuzano, V., Montermini, L., Molto, M.D. *et al.* (1996) *Science*, **271**, 1423–1427.

Campuzano, V., Montermini, L., Lutz, Y., Cova, L. *et al.* (1997), *Hum. Mol. Genet.*, **6**, 1771–1780.

Cavadini, P., Gellera, C., Patel, P.I. and Isaya, G. (2000) *Hum. Mol. Genet.*, **9**, 2523–2530.

Chamberlain, S., Shaw, J., Rowland, A., Wallis, J., *et al.* (1988) *Nature*, **334**, 248–250.

Cho, S.-J., Lee, M.G., Yang, L.K., Lee, J.Y. *et al.* (2000) *Proc. Natl. Acad. Sci., USA*, **97**, 8932–8937.

Corbin, F., Bouillon, M. Fortin, A., Morin, S. *et al.* (1997) *Hum. Mol. Genet.*, **6**, 1465–1472.

Cossée, M., Dürr, A., Schmitt, M. *et al.* (1999) *Ann. Neurol.*, **45**, 200–206.

Cossée, M., Puccio, H., Gansmuller, A., Koutnikova, H. *et al.* (2000) *Hum. Mol. Genet.*, **9**, 1219–1226.

Cummings, C.J. and Zohgbi, H.Y. (2000) *Hum. Mol. Genet.*, **9**, 909–916.

Delatycki, M.B., Williamson, R. and Forrest, S.M. (2000) *J. Med. Genet.*, **37**, 1–8.

Dhe-Paganon, S., Shigeta, R., Chi, Y.-I., Ristow, M. and Shoelson, S.E. (2000) *J. Biol. Chem.*, **275**, 30753–30756.

Dürr, A. (2002) *Lancet Neurol.*, **1**, 370–374.

Dürr, A., Cossee, M., Agid, Y., Campuzano, V., *et al.* (1996) *N. Engl. J. Med.*, **335**, 1169–1175.

Epplen, C., Epplen, J.T., Frank, G., Miterski, B. *et al.* (1997) *Hum. Genet.*, **99**, 834–836.

Feng, Y., Absher, D., Eberhart, D.E., Brown, V. *et al.* (1997a) *Mol. Cell*, **1**, 109–118.

Feng, Y., Gutekunst, C.A., Eberhart, D.E., Yi, H. *et al.* (1997b) *J. Neurosci.*, **17**, 1539–1547.

Foury, F. and Cazzalini, O. (1997) *FEBS Lett.*, **411**, 373–377.

Foury, F. (1999) *FEBS Lett.*, **456**, 281–284.

Friedreich, N. (1863) *Virchow's Arch. Pathol. Anat.*, **26**, 391–419, 433–359.

Friedreich, N. (1863) *Virchow's Arch. Pathol. Anat.*, **27**, 1–26.

Gabus, C., Mazroui, R., Tremblay, S., Khandjian, E.W. and Darlix, J.L. (2004) *Nucleic Acids Res.*, **32**, 2129–2137.

Gerber, J., Mühlenhoff, U. and Lill, R. (2003) *EMBO Rep.*, **4**, 906–911.

Gibson, T.J., Koonin, E.V., Musco, G., Pastore, A. and Bork, P. (1996) *Trends Neurosci.*, **19**, 465–468.

Grabcyk, E. and Usdin, K. (2000) *Nucleic Acids Res.*, **28**, 2815–2822.

Hagerman, R.J. (1991) in *Fragile X syndrome: Diagnosis, treatment and research.* (eds. Hagerman, R.J. and Silverman, A.C.) John Hopkins University Press, Baltimore, 3–68.

Harding, A.E. (1981) *Brain*, **104**, 589–620.

Huynen, M.A., Snel, B., Bork, P. and Gibson, T.J. (2001) *Hum. Mol. Genet.*, **10**, 2463–2468.

Jin, P., Warren, S.T. and Warren, S. (2000) *Hum. Mol. Genet.*, **9**, 901–908.

Koutnikova, H., Campuzano, V., Foury, F., Dolle, P. *et al.* (1997) *Nat. Genet.*, **16**, 345–351.

Lesuisse, E., Santos, R., Matzanke, B.F., Knight, S.A. *et al.* (2003) *Hum. Mol. Genet.*, **12**, 879–889.

Lutz, T., Westermann, B., Neupert, W. and Herrmann, J.M. (2001) *J. Mol. Biol.*, **307**, 815–825.

Masino, L. and Pastore, A. (2001) *Brain Res. Bull.*, **56**, 183–189.

Mühlenhoff, U., Richhardt, N., Gerber, J. and Lill, R. (2002) *J. Biol. Chem.*, **277**, 29810–29816.

Musco, G., Stier, G., Kolmerer, B., Adinolfi, S. *et al.*, (2000) *Structure Fold. Des.*, **8**, 695–707.

Nichol, H., Gakh, O., O'Neill, H.A., Pickering, I.J. *et al.* (2003) *Biochem.*, **42**, 5971–5976.

Ohshima, K., Motermini, L., Wells, R.D. and Pandolfo, M. (1998) *J. Biol. Chem.*, **273**, 14588–14595.

Pandolfo, M. (1999) *Arch. Neurol.*, **104**, 1201–1208.

Park, S., Gakh, O., O'Neill, H.A., Mangravita, A. *et al.* (2003) *J. Biol. Chem.*, **278**, 31340–31351.

Pieretti, M., Zhang, F., Fu, Y.H., Warren, S.T. *et al.* (1991) *Cell*, **66**, 817–822.

Priller, J., Scherzer, C.R., Faber, P.W., MacDonald, M.E. and Young, A.B. (1997) *Ann. Neurol.*, **42**, 265–269.

Puccio, H., Simon, D., Cossee, M., Criqui-Filipe, P., *et al.* (2001) *Nature Genet.*, **27**, 181–186.

Ramazzotti, A., Vanmansart, V. and Foury, F. (2004) *FEBS Lett.*, **557**, 215–220.

Rötig, A., de Lonlay, P., Chretien, D., Foury, F. *et al.* (1997) *Nat. Genet.*, **17**, 215–217.

Sakamoto, N., Chastain, P.D., Parniewski, P. *et al.* (1999) *Mol. Cell*, **3**, 465–475.

Siomi, H., Siomi, M.C., Choi, M.C., Nussbaum, R.L. and Dreyfuss, G. (1993) *Cell*, **74**, 1193–1198.

Verkerk, A.J.M.H., Pieretti, M., Sutcliffe, J.S., Fu, Y.H. *et al.* (1991) *Cell*, **65**, 905–914.

Yoon, T. and Cowan, J.A. (2003) *J. Am. Chem. Soc.*, **125**, 6078–6084.

Yoon, T. and Cowan, J.A. (2004) *J. Biol. Chem.*, **279**, 25943–25946.

Zoghbi, H.Y. and Orr, H.T. (2000) *Annu. Rev. Neurosci.*, **23**, 217–247.

7

Creutzfeldt-Jakob and Other Prion Diseases

7.1 INTRODUCTION

There are a number of transmissible infectious degenerative diseases which affect the central nervous system of mammals, all of which are ultimately fatal. These take a long period of time to develop such that they were initially classified as being due to 'slow viruses'. It turned out subsequently that these disorders are characterized by the development within neurons of large vacuoles, which give the brain tissue a sponge-like microscopic appearance, hence the term transmissible spongiform encephalopathies (TSEs), now known as prion[1] diseases. They are all accompanied by motor dysfunction resulting in ataxia, dementia and death.

Among animal species (**Table 7.1**), they include scrapie in sheep and goats, BSE (bovine spongiform encephalopathy), often termed mad cow disease, in cattle, feline spongiform encephalopathy in zoological and domestic cats, chronic wasting disease in North American cervids (deer and elk), transmissible spongiform encephalopathy of zoological ruminants and non-human primates, and transmissible mink encephalopathy of farmed mink (Sigurdson and Miller, 2003). In humans three groups of TSEs have been identified (**Table 7.1**): those which are inherited (familial), those which arise spontaneously (sporadic), and those which are infectious. The first group concerns three rare, dominantly inherited human neurodegenerative disorders which have been traced to mutations in the prion protein (*PRNP*) gene (see section **7.2** below). They are familial Creutzfeldt-Jakob disease (fCJD), Gerstmann-Sträussler-Scheinker syndrome, and Fatal Familial Insomnia. In sporadic cases of TSEs (sCJDs), prions seem to occur spontaneously in the brain of the patients, by modes of transmission which are not understood. The infectious forms of CJD include iatrogenic CJD (iCJD), attributed to surgical procedures, which include cerebral contamination by instruments or dura mater grafts, and extracerebral transmission by injection of hormones extracted from infected humans (Brown et al., 2000); variant CJD (vCJD) and Kuru, both of which are described in section **7.3** below.

---

[1] Prion. The term was introduced by Stanley Prusiner in 1982 to define a proteinaceous infectious particle which lacks nucleic acid.

Table 7.1: Spectrum of prion diseases of humans and animals

Prion disease	Natural host species	Etiology
sCJD	Humans	Unknown (somatic *PRNP* mutation?)
Familial Creutzfeldt-Jakob disease (fCJD)	Humans	Familial (germ line *PRNP* mutation)
Iatrogenic Creutzfeldt-Jakob disease (iCJD)	Humans	Surgical procedures (infection)
vCJD	Humans	Ingestion of BSE-contaminated food; transfusion medicine (infection)
Kuru	Humans	Ingestion, ritualistic cannibalism (infection)
Fatal Familial Insomnia (FFI)	Humans	Familial (germ line *PRNP* mutation)
Gerstmann-Sträussler-Scheinker Syndrome	Humans	Familial (germ line *PRNP* mutation)
Scrapie	Sheep, goats	Infection, natural; mode of transmission unclear
Chronic Wasting Disease (CWD)	Deer, Elk	Infection; mode of transmission unclear
BSE	Cattle	Ingestion of BSE-contaminated feed (infection)
Transmissible mink encephalopathy	Mink	Ingestion (infection); Origin unclear
Feline spongiform encephalopathy	Cats	Iingestion of BSE-contaminated feed (infection)
Spongiform encephalopathy of zoo animals	Zoologic bovids, primates	Ingestion of BSE-contaminated feed (infection)

7.2 A BRIEF HISTORY OF PRION DISEASES

The first cases of Creutzfeldt-Jacob disease in humans were described by Creutzfeldt (1920) and Jakob (1921) over eighty years ago. Although scrapie was known as a fatal neurological disorder of sheep as early as the 1700s, its transmissibility was first demonstrated in 1939 (Cuille and Chelle, 1939). The disease gets its name because of the tendency for affected sheep to attempt to scrape off their wool by rubbing against fences. This is, in fact, a response to their ataxia, since leaning against the fence enables them to remain upright. The causative agent, which we now call prion, was extremely resistant, as was shown by a study in which 10% of a flock of Scottish sheep came down with scrapie after being vaccinated with a formaldehyde-treated sheep brain extract (Gordon, 1946). The similarity between the brain pathology of scrapie and the then recently discovered human disease Kuru, led to the suggestion that the two diseases might be related (Hadlow, 1959). An association between ritual cannibalism among the Fore natives of New Guinea and the Kuru epidemic had led to the suggestion that the disease could be orally transmitted (Gajdusek, 1977). Suspicions that the probable route of transmission was the ritual consumption of the brain of deceased tribal members, were essentially confirmed by the progressive disappearance of the Kuru epidemic after ritual cannibalism was abandoned by the late 1950s. This then served as the model for the BSE epidemic in cattle which emerged in the mid-eighties, leading to about 180,000 diagnosed cases. The outbreak was attributed to the feeding of BSE-prion-contaminated bone-and-meat to cattle (Kimberlin and Wilesmith, 1994). In the case of the recent CJD epidemic in Europe, it is thought that the vCJD resulted from the contamination of humans by the agent of BSE (Collinge et al., 1996; Bruce et al., 1997). The epidemic is thought to have arisen by the consumption of BSE-contaminated beef from the process of recycling contaminated carcasses to produce industrial feed for cattle (Prusiner, 1997). The BSE agent can experimentally infect mice, sheep, calves and non-human primates by the oral route, while scrapie in sheep is probably also transmitted by ingestion of the infectious agent (reviewed in Weissmann et al., 2002). In section **7.5**, we will discuss how prions can make their way from the digestive tract to the central nervous system.

The study of prion behaviour has been greatly facilitated by the discovery of prions in yeast and other fungi, which are genetically and biochemically more tractable for studies on the mechanism of conformation based inheritance and infection (reviewed in Uptain and Lindquist, 2002).

7.3 THE 'PRION' OR 'PROTEIN-ONLY' HYPOTHESIS AND CONFORMATION-BASED PRION INHERITANCE

Using mice as host it was shown that the infectious agent of scrapie was remarkably resistant to UV irradiation, even compared with small viruses and bacteriophages, suggesting that it was not a nucleic acid (Alper et al., 1967). In order to account for this observation, and more importantly, to reconcile it with the newly emerging central dogma[2] of molecular biology, Griffith (1967) suggested three mechanisms for the replication of a protein so that 'the occurrence of a protein agent would not necessarily be embarassing'. The second of these essentially suggested that an altered protein in an oligomer together with unaltered protein subunits could drive the conversion of the unaltered to the altered form; this is essentially the modern prion model for scrapie. The idea that a protein conformation can replicate itself, and in that sense, function as a genetic element, was formalized by the prion hypothesis.

This 'protein-only' hypothesis (Griffith, 1967) was refined, stating that mammalian TSEs are due to conformational changes in a normal host protein, and the term 'prion' was introduced (Prusiner, 1982, 1989). The prion is a conformational isoform of a normal host glycoprotein PrP^C (Basler et al.,1986; Oesch et al., 1985). PrP^C is normally attached to the outer leaflet of the plasma membrane via its C-terminal glycophosphatidylinositol (GPI) anchor (Stahl et al., 1990). The exact function of PrP^C remains unknown. While it is expressed in many non-neuronal tissues, it is abundant in the CNS, where it is particularly localized to synaptic membranes, suggestive of a role in synaptic transmission and neuronal excitability.

The primary structure of the prion protein is presented schematically in **Figure 7.1** (Milhavet and Lehmann, 2002). The first 22 amino acids form a signal peptide which is cleaved after translation into the endoplasmic reticulum, while the last 23 amino acids are also cleaved with the fixation of the GPI anchor on the serine residue at position 230. The two cysteine residues at positions 179 and 214 form a disulphide bridge, while there are two glycosylation sites at positions 182 and 198. In the amino-terminal region, a repeated sequence of five octapeptides is present, which can bind copper. In its fully mature form, PrP^C is a diglycosylated protein of 33-35kD localized and anchored through its GPI anchor

---

[2] The central dogma states that genetic information flows from DNA to RNA to protein.

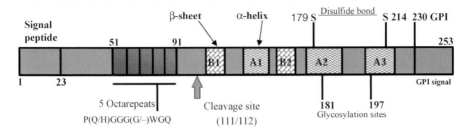

Figure 7.1: Primary structure of PrP^C (reprinted *Brain Research Reviews*, Vol 38, from Milhavet and Lehmann, Oxidative stress and the prior protein in transmissible spongiform encephalopathies, pp 328–339, Copyright 2002, with permission from Elsevier).

in specific regions of the plasma membrane, known as lipid rafts (often referred to as detergent-resistant membranes, or DRMs). These structures, rich in cholesterol, glyco-sphingolipids and acylated proteins, seem to be the target for delivery of PrP^C, β-amyloid peptide and the surface envelope glycoprotein gp120 of human immunodeficiency virus (HIV)-1, through a common sphingolipid-binding domain (Mahfoud et al., 2002). The protein is cleaved around residues 111–112 in the course of its normal metabolism.

The first evidence that a conformational change was involved in prion diseases was found during the purification of the infectious scrapie agent. A protease-resistant fragment copurified with infectivity (Bolton et al., 1982; Prusiner et al., 1982): subsequent cloning revealed that it was part of a larger 33-35kDa host glycoprotein, encoded by the *PRNP* gene (Prusiner et al., 1984; Oesch et al., 1985; Chesebro et al., 1985). This protein, PrP^{C},[3] is widely distributed in tissues, although its function is unknown, and is both soluble and highly sensitive to proteinase K digestion. In infected animals an insoluble form of PrP, designated PrP^{Sc}, is present and is found to accumulate in aggregates and plaques in the brain. Digestion with proteinase K cleaves only its first 66 amino-terminal residues leaving a fragment referred to as PrP$^{Sc27-30}$, with an apparent molecular weight of 27-30kD. No differences in primary structure of PrP^C and PrP^{Sc} were detected (Stahl et al., 1993), suggesting that they differ in conformation, as predicted by the prion hypothesis. More recently evidence has been found in human and animal TSEs for covalent modification of Lys and Arg residues in PrP^{Sc} with advanced glycosylation end products (Choi et al., 2004). Immunostaining studies indicate that, at least in clinically affected hamsters, astrocytes are the first site of this glycation process.

Extensive evidence now shows that PrP^C and PrP^{Sc} have distinctly different conforma-tions. The structures of human, hamster, bovine and mouse PrP^C have been solved by NMR, and are all very similar. They consist of a C-terminal globular domain consisting of predominantly α-helical protein folds, with a flexible, unstructured amino terminus compris-ing about 100 amino acid residues (**Figure 7.2**). The globular domain consists of three α-helices A, B and C, with a short two-stranded anti-parallel β-sheet (S1 and S2) made up of residues on the amino-terminal side of helix A and situated between, helix A and B, respectively. PrP^{Sc}, in contrast, is predominantly β-sheet as determined by Fourier transform IR spectroscopy (Pan et al., 1993) and is present in insoluble protease-resistant high molecular weight aggregates (**Figure 7.2**).

There is a considerable body of evidence which indicates that the progression of mammalian prion diseases involves a process in which the normal cellular PrP (PrP^C) is

---

[3] In the text the terms PrP^C and PrPS^C are used to designate the cellular prion protein and the disease-associated prion protein respectively, regardless of their origins.

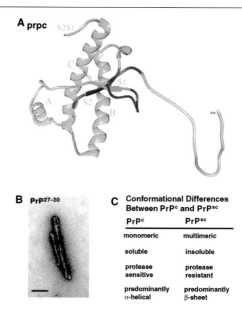

Figure 7.2: PrP^C and PrP^{Sc} are conformationally distinct. (A) Solution NMR structure of Syrian hamster PrP^C, residues 90–231. The structure is predominantly α-helical, with an unstructured amino terminus (from Liu et al., 1999). (B) Negatively stained EM image of Syrian hamster PrP$^{Sc27-30}$ stained with uranyl acetate. The material is in insoluble protease-resistant high molecular weight aggregates which are predominantly β-sheet. Scale bar is 100 nm. (C) Summary of differences between PrP^C and PrP^{Sc} (from Chien et al., reprinted, with permission, from the *Annual Review of Biochemistry*, Volume 73, Copyright 2004 by Annual Reviews, www.annualreviews.org).

converted into PrP^{Sc} through a post-translational process during which it acquires a high β-sheet content (reviewed in Prusiner, 1998). *In vivo*, PrP knock-out (*PRNP$^{0/0}$*) mice are completely protected against prion infection and fail to propagate prions (Büeler et al., 1993; Prusiner et al., 1993), and the introduction of murine *PRNP* transgenes into these mice restores susceptibility to prions (Fischer et al., 1996). This argues convincingly that conversion of the endogenous protein is required to develop the disease.

7.4 MECHANISM OF CONFORMATION-BASED PRION TRANSMISSION

7.4.1 Models of PrP^C to PrP^{Sc} Conversion

As we have outlined above, the propagation of prion diseases involves the conversion of the predominantly α-helical normal form of PrP into the prion form with its high β-sheet conformation. This initial event is then followed (**Figure 7.3**) by the spontaneous formation of a self-propagating aggregate. Finally, the newly formed prion must replicate itself in a process which involves two separate steps: growth of the infectious particle by addition of the aggregate and amplification of the number of infectious particles.

Two models have been proposed for the conversion of PrP^C to PrP^{Sc} which are illustrated in **Figure 7.4**. The "**Refolding**" or heterodimer model (Prusiner, 1991) proposes that the

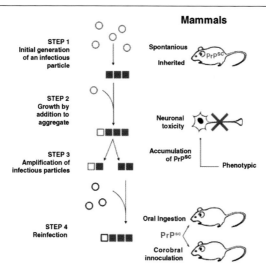

Figure 7.3: Steps in prion transmission. A general replication cycle for self-propagating conformationally based prion protein is shown on the left. The corresponding steps during prion infection in mammals are shown on the right (from Chien et al., reprinted, with permission, from the *Annual Review of Biochemistry*, Volume 73, Copyright 2004 by Annual Reviews, www.annualreviews.org).

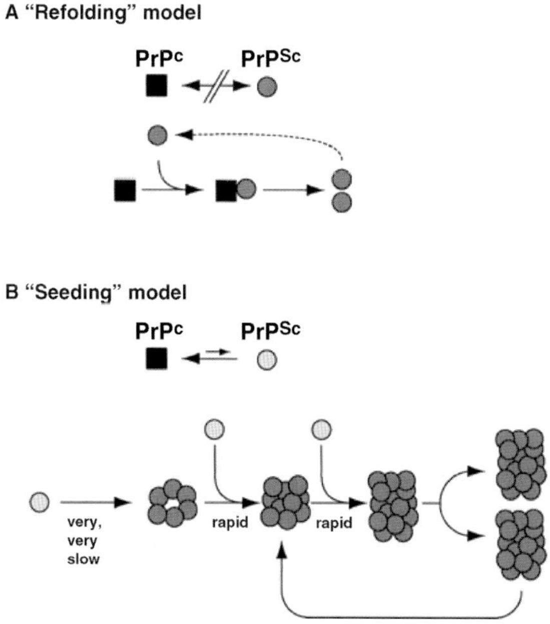

Figure 7.4: Models for the conversion of PrP^C to PrP^{Sc}. (**A**) The "**Refolding**" model; (**B**) the "**Seeding**" model (reprinted from Weissmann et al., *Proc Natl Acad Sci*, 99, pp 16378–16383, Copyright 2002, with permission from National Academy of Sciences, USA).

conformational change involving direct conversion of PrP^C to PrP^{Sc} is kinetically controlled, with a high activation energy barrier preventing spontaneous conversion at detectable rates. The interaction of PrP^C with exogenously introduced PrP^{Sc} causes PrP^C to undergo an induced conformational change to a partially unfolded form, which refolds to form PrP^{Sc}. It is possible that an enzyme or a chaperone could facilitate this reaction. The occurrence of certain mutations in PrP^C might result in spontaneous conversion to PrP^{Sc} which, albeit a rare event (occurring in about 1 in 10^6 individuals per year and late in life) could explain sporadic CJD.

In contrast, the "**Seeding**" or nucleation model (Jarret and Lansbury, 1993) postulates that PrP^C and PrP^{Sc} (or a PrP^{Sc}-like molecule, light coloured spheres) are in equilibrium, with the equilibrium largely in favour of PrP^C. PrP^{Sc} is only stable when it forms a multimer, hence PrP^{Sc} is stabilized when it adds onto a crystal-like seed or aggregate of PrP^{Sc} (dark spheres). Seed formation is an extremely rare event: however, once a seed is present, monomer addition ensues rapidly.

7.4.2 Formation of Prion Aggregates

A wide range of unrelated proteins, including PrP, or fragments of these proteins convert from their soluble forms to insoluble fibrils or plaques, which are known in their final form as amyloid[4]. Amyloids are associated with a wide number of protein misfolding diseases, including as we have seen in earlier chapters neurodegenerative diseases such as Alzheimer's, Parkinson's and Huntington's, as well as the prion diseases. They are also found in a number of systemic amyloidoses, characterized by peripheral deposition of a number of aggregated proteins such as lysozyme, transthyretin, immunoglobulin light chain and β2-microglobulin (Kelly, 1996). However, it has become apparent that amyloid can be formed from proteins which are not associated with any disease, such as acylphosphatase (Chiti et al., 1999) and the SH3 domain of PIP$_3$ kinase (Guijarro et al., 1998). That so many different polypeptides can form amyloid strongly supports the idea that this fold is generally accessible, perhaps because it is stabilized by hydrogen bonds between main chain residues (Dobson, 1999).

The β-sheets in amyloid fibres appear to be organized in a cross β-fold in which individual β strands are oriented perpendicular to the fibre axis, whereas β-sheets are oriented parallel to it (Sunde et al., 1997; Perutz et al., 2002; Wetzel, 2002). The repeating β-sheet structure allows hydrophobic dyes like Congo red to interact with the regularly spaced protein chains, which is commonly used to monitor amyloid formation *in vitro*. Reconstruction from electron micrographs of two-dimensional crystals of PrP^{Sc} from infectious preparations (Wille et al., 2002) and the determination of the crystal structure of a PrP dimer (Knaus et al., 2001) have led to structural proposals of how subunits might assemble into a fibre. Careful analysis of the fibrils grown from the SH3 domain of PIP$_3$ kinase by cryo-electron microscopy and image reconstruction techniques (Jimenez et al., 1999) show that the fibrils consist (**Figure 7.5A**) of four protofilaments containing specific segments of β-sheet, wound around each other in a helical array forming a hollow tube of diameter approximately 6 nm. The constraints of the cross-β-sheet structure (Wetzel, 2002) can be satisfied by multiple folds, such as the left-handed β-helix shown in **Figure 7.5B**. Amyloids can incorporate new protein to form fibres of defined diameter, but unlimited length. Although high-resolution structural studies of prion aggregates are difficult on account of their heterogeneity and insolubility, they are known to share many features with amyloids. Given the structural similarities between amyloid and prion aggregates, the

---

[4] We have defined amyloid earlier in Chapter 2.

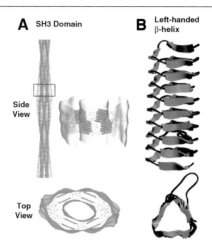

A SH3 Domain   **B** Left-handed β-helix

Side View

Top View

Figure 7.5: Two models for amyloid structure which both fulfil the requirements of the cross-β fold in which individual β strands are oriented perpendicular to the fibre axis, whereas β-sheets are oriented parallel to it. (**A**) Model from cryo-EM studies of amyloid formed by the SH3 domain of PIP_3 kinase (from Jimenez et al., 1999). (**B**) An example of a left-handed β-helix (from UDP-N-acetylglucosamine pyrophosphorylase of *Streptococcus pneumoniae*, which has been proposed to resemble PrP^{Sc} (from Wille et al., 2002). Figure from Chien et al., reprinted with permission from the *Annual Review of Biochemistry*, Volume 73, Copyright 2004 by Annual Reviews, www.annualreviews.org.

propagation of β-sheet-rich amyloid cores could provide the molecular mechanism involved in prion growth (Chien et al., 2004).

7.4.3 Steps in Prion Transmission

As was described above, the prion, a self-propagating aggregate, must form spontaneously. This is a step common to all of the amyloid diseases. In the next part of the process the prion must replicate itself. This involves two distinct steps, the growth of the infectious particle, by addition to the aggregate and amplification of the number of infectious particles (**Figure 7.3**). The first of these two steps results from recruitment and assembly of new protein onto the prion. Mutations can accelerate the rate of spontaneous aggregation, as can over-expression of the aggregation-prone protein. Likewise, exposure to environmental factors, such as pesticides, or to increased levels of metals, may also facilitate protein aggregation (Yamin et al., 2003; Uversky et al., 2002).

However, growth of the aggregate alone would not result in an increase in the number of infectious particles, only an increase in the mass of protein in the prion form. To explain the exponential increase of PrP^{Sc} during infection (**Figure 7.3**), aggregates must be continuously fragmented ('breakage' of aggregates), thereby generating increasing surface areas for further accretion (Orgel, 1996). It has been shown that shearing aggregates during the polymerization reaction increases the yield of protease-resistant material (Saborio et al., 2001; Lucassen et al., 2003). However, to date such material created *in vitro* has not been shown to cause *de novo* infection. Transmissible and non-transmissible aggregates may differ at the step of division. If the aggregates are too stable to release smaller units or to be degraded, they would never be able to amplify exponentially during infection. How this step of division is achieved *in vivo* by mammalian prions is not known, but in the case of the yeast prion [*PSI*⁺], division of prion aggregates appears to require the chaperone Hsp104p (Chernoff et al., 1995).

7.5 PATHWAYS OF PRION PATHOGENESIS

Infectious prion aggregates must be transmitted into a naïve host and reach a pool of substrate protein. Mammalian prions can be ingested orally, as we saw in section **7.2** in the case of BSE in cattle and vCJD and Kuru in humans. The pathway of prion pathogenesis can be broken down into spatially and temporally distinct phases, consisting initially of infection and peripheral replication, followed by transmigration of the infectious agent from the periphery to the CNS (often referred to as "neuroinvasion"), and finally the process of neurodegeneration (reviewed in Aguzzi et al., 2004).

7.5.1 Peripheral Replication

One important difference between patients with vCJD compared to those with sCJD is the presence of PrP^{Sc} and infectivity within lymphoid follicles (Wadsworth et al., 2001; Bruce et al., 2001); this is illustrated in **Figure 7.6** (Haïk et al., 2004). Indeed, the major criterion for pre-mortem diagnosis of vCJD is the demonstration of PrP^{Sc} in tonsil (Hill et al., 1999). It is now well established that peripheral replication of the prion agent occurs in lymphoid

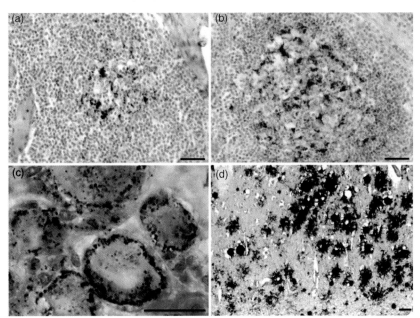

Figure 7.6: Distribution of PrP^{Sc} in patients with variant Creuzfeldt-Jakob disease (vCJD). Deposits of PrP^{Sc} within (**a**) germinal centres of a mesenteric lymph node, (**b**) the tonsil, and (**c**) noradrenergic neurons of the celiac ganglia. (**d**) Isocortical devastation with massive PrP^{Sc} accumulation. PrP^{Sc} deposits detected using a specific antibody, visible as a brown precipitate. Reprinted from *Trends in Molecular Medicine*, Vol 10, Haïk et al., Brain targeting through the autonomous nervous system: Lessons from prior disease, pp 109–112, Copyright 2004, with permission from Elsevier.

tissues such as spleen and lymph nodes, well before neuroinvasion and subsequent detection in the CNS (Aguzzi, 2003). Following an oral challenge, an early rise in prion infectivity is observed in the distal ileum of infected organisms. Prions must then make their way across the digestive tract and into the central nervous system (**Figure 7.7a**). It is likely that the relative resistance of prion protein to proteolytic digestion (Bolton et al., 1982) allows a significant amount of the infectious agent to survive its passage through the intestinal tract. M cells, which allow antigens and pathogens to cross the intestinal tract, are able to mediate the transport of prions (Heppner et al., 2001). When scrapie or BSE are administered to mice PrP^{Sc} first accumulates in gut-associated lymphoid tissue (mesenteric lymph nodes and Peyer's patches (Maignien et al., 1999)). One possible route for the infectious prions would be to penetrate the mucosa through M cells and reach Peyer's patches (**Figure 7.7b**), where they are found early on (Maignien et al., 1999), as well as in the enteric nervous system (Beekes and McBride, 2000). Immune cells appear to be crucially involved in the process of neuroinvasion following oral application. Mature follicular dendritic cells (FDCs) located in Peyer's patches, may play an important role in the transmission of scrapie from the gastrointestinal tract (Aguzzi, 2003; Prinz et al., 2003a). Other tissues of the lympho-reticular system, particularly the spleen but also lymph nodes (Prinz et al., 2002), are sites where prions replicate and accumulate. This is the case for scrapie and BSE in sheep, vCJD in man and experimental mouse scrapie, but not for BSE in cattle (Bradley, 1999). Myeloid dendritic cells are thought to mediate transport within the lymphoreticular system (LRS).

7.5.2 Transmigration from the Periphery to the CNS

Once prions have crossed the gut and reached associated lymphoid structures, the most logical route for them to reach the CNS is to proceed along the peripheral nervous system (PNS). Experimental studies using peripheral inoculation indicate that the time between prion replication in lymphoid structures and CNS neuroinvasion is consistent with propagation along this pathway (Kimberlin and Walker, 1986). The sympathetic system is one of the components of the PNS which innervates the gastrointestinal tract, associated lymph nodes and the spleen, and appeared from previous data, to be the most relevant for prion neuroinvasion (Glatzel et al., 2001). This view has been reinforced by recent data. In a transgenic mouse line, in which the distance between follicular dendritic cells and nerve ending is decreased, the neuro-immune transfer following an intraperitoneal challenge with scrapie is accelerated relative to control animals (Prinz et al., 2003b). The presence of PrP^{Sc} in noradrenergic neurons from celiac and stellate ganglia, two major components of the sympathetic system that enervate almost all parts of the gut and its lymphoid tissue, has been demonstrated in patients with vCJD (Haïk et al., 2004). No positive result was found in patients with sporadic CJD. These observations indicate that sympathetic neurons are involved in neuroinvasion in humans and also provide indirect evidence of oral prion uptake in vCJD (**Figure 7.7a**).

The precise way in which PrP^{Sc} transits between prion presenting follicular dendritic cells of the lymphoid system and sympathetic neurons is not known. It is, however, clear that the neuro-immunological junction constitutes the first step in a multisynaptic pathway which transports prions from the LRS and possibly from other sites. They proceed along the peripheral nervous system through sympathetic ganglia neurons, spinal cord and medulla

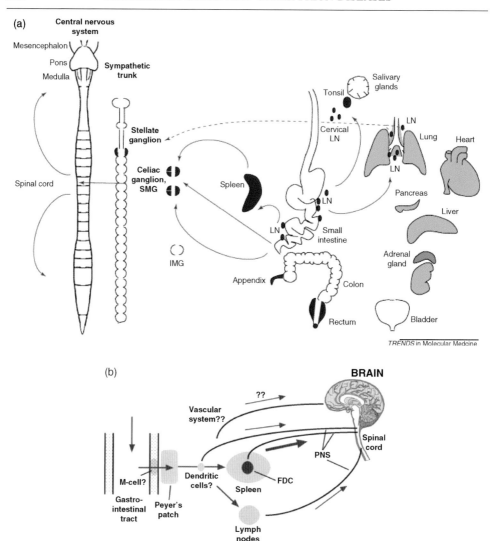

Figure 7.7: (**a**) Scheme of the route taken by prions through the sympathetic nervous system in patients with variant Creuzfeldt-Jakob disease (vCJD). Anatomic structures in red: structures in which PrP^{Sc} or infectivity could be detected. Anatomic strctures in green: structures in which PrP^{Sc} or infectivity was not found (results for adrenal gland were diverging). Unbroken lines: most likely route of prions. Broken line: possible but unlikely route of prions. Abbreviations: IMG inferior mesenteric ganglia; LN, cervical, madiastinal or mesenteric lymph nodes; SMG, superior mesenteric ganglia. Reprinted from *Trends in Molecular Medicine*, Vol 10, Haïk et al., Brain targeting through the autonomous nervous system: Lessons from prior disease, pp 109–112, Copyright 2004, with permission from Elsevier. (**b**) Possible routes of ingested prions. After oral intake, prions may penetrate the intestinal mucosa through M cells and reach Peyer's patches as well as the enteric nervous system. Prions may replicate in spleen and lymph nodes. Myeloid dendritic cells are thought to mediate transport within the lymphoreticular system (LRS). From the LRS and likely from other sites, prions proceed along the peripheral nervous system to finally reach the brain, either directly via the vagus nerve or via the spinal cord, under involvement of the sympathetic nervous system (reprinted from Weissmann et al., *Proc Natl Acad Sci*, 99, pp 16378–16383, Copyright 2002, with permission from National Academy of Sciences, USA).

neurons, and interneurons to finally reach the brain, either directly via the vagus nerve or via the spinal cord.

7.6 PRION-METAL INTERACTIONS

It has been well documented that the prion protein binds copper (II) ions and that, among divalent metal ions, PrP^C selectively binds Cu(II) (Stockel et al., 1998). The major copper(II)-binding site has been identified as being within the unstructured amino terminal region (encompassing residues 60–91 of human PrP^C). Specifically, copper binds to a highly conserved octapeptide repeat domain, consisting of four sequential repeats of the sequence ProHisGlyGlyGlyTrpGlyAsn (Hornshaw et al., 1995; Brown et al., 1997). The Cu(II) to octapeptide binding stoichiometry is 1:1, i.e. the octapeptide repeat region binds four Cu(II) ions (Hornshaw et al., 1995; Brown et al., 1997; Miura et al., 1999; Viles et al., 1999; Kramer et al., 2001; Garnett and Viles, 2003), and copper binding is most favoured at physiological pH, falling off sharply under mildly acidic conditions. While most studies of copper binding have focused on the octarepeat region, evidence has been found for a fifth preferential Cu(II) coordination site, between residues His96 and His111, outside of the octarepeat domain (Jones et al., 2004), with a nanomolar dissociation constant. Interestingly,

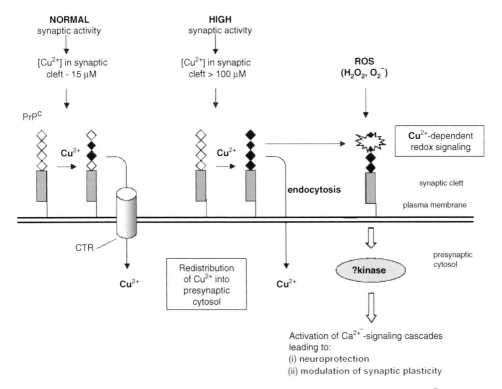

Figure 7.8: Schematic representation of the physiological role of prion proteins (PrP^C) in copper homeostasis and redox signaling. Open diamonds represent octarepeats; filled diamonds octarepeat bound to Cu(II) ion; CTR – copper transport proteins (reprinted from Vassallo and Herms, in copper homeostasis and redox signalling at the synapse, pp 538–544, *J Neurochem*, Vol 86, Copyright 2003, with permission from Blackwell Publishing Ltd).

circular dichroism studies show that copper coordination is associated with a loss of irregular structure and an increase in beta-sheet conformation.

Evidence is also growing that PrP^C plays an important role in copper homeostasis, in particular at the pre-synaptic membrane; that it may be involved in triggering intracellular calcium signals; and that it may play a neuroprotective role in response to copper and oxidative stress. Exposure of neuroblastoma cells to high Cu(II) concentrations (mM) stimulated endocytosis of PrP^C (Pauly and Harris, 1998), whereas deletion of the four octarepeats or mutation of the histidine residues in the central two repeats abolished endocytosis of PrP^C (Perera and Hooper, 2001). However, studies at physiological concentrations of copper, led to the conclusion that PrP^C does not participate in the uptake of extracellular Cu(II) (Rachidi et al., 2003). It has been suggested (**Figure 7.8**) that in the unique setting of the synapse, PrP^C acts to buffer Cu(II) levels in the synaptic cleft, following the release of copper ions as a result of synaptic vesicle fusion (Vassallo and Herms, 2003). Cu^{2+} ions released during neurotransmitter vesicle exocytosis are buffered by PrP^C, and subsequently returned to the pre-synaptic cytosol. This can occur either by transfer of copper to copper transport proteins (CTR) within the membrane, or in the case of higher copper concentrations, by PrP^C-mediated endocytosis. Copper-loaded PrP^C may interact with ROS, triggering redox signaling and subsequently activation of Ca^{2+}-dependent signalling cascades. These changes in intracellular Ca^{2+} levels lead to modulation of synaptic activity and to neuroprotection.

REFERENCES

Alper, T., Cramp, W.A., Haig, D.A. and Clarke, M.C. (1967) *Nature*, **214**, 764–766.

Aguzzi, A. (2003) *Adv. Immunol.*, **81**, 118–171.

Aguzzi, A., Heikenwalder, M. and Miele, G. (2004) *J. Clin. Invest.*, **114**, 153–160.

Basler, K., Oesch, B., Scott, M., Westaway, D. *et al.* (1986) *Cell*, **46**, 417–428.

Beekes, M. and McBride, P.A. (2000) *Neurosci. Lett.*, **278**, 181–184.

Bolton, D.C., McKinley, M.P. and Prusiner, S.B. (1982) *Science*, **218**, 1309–1311.

Bradley, R. (1999) *Dev. Biol.*, **99**, 35–40.

Brown, D.R., Qin, K., Herms, J.W., Madlung, A. *et al.* (1997) *Nature*, **390**, 684–687.

Brown, P., Preece, M., Brandel, J.P., Sato, T. *et al.* (2000) *Neurology*, **55**, 1075–1081.

Bruce, M.E., Will R.G., Ironside, J.W., McConnell, I. *et al.* (1997) *Nature*, **389**, 498–501.

Bruce, M.E., McConnell, I., Will R.G. and Ironside, J.W. (2001) *Lancet*, **358**, 208–209.

Büeler, H., Aguzzi, A., Sailer, A., Greiner, R.A. *et al.* (1993) *Cell*, **73**, 1339–1347.

Chernoff, Y.O., Lindquist, S.L., Ono, B., Inge-Vechtomov, S.G. and Liebman, S.W. (1995) *Science*, **268**, 880–884.

Chesebro, B., Race, R., Wehrly, K., Nishio, J. *et al.* (1985) *Nature*, **315**, 331–333.

Chien, P., Weissman, J.S. and De Pace, A.H. (2004) *Annu. Rev. Biochem.*, **73**, 617–656.

Chiti, F., Webster, P., Taddei, N., Clark, A. *et al.* (1999) *Proc. Natl. Acad. Sci. USA*, **96**, 3590–3594.

Choi, Y.G., Kim, J.I., Jeon, Y.C., Park, S.J. *et al.* (2004) *J. Biol. Chem.*, **279**, 30402–30409.

Collinge, J., Sidle, K.C., Meads, J., Ironside, J. and Hill, A.F. (1996) *Nature*, **383**, 685–690.

Creutzfeldt, H.G. (1920) *Zeitschr. gesamte Neurol. Psychiatr.*, **64**, 1–19.

Cuille, J. and Chelle, P.l. (1939) *C.R. Séances Acad. Sci.*, **208**, 1058–1060.

Dobson, C.M. (1999) *Trends Biochem. Sci.*, **24**, 329332.

Fischer, M., Rülicke, T., Raeber, A., Sailer, A. *et al.* (1996) *EMBO J.*, **15**, 1255–1264.

Gajdusek, D.C. (1977) *Science*, **197**, 943–960.

Garnett, A.P. and Viles, J.H. (2003) *J. Biol. Chem.*, **278**, 6795–6802.

Glatzel, M., Heppner, F.L., Albers, K.M. and Aguzzi, A. (2001) *Neuron*, **31**, 25–34.

Gordon, W.S. (1946) *Vet. Rec.*, **58**, 516–520.

Griffith, J.S. (1967) *Nature*, **215**, 1043–1044.

Guijarro, J.I., Sunde, M., Jones, M.A., Campbell, I.D. and Dobson, C.M. (1998) *Proc. Natl. Acad. Sci. USA*, **95**, 4224–4228.

Hadlow, W.J. (1959) *Lancet*, **2**, 289–290.

Haïk, S., Faucheux, B.A. and Hauw, J.-J. (2004) *TRENDS Molec. Med.*, **10**, 109–112.

Heppner, F.L., Christ, A.D., Klein, M.A., Prinz, M. *et al.* (2001) *Nat. Med.*, **7**, 976–977.

Hill, A.F. *et al.* (1999) *Lancet*, **353**, 183–189.

Hornshaw, M.P., McDermott, J.R. and Candy, J.M. (1995) *Biochem. Biophys. Res. Commun.*, **207**, 621–629.

Jakob, A. (1921) *Zeitschr. gesamte Neurol. Psychiatr.*, **57**, 147–228.

Jarrett, J.T. and Lansbury, P.J. (1993) *Cell*, **73**, 1055–1058.

Jimenez, J.L., Guijarro, J.I., Orlova, E., Zurdo, J. *et al.* (1999) *EMBO J.*, **18**, 815–821.

Jones, C.E., Abdelraheim, S.R., Brown, D.R. and Viles, J.H. (2004) *J. Biol. Chem.*, **279**, 32018–32027.

Kelly, J.W. (1996) *Curr. Opin. Struct. Biol.*, **6**, 11–17.

Kimberlin, R.H. and Walker, C.A. (1986) *J. Gen. Virol.*, **67**, 255–263.

Kimberlin, R.H. and Wilesmith, J.W. (1994) *Ann. N. Y. Acad. Sci.*, **724**, 210–220.

Knaus, K.J., Morillas, M.D., Swietnicki, W., Malone, M. *et al.* (2001) *Nat. Struct. Biol.*, **8**, 770–774.

Kramer, M.L., Kratzin, H.D., Schmidt, B., Romer, A. *et al.* (2001) *J. Biol. Chem.*, **276**, 16711–16719.

Liu, H., Farr-Jones, S., Ulyanov, N.B., Llinas, M., Marqusee, S. *et al.* (1999) *Biochemistry*, **38**, 5362–5377.

Lucassen; R., Nishina, K. and Supattapone, S. (2003) *Biochem.*, **42**, 4127–4135.

Mahfoud, R., Garmy, N., Maresca, M., Yahi, N. *et al.* (2002) *J. Biol. Chem.*, **277**, 11292–11296.

Maignien, T., Lasmezas, C.I., Beringue, V., Dormont, D. and Deslys, J.P. (1999) *J. Gen. Virol.*, **80**, 3035–3042.

Milhavet, O. and Lehmann, S. (2002) *Brain. Res. Rev.*, **38**, 328–339.

Miura, T., Hori, I.A., Mototani, H. and Takeuchi, H. (1999) *Biochem.*, **38**, 11560–11569.

Oesch, B., Westaway, D., Wälchi, M., McKinley, M.P. *et al.* (1985) *Cell*, **40**, 735–746.

Orgel, L.E. (1996) *Chem. Biol.*, **3**, 413–414.

Pan, K.M., Baldwin, M., Nguyen, J., Gasset, M. *et al.* (1993) *Proc. Natl. Acad. Sci. USA*, **90**, 10962–10966.

Pauly, P.C. and Harris, D.A. (1998) *J. Biol. Chem.*, **273**, 33107–33110.

Perera, W.S. and Hooper, N.M. (2001) *Curr. Biol.*, **11**, 519–523.

Perutz, M.F., Finch, J.T., Berriman, J. and Lesk, A. (2002) *Proc. Natl. Acad. Sci. USA*, **99**, 5591–5595.

Prinz, M., Montrasio, F., Klein, M.A., Schwartz, P. *et al.* (2002) *Proc. Natl. Acad. Sci. USA*, **99**, 919–924.

Prinz, M., Huber, G., Macpherson, A.J., Heppner, F.L. *et al.* (2003a) *Am. J. Pathol.*, **162**, 1103–1111.

Prinz, M., Heikenwalder, M., Junt, T., Schwarz, P. *et al.* (2003b) *Nature*, **425**, 957–962.

Prusiner, S.B. (1982) *Science*, **216**, 136–144.

Prusiner, S.B. (1989) *Annu. Rev. Microbiol.*, **43**, 345–374.

Prusiner, S.B. (1991) *Science*, **252**, 1515–1522.

Prusiner, S.B. (1997) *Science*, **278**, 245–251.

Prusiner, S.B. (1998) *Proc. Natl. Acad. Sci. USA*, **95**, 13363–13383.

Prusiner, S.B., Bolton, D.C., Groth, D.F., Bowman, K.A. *et al.* (1982) *Biochem.*, **21**, 6942–6950.

Prusiner, S.B., Groth, D.F., Bolton, D.C., Kent, M.P. and Hood, L.E. (1984) *Cell*, **38**, 127–134.

Prusiner, S.B., Groth, D.F., Serban, A., Koehler, R. *et al.* (1993) *Proc. Natl. Acad. Sci. USA*, **90**, 10608–10612.

Rachidi, W., Vilette, D., Guiraud, P., Arlotto, M. *et al.* (2003) *J. Biol. Chem.*, **278**, 9064–9072.

Saborio, G.P., Permanne, B. and Soto, C. (2001) *Nature*, **411**, 810–813.

Sigurdson, C.J. and Miller, M.W. (2003) *Br. Med Bull.*, **66**, 199–212.

Stahl, N., Borchelt, D.R. and Prusiner, S.B. (1990) *Biochem.*, **29**, 5405–5412.

Stahl, N., Baldwin, M.A., Teplow, D.B., Hood, L. *et al.* (1993) *Biochem.*, **32**, 1991–2002.

Stockel, J., Safar, J., Wallace, A.C., Cohen, F.E. and Prusiner, S.B. (1998) *Biochem.*, **37**, 7185–7193.

Sunde, M., Serpell, L.C., Bartlam, M., Fraser, P.E. *et al.* (1997) *J. Mol. Biol.*, **273**, 729–739.

Uptain, S.M. and Lindquist, S. (2002) *Annu. Rev. Microbiol.*, **56**, 703–741.

Uversky, V.N., Li, J., Bower, K. and Fink, A.L. (2002) *Neurotoxicology*, **23**, 527–536.

Vassallo, N. and Herms, J. (2003) *J. Neurochem.*, **86**, 538–544.

Viles, J.H., Cohen, F.E., Prusiner, S.B., Goodin, D.B. *et al.* (1999) *Proc. Natl. Acad. Sci. USA*, **96**, 2042–2047.

Wadsworth, J.D., Joiner, S., Hill, A.F., Campbell, T.A. *et al.* (2001) *Lancet*, **358**, 171–180.

Weissmann, C., Enari, M., Klöhn, P.-C., Rossi, D. and Flechsig, E. (2002) *Proc. Natl. Acad. Sci. USA*, **99**, 16378–16383.

Wetzel, R. (2002) *Structure*, **10**, 1031–1036.

Wille, H., Michelitsch, M.D., Guenebaut, V., Supattapone, S. *et al.* (2002) *Proc. Natl. Acad. Sci. USA*, **99**, 3563–3568.

Yamin, G., Glaser, C.B., Uversky, V.N. and Fink, A.L. (2003) *J. Biol. Chem.*, **278**, 27630–27635.

8
Amyotrophic Lateral Sclerosis

8.1 INTRODUCTION

Charcot described amyotrophic lateral sclerosis (ALS, also referred to as motor neurone disease or Lou Gehrig's disease[1]), a late onset, rapidly progressive neurological disorder, for the first time in 1874. ALS is one of the most common neurodegenerative disorders with an incidence of 4–6 per 100,000. The primary characteristic is the selective degeneration and death of upper (cortico-spinal) and lower (spinal) motor neurones. The disease typically initiates in mid adult life, and almost invariably progresses to paralysis and death. It is a particularly hideous disease, "in that preservation of cognitive function leaves the victim fully aware of the progressive muscle wasting and loss of motor function, culminating in death within 1–5 years of diagnosis" (Xiong and McNamara, 2002). Most instances have no apparent genetic linkage (sporadic ALS), but the disease is inherited in a dominant manner in the some 5–10% of cases (familial ALS, or FALS). A third form of ALS (Guamanian), is found with a high prevalence in the island of Guam and other Pacific countries.

8.2 MAJOR GENES INVOLVED IN ALS

The prevalence of ALS is estimated to be 4–6 per 100,000 of the population, increasing with age, to reach a peak in the age range 60–75 years of age, with a male preponderanceof 1.5:1. The importance of environmental risk factors in ALS is largely unknown, although it is clear that the endemic occurrence of ALS in specific regions of the South Pacific, where ALS accounts for about one in ten deaths cannot fully be explained by genetic factors. Attention has focused particularly on the fruit of the local cycad palms, described by the neurologist Oliver Sachs in his book 'Cycad Island' (Sacks, 1996): the pathogenic effect of the principal

---

[1] **Henry Louis Gehrig**, born **Ludwig Heinrich Gehrig** (June 19, 1903–June 2, 1941), was an American first baseman in Major League Baseball who played his entire career for the New York Yankees and was elected to the Baseball Hall of Fame in 1939. His career was prematurely ended by illness, and he retired from the sport later that year after learning he had amyotrophic sclerosis, a degenerative terminal diseases so rare that it first became widely known due to him, and is today widely known as "Lou Gherig's disease".

Metal-based Neurodegeneration: From Molecular Mechanisms to Therapeutic Strategies   R. R. Crichton and R. J. Ward
© 2006 John Wiley & Sons, Ltd

Table 8.1   Genetics of amyotrophic lateral sclerosis (ALS). From Majoor-Krakauer et al. (2003), reproduced by permission of Blackwell Publishing Ltd

Classification	Gene	Localization	Inheritance
ALS1	*SOD-1*	21q22	AD/AR
ALS2	*ALSin*	2q33-34	AR
ALS3		Unknown	AD
ALS4		9q34	AD
ALS5		15q12-21	AR
ALS6		18q21	AD
FTDP	*TAu*	17q	AD
FTD		9q21-22	AD
Neurofilament heavy chain	*NF-H*	22q12.2	
Neurofilament light chain	*NF-L*	8p21	
Peripherin	*PRPH*	12q12-13	
Glutamate transporter	*EAAT2*	11p13-12	
Glutamate receptor	*AMPA*	5p33	
Apolipoprotein E	*ApoE*	19q13.2	
Ciliairy neurotrophic factor	*CNTF*	11q12.2	
Debrisoquine hydroxylase	*CYP2D*	22q13.1	
Apurinic apyrimidinic endonuclease	*APEX*	14q11-12	
Mitochondrial DNA	*COX*		
Manganese superoxide dismutase	*SOD-2*	6q25	
P2 blood group	*P2*	22q11	

toxin, cycasin, seems to be mediated by damage to neuronal DNA, up-regulation of Tau mRNA expression and enhancement of excitatory neurotoxicity (Esclaire et al., 1999).

Genetic risk factors for ALS have been extensively studied, and although they only represent 10% of all ALS, molecular genetic analysis of familial ALS (FALS), a clinically and genetically heterogeneous form of ALS, has led to the discovery of several genes involved in FALS (**Table 8.1**). Seven genetic loci have been reported, and three major genes have been identified (*SOD-1, AlSin* and *Tau*). A number of other genes, called 'suscept-ibility' genes, may trigger the neurodegenerative cascade, or act as susceptibility factors together with environmental or other risk factors for ALS, and they include genes with clearly defined biochemical functions (**Table 8.1**). A first class of genes that may play a role in the development of ALS, associated with the abnormal accumulation of intermediate filaments within affected motor neurons, are genes involved in neurofilament formation (both heavy and light chains of neurofilaments and peripherin, another intermediate filament found in degenerating motor neurons of patients with ALS). A second group involves excitotoxicity genes. Excitotoxicity is a phenomenon associated with excessive or prolonged activation of excitatory amino acid receptors (notably glutamate), which results in damage and eventually death of the neurons expressing these receptors. Indeed, riluzole, an antiglutamate drug, is to date the only drug shown to provide some therapeutic effect in ALS. There are a number of other candidate genes, indicated in **Table 8.1**, which appear to be involved in predisposition to expression of the ALS phenotype.

The first ALS gene (ALS1) was mapped to chromosome 21q (Siddique et al., 1991) and two years later it was shown to be the *SOD-1* gene (Rosen et al., 1993). We will discuss the possible mechanisms whereby mutations in the *SOD-1* gene, which encodes copper-zinc superoxide dismutase may cause neurodegeneration later. Mutations in SOD-1 account for some 21% of dominant FALS, while around 12% of apparently sporadic ALS patients are also heterozygous for mutations in SOD-1 (reviewed in Majoor-Krakauer et al., 2003).

Mutations in a gene (ALS2) with linkage to chromosome 2q33-34 are associated with autosomal recessive FALS. The ALS2 gene has been designated *alsin*: alternative splicing of this gene and deletions in both transcripts results in the ALS2 phenotype. The mouse orthologue is found in neuronal cells throughout the brain and spinal cord, and the protein is thought to be a regulator/activator of GTPases, perhaps involved in the modulation of microtubule assembly, membrane organization and trafficking in neurons.

ALS can also be part of a multisystem neurodegeneration, including the Tauopathies and the combination of ALS with dementia and parkinsonism. Mutations in the *tau* gene are associated with a wide range of clinical phenotypes, and one particular class of mutations in Tau protein were recognized in a syndrome termed frontotemporal dementia and parkinsonism complex (Wilhelmsen et al., 1994; Hutton et al., 1998), which is now classed as a form of ALS. The mutations involve alternative splicing of exon 10 of the *tau* gene.

8.3 SUPEROXIDE DISMUTASE AND ALS

Superoxide dismutase 1 is a ubiquitous dimeric metalloenzyme localized in the cytosol, with a high expression in nervous tissue, liver and erythrocytes, which catalyses the dismutation of two molecules of superoxide anion into hydrogen peroxide and oxygen (**Figure 8.1**). It contains one atom of Zn^{2+} and one atom of redox-active copper in its catalytic site

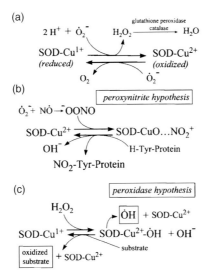

Figure 8.1: SOD-1 chemistry. (**a**) The chemistry of superoxide dismutation by SOD-1 involving two asymmetric steps. (**b**) Protein nitration from peroxynitrite. (**c**) Hydroxyl radical formation from hydrogen peroxide. Reprinted from *Neuron*, Vol 24, Cleveland, From charcot to SOD1: mechanisms of selective motor neuron death in ALS, pp 515–520, Copyright 1999, with permission from Elsevier.

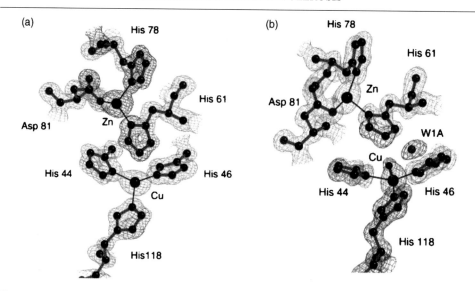

Figure 8.2: The structure of the copper and zinc sites in monomers A (**a**) and B (**b**) of fully reduced bovine superoxide dismutase at a resolution of 0.115 nm. In both subunits Cu (I) is bound to three nitrogen atoms from His 44, His 46 and His 118 in a distorted trigonal planar geometry. In subunit B, a low (10%) occupancy copper ion has been modelled in a position consistent with Cu(II) (shown as smaller purple sphere). Reprinted from *Structure*, Vol 11, Hough and Hasnain, structue of fully reduced bovine copper zinc superoxide dismutase at 1.15A, pp 937–946, Copyright 2003, with permission from Elsevier.

(**Figure 8.2**) and its structure consists of an eight-stranded β-barrel, with three extended loops. More than 100 point mutations (Bendotti and Carri, 2004) have been found in families with FALS (**Figure 8.3**), most of them autosomal dominant, although those causing the substitutions D90A and N86S are recessive. The mutations are distributed among all five

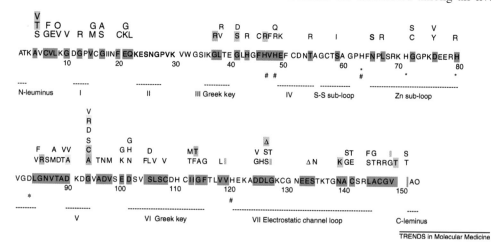

Figure 8.3: Mutations of superoxide dismutase 1 (SOD-1) observed in patients with familial amyotrophic lateral sclerosis. Mutations are indicated above the wild type sequence. Copper-binding residues are indicated by #, zinc-binding residues by *. The vertical arrow indicates a point where an insertion has been observed in some patients; Δ indicates a deletion; ST indicates stop codon generating a truncated protein. Reprinted from *Trends in Molecular Medicine*, Vol 10, Bendotti and Carri, Lessons from models of SOD1-linked familial ALS, pp 393–400, Copyright 2004, with permission from Elsevier.

exons of the gene and are scattered throughout the protein structure, some in the copper and zinc sites, others in the dimer interface, within β-strands, or in connecting loops. It is widely accepted that these mutations exert their toxic effects by a gain-of function mechanism, and one of the most attractive hypotheses is that the mutant proteins have the propensity to form insoluble aggregates. This is supported by the demonstration that mutant SOD-1 can form amyloid-like fibrillary structures (Elam et al., 2003). The Ala4Val (A4V) mutant of SOD-1 is the most common mutation found to date, accounting for about 50% of SOD-1-linked FALS cases (Cudkowicz et al., 1997), and is associated with a particularly rapid rate of disease progression, resulting in death within an average of 1.2 years after onset of symptoms (Rosen et al., 1994). The Ile113Thr mutant of SOD-1 is less frequent, but is characterized by the observation of massive neurofilament aggregation in affected motor neurons (Kokubo et al., 1999). The structures of these two mutant enzymes have been recently determined (Hough et al., 2004), and while both proteins retain the same subunit fold and geometry of the active site as the wild type enzyme (**Figure 8.4**), they are twisted in a corkscrew fashion

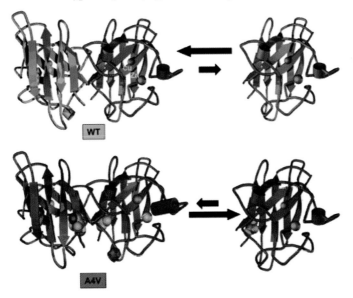

Figure 8.4: The wild type (WT) and A4V SOD-1 dimers differ slightly at the dimer interface. Ribbon diagrams of WT (upper) and A4V (lower) (Hough et al., 2004). Dimers are depicted as being in equilibrium with a structured monomer which, in the absence of the other subunit, is likely to unfold partially or completely. The WT dimer is much more stable than the AV4 dimer (Ray et al., 2004). From Ray and Lansbury, *Proc Natl Acad Sci USA* 101, 2, pp 5701–5702, Copyright 2004, reproduced with permission of National Academy of Sciences, USA.

relative to each other, consistent with destabilization of the dimer interface. A number of studies indicate that dissociation of the dimer of SOD-1 into the monomeric form could be the key intermediate in the pathway that leads to formation of aggregates as indicated in **Figure 8.5** (Ray and Lansbury, 2004). Copper-catalysed oxidation of either mutant or wild type SOD-1 causes the enzyme to dissociate to monomers prior to the formation of aggregates (Rakhit et al., 2004), and copper-induced oxidation of metal-depleted SOD causes its aggregation into pore-like structures (Chung et al., 2003). The metal content of some FALS SOD-1 is very low (Hayward et al., 2002) and zinc-deficient SOD-1 is known to aggregate upon oxidation (Rakhit et al., 2002). A covalently linked variant of A4V SOD-1 in

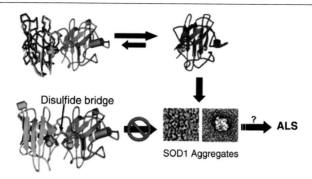

Disulfide bridge

SOD1 Aggregates

? ALS

Figure 8.5: SOD-1 dimer dissociation may be the first step in ALS pathogenesis. (*Upper*) A4V dimer (left subunit shows overlay of WT and A4V backbones) dissociation is the first step in SOD-1 aggregation (an electron microscopy image of A4V aggregates including pore-like and large spherical structures formed *in vitro* is shown. It is proposed that SOD-1 aggregates initiate motor neuron death and ALS. (*Lower Left*) The disulphide-bonded variant of A4V (perspective is different from A4V dimer at top in order to show the disulphide bond) does not aggregate. From Ray and Lansbury, *Proc Natl Acad Sci USA* 101, 1, pp 5701–5702, Copyright 2004, reproduced with permission of National Academy of Sciences, USA.

which an intersubunit disulphide bond had been engineered across the A4V dimer interface (**Figure 8.5**) formed a stable disulphide-linked dimer, which did not aggregate *in vitro* (Ray et al., 2004). Thus, a drug molecule that was able to stabilize the SOD-1 dimer, could be a useful tool in delaying the onset and slowing the progression of FALS.

8.4 CONTRIBUTORS TO DISEASE MECHANISMS IN ALS

Four principal causes have been advanced to explain motor neuron death in ALS (Cleveland, 1999): (i) oxidative damage, prompted by the discovery that mutations in superoxide dismutase are associated with the disease, and that aberrant copper-mediated chemistry could be responsible; (ii) axonal strangulation, supported by the massive conglomeration of neurofilaments found in motor neurons as a hallmark of disease pathology; (iii) toxicity arising from intracellular protein aggregates and/or a failure of protein folding; (iv) repetitive motor neuron firing resulting in excitotoxic death if glutamate release is not handled properly at the dendrites of upper or lower motor neurons. These arguments have been further developed in a recent review (Bruijn et al., 2004).

8.4.1 Oxidative Damage

The first of these, namely that aberrant copper-mediated oxidative damage, either through nitrogen free radicals (peroxynitrite) or peroxide-derived ROS (hydroxyl radical), causes the disease (**Figure 8.1B, C**), does not hold up, for several reasons. SOD-1 mutants lacking the copper-coordinating histidines still cause progressive motor neuron disease (Wang et al., 2003). No increased levels of nitration products in proteins are observed in ALS patients (Bruijn et al., 1997), nor in neurofilaments isolated from transgenic mice expressing SOD-1 mutations (Williamson et al., 2000). Since NO is essential for peroxynitrite formation, one would expect alterations in NO synthesis to alter the course of the disease, if peroxynitrite were involved. However, reduction of either neuronal nitric oxide synthase (nNOS) (Dawson, 2000) or of inducible NOS (iNOS) in astrocytes and microglia (Son et al., 2001) did not affect disease progression. While increases in hydroxyl radicals have been measured in some transgenic SOD-1 mice models, they have not been found in others. Although copper acquisition by SOD-1 in yeast requires CCS, a specific copper chaperone (Culotta et al., 1997), elimination of CCS in mutant SOD-1 mice, while significantly lowering copper loading into mutant SOD-1, did not affect onset or progression of motor neuron disease (Subramaniam et al., 2002). A final hypothesis was that copper might contribute to toxicity through aberrant chemistry of copper bound to sites on the surface of SOD-1 subunits (Bush, 2002). While this cannot be formally excluded, given that the average pool of free copper is only a fraction of a copper atom per cell (Rae et al., 1999), the source of such copper is hard to envisage.

8.4.2 Neurofilament Disorganization

Neurofilament proteins are synthesized in the cell body of neurons and then assembled and transported into the axons, where they influence proper axonal diameters, transport along the axons and nerve conduction velocities. Both affected familial and sporadic ALS patients and transgenic mice expressing the SOD-1 mutation accumulate neurofilaments in the perikarya and axons of motor neurons (reviewed in Julien, 2001). Neurofilaments, like other components of the cytoskeleton, are continually renewed and require transport from the cell body, where they are synthesized, into and through the axon. These large neurofilaments are normally transported by microtubule-based anterograde transport at a rate an order of magnitude slower than the rate of transport of organelles. Of the five major types of intermediate filament proteins expressed in mature neurons, four, namely the three neurofilament proteins, NF-H, NF-M and NF-L and the intermediate protein, peripherin, are found in the majority of axonal inclusions of motor neurons of ALS patients (Corbo and Hays, 1992). Mutations in the NF-H genes have been identified in sporadic ALS and a dominant mutation in NF-L has been found to be a primary cause of the motor neuropathy Charcot-Marie-Tooth disease, type II (reviewed in Bruijn et al., 2004).

8.4.3 Intracellular Protein Aggregates

As in many other neurodegenerative diseases, intracellular cytoplasmic inclusions of abnormal protein aggregates are found in motor neurons, and in some cases within the astrocytes surrounding them, in mouse models of SOD-1-mediated disease and in all reported instances of human ALS (Bruijn et al., 1998). Whether these aggregates damage neurons remains unknown, although several possible toxicities of protein aggregates have been proposed (**Figure 8.6**). These include aberrant chemistry; loss of protein function through co-aggregation; depletion of chaperones required for protein folding (such as the heat shock protein Hsp-70); loss of correct functioning of the proteosome, overwhelmed with misfolded proteins; and inhibition of specific cell organelles, including mitochondria and peroxisomes, through aggregation on or within such organelles. That the ubiquitin-proteasome system is involved is underlined by the finding that the aggregates are highly immunoreactive with antibodies to ubiquitin. Dorfin, an E3 ubiquitin ligase, can ubiquitinate mutant superoxide dismutase 1, and prevents mutant SOD-1-mediated neurotoxicity (Niwa

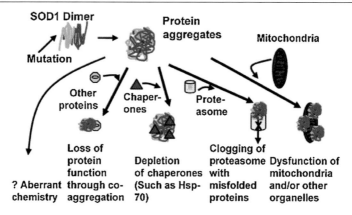

Figure 8.6: Putative toxicities of protein aggregates. Reprinted with permission from Bruijn et al., from the *Annual Review of Neuroscicence*; Volume 27, © 2004 by Annual Reviews, www.annualreviews.org.

Parkin and Dorfin Have Four Blocks of Conserved Sequences

[1]	*parkin*	SSVLPGDSVGLAVILHTDSRKDSPPAGSPAGRS
	dorfin	SSVDDGSA--------TRSHAGGSSSGLPEGKS
	consensus 1	* * * * . : * *: ....:* * *:*

[2]	*parkin*	EREPQSLTRVDLS
	dorfin	ESKPSKFRHNSGS
	consensus 2	* :*..: : . *

[3]	*parkin*	EQARWEAASKET
	dorfin	SATKW---SKEA
	consensus 3	. : :* ***:

[4]	*parkin*	HGFPVEVDSD
	dorfin	EGNSMEVQVD
	consensus 4	.* .:**: *

Symbols
* identical
: strongly conserved
. weakly conserved

Figure 8.7: Sequence alignment between parkin and dorfin. Reprinted from *Neuroscience Research*, Vol 44, Gearhart et al., Identification of brain proteins that interact with 2-methylnorharman: An analog of the Parkinsonian-inducing toxic, MPP+, pp 255–265, Copyright 2002, with permission of Elsevier.

et al., 2002). It is located in ubiquitinated inclusions (UBIs) in various neurodegenerative disorders, including both familial and sporadic ALS and Parkinson's disease (Hishikawa et al., 2003), where it localizes to Lewy bodies and ubiquitinates synphilin-1 (Ito et al., 2003). Dorfin has sequence homology with parkin (**Figure 8.7**), and interacts with an analogue of the parkinsonian-inducing toxin MPP^+ (Gearhart et al., 2002).

Aggregates could also affect the function of chaperones in protein folding as the co-immunoprecipitation of Hsp-70, Hsp-40 and $\alpha\beta$-crystallin with mutant SOD-1 confirms (Shinder et al., 2001). Up-regulation of the protein chaperone Hsp-70 preserves the viability of cells expressing toxic SOD-1 mutants (Bruening et al., 1999).

8.4.4 Activation of Caspases

In order to understand the molecular basis for the selective vulnerability of motor neurons in ALS it is important to identify the key mediators of programmed cell death which affect motor, but not other, neurons. Using a preparation of cultured embryonic motor neurons, a novel Fas signaling pathway has been identified which requires NO for cytotoxicity, and seems to be specific to motor neurons (Raoul et al., 2002). Fas-triggered apoptosis of these normal embryonic motor neurons requires transcriptional up-regulation of neuronal NOS (nNOS), and is abolished by nNOS inhibitors. Motor neurons from transgenic mice expressing the SOD-1 mutant genes show increased susceptibility to activation of this pathway and were more sensitive to Fas- or NO-triggered cell death. Since (Chapter 2) Fas-triggered apoptosis involves the external pathway, activation of the motor neuron-restricted cell death pathway by neighbouring cells could contribute to motor neuron loss in ALS. Whether Fas activation is important in the survival of adult motor neurons in ALS remains to be established.

8.4.5 Mitochondrial Damage

The evidence that mitochondria are important targets for damage common to SOD-1 mutants remains controversial. The presence of what appear to be vacuolated mitochondrial remnants in spinal motor neurons from lines of mice with mutant SOD-1 was not confirmed in other rodent models (reviewed in Bruijn et al., 2004).

8.4.6 Excitotocity and Decreased Glutamate Uptake by Astroglia

Neuronal cell death has been associated for a long time with excitotoxicity mediated by glutamate, either from excessive firing of the neurons and/or elevation of intracellular calcium, via calcium-permeable glutamate receptors. Glutamate is normally actively cleared from the synapse of motor neurons by the glial glutamate transporter EAAT2 (Rothstein et al., 1996; Tanaka et al., 1997), but increased levels of glutamate in cerebrospinal fluid of ALS patients (Rothstein et al., 1990; Rothstein et al., 1991; Shaw et al., 1995) together with a pronounced loss of astroglial EAAT2 protein (Rothstein et al., 1995) in affected brain regions, led to the recognition that abnormal glutamate handling was possibly involved in ALS. By lowering EAAT2 levels with an antisense oligonucleotide it was shown that loss of transport activity directly causes neuronal death (Rothstein et al., 1996). A patient with sporadic ALS was found to have a mutation in a putative glycosylation site in EAAT2, which resulted in aberrant transfer to the membrane, and decreased glutamate uptake (Trotti et al., 2001). Finally, in human autopsy specimens, the intracellular calcium binding proteins calbindin-D28k and parvalbumin were absent in motoneuron populations lost early in ALS (i.e., cortical and spinal motoneurons, lower cranial nerve motoneurons), while motoneurons damaged late or infrequently in the disease (i.e., Onuf's nucleus motoneurons, oculomotor, trochlear, and abducens nerve neurons) expressed markedly higher levels of immunoreactive calbindin-D28K and/or parvalbumin (Alexianu et al., 1994; Ince et al., 1993).

Excitotoxicity is also an important factor in common between sporadic and SOD-1 mutant-mediated ALS, since it has been shown that SOD-1 mutant animal models show a selective focal loss (**Figure 8.8**) of EAAT3 from the astrocytes within the region of the spinal cord containing the motor neuron cell bodies (Howland et al., 2002). It seems therefore that glutamate excitotoxicity is an important contributor to motor neuron death in ALS, which is reflected by the fact that the only FDA-approved drug therapy in ALS, Riluzole, acts by decreasing glutamate toxicity.

nontransgenic   SOD1^{G931} end stage

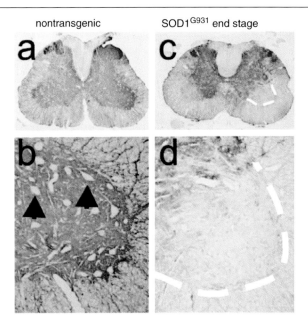

Figure 8.8: Excitotoxicity in ALS. Selective loss of the glial glutamate transporter EAAT2 during disease within an ALS-linked SOD-1 mutant. (**a**) Nearly ubiquitous expression (*brown*) of the glutamate transporter EAAT2 in the gray matter of the spinal cord in nontransgenic animals. (**b**) Higher magnification view, showing EAAT2 staining surrounding the motor neurons (*arrows*). (**c–d**) Striking loss of EAAT2 staining in the anterior horn of end-stage SOD-1^{G93A} rats. Reprinted from Howland et al., Focal loss of the glutamate transporter EAAT2 in a transgenic rate model of SOD1, pp 1604–1609, Vol 99, *PNAS*, Copyright 2002 with permission of National Academy of Sciences, USA.

8.5 OTHER PATHWAYS THAT MAY CAUSE DAMAGE TO MOTOR NEURONS

Motor neurons of the brain and spinal cord have extremely long axons – up to one metre long in adult humans. This means that active axonal transport, which is dependent on micro-tubules, is essential for normal cellular function. Axonal transport involves the anterograde transport of organelles and neurofilaments synthesized in the cell body into the extended axon. Then via fast (in the case of organelles) and slow (for neurofilaments) processes components move toward the synapse. There is also fast retrograde transport of multi-vesicular bodies and trophic factors, like nerve growth factor, back to the cell body. SOD-1 mutants impair slow axonal travel months prior to disease onset (Williamson et al., 1998), which led to the conclusion that there was a correlation between development of motor neuron disease and diminished axonal transport.

The cytoplasmic protein dynein plays an important role in many cellular processes, including positioning the endoplasmic reticulum and the Golgi apparatus, as well as in assembly of the mitotic spindle. In neurons, it is the only known motor for retrograde transport (Paschal and Vallee, 1987; Hirokawa, 1990). Dynein has also been proposed to be a participant in slow anterograde transport of neurofilaments together with the associated multiprotein complex dynactin (Shah et al., 2000; Wang et al., 2000). Two mis-sense point mutations in dynein cause a progressive motor neuron disease in mice (Hafezparast et al., 2003), accompanied by the formation of inclusion bodies. Disruption of the dynein/dynactin complex inhibits retrograde axonal transport in motor neurons and causes late-onset progressive degeneration (LaMonte et al., 2002).

The role of microglia in ALS is unclear. In regions of motor neuron loss in ALS, microglia are activated and proliferate (Kawamata et al., 1992; Ince et al., 1996). The expression of proinflammatory mediators, such as TNF-α, interleukin-1B and cyclooxygenase 2, is an early event in SOD-1 mutant mouse models, while both minocycline, an antibiotic which blocks microglial activation, and celecoxib, an inhibitor of COX-2, slow the disease in animal models (reviewed in Bruijn et al., 2004): both are currently in human clinical trials.

The targeted deletion of the hypoxia response element in the vascular endothelial cell growth factor (VEGF) gene in mice results in normal baseline levels of VEGF, but a decreased ability to induce VEGF in response to hypoxia. The mice developed motor neuron deficits, with all the classic features of ALS (Oosthuyse et al., 2001). In a large population study mutations in the VEGF gene were found: subjects homozygous with mutations in the VEGF promoter/leader sequence had a 1.8 times greater risk of ALS (Lambrechts et al., 2003). These findings indicate that VEGF is a modifier of motor neuron degeneration in human ALS and indicate the therapeutic potential of VEGF for stressed motor neurons in mice. Further studies to establish the potential role of VEGF in motor neuron survival are under way. Whether other neurotrophic factors might be important in ALS is not clear, although human trials with neurotrophic factors have been disappointing, perhaps because the factors have not been delivered effectively to the target neurons. Although chronic delivery of molecules to the central nervous system has proven difficult, it was recently found that adeno-associated virus can be retrogradely transported efficiently from muscle to motor neurons of the spinal cord. Using this approach it was shown that insulin-like growth factor 1 prolongs life and delays disease progression in a SOD-1 mouse model, even when delivered at the time of overt disease symptoms (Kaspar et al., 2003).

8.6 CONCLUSIONS

As we have seen the different possibilities that might be involved in ALS are many (**Figure 8.9**). However, it may be that the selective killing of motor neurons results from the convergence of a series of factors, rather from a single factor (**Figure 8.9**). In the SOD-1

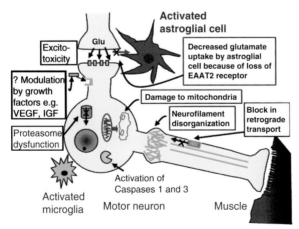

Figure 8.9: Convergence of multiple pathways that may damage the motor neuron. From Bruijn et al., reprinted, with permission, from the *Annual Review of Neuroscience*, Volume 27, © 2004 by Annual Reviews www.annualreviews.org.

familial ALS the disease is the consequence of acquired toxicity of mutant SOD-1 rather than loss of function. The toxic property affects neurons and glia, and in neurons it probably disrupts protein breakdown by the ubiquitin-proteasome system, affects slow anterograde transport, fast retrograde axonal transport, calcium homeostasis, mitochondrial function and the maintenance of cytoskeletal architecture. While aggregates are clearly present it is impossible to determine whether they are protective or pathogenic. There is certainly concurrent damage to astrocytes and microglia, and the loss of glutamate transporters in the astroglial cells is the likely cause of excitotoxic stress to the already damaged motor neurons. Inflammatory cytokines produced by the activation of microglia may contribute to the death of the motor neurons, ultimately the victim of the caspase executioner caspase-3.

However, we would do well to remember that SOD-1 mutations only account for 2% of ALS, and our understanding of the nature of the toxicity in the sporadic and non-SOD-1 familial forms of ALS remains relatively limited. It seems likely that these forms of ALS also result from the convergence of a number of factors, some of them similar to those described above. However, there are probably genetic and also environmental factors. With regard to the latter, we mentioned the clusters of ALS in the Guamanian form of ALS, and more recently the importance of environmental factors has been underlined by the recognition of a twofold increased risk of ALS in veterans of the Gulf war (Haley, 2003; Horner et al., 2003).

REFERENCES

Alexianu, M.E., Ho, B.K., Mohamed, A.H. La Bella, V. *et al.* (1994) *Ann. Neurol.*, **36**, 846–858.

Bendotti, C. and Carri, M.T. (2004) *TRENDS Molec. Med.*, **10**, 393–400.

Bruening, W., Roy, J., Giasson, B., Figlewicz, D.A. *et al.* (1999) *J. Neurochem.*, **72**, 693–699.

Bruijn, L.I., Beal, M.F., Beecher, M.W., Schultz, J.B. *et al.* (1997) *Proc. Natl. Acad. Sci. USA*, **94**, 7606–7611.

Bruijn, L.I., Houseweart, M.K., Kato, S., Anderson, K.L. *et al.* (1998) *Science*, **281**, 1851–1854.

Bruijn, L.I., Miller, T.M. and Cleveland, D.W. (2004) *Annu. Rev. Neurosci.*, **27**, 723–749.

Bush, A.I. (2002) *Nat. Neurosci.*, **5**, 919.

Chung, J., Yang, H., de Beus, M.D., Ryu, C.Y. *et al.* (2003) *Biochem. Biophys. Res. Commun.*, **312**, 873–876.

Cleveland, D.W. (1999) *Neuron*, **24**, 515–520.

Corbo, M. and Hays, A.P. (1992) *J. Neuropathol. Exp. Neurol.*, **51**, 531–537.

Cudkowicz, M.E., McKenna-Jasek, D., Sapp, P.E., Chin, W. *et al.* (1997) *Ann. Neurol.*, **41**, 210–221.

Culotta, V.C., Klomp, L.W., Strain, J., Casareno, R.L. *et al.* (1997) *J. Biol. Chem.*, **272**, 23469–23472.

Dawson, T.M. (2000) *Cell*, **101**, 115–118.

Elam, J.S., Taylor, A.B., Strange, R., Antonyuk, S. *et al.* (2003) *Nat. Struct. Biol.*, **10**, 461–467.

Esclaire, F., Kisby, G.E., Spencer, P., Milne, J. *et al.* (1999) *Exp. Neurol.*, **155**, 11–21.

Gearhart, D.A., Toole, P.F. and Warren Beach, J. (2002) *Neurosci. Res.*, **44**, 255–265.

Hafezparast, M., Klocke, R., Ruhrberg, C., Marquardt, A. *et al.* (2003) *Science*, **300**, 808–812.

Haley, R.W. (2003) *Neurology*, **61**, 750–756.

Hayward, L.J., Rodriguez, J.A., Kim, J.W., Tiwari, A. *et al.* (2002) *J. Biol. Chem.*, **277**, 15923–15931.

Hirokawa, N., Sato-Yoshitake, R., Yoshida, T. and Kawashima, T. (1990) *J. Cell Biol.*, **111**, 1027–1037.

Hishikawa, N., Niwa, J., Doyu, M., Ito, T. *et al.* (2003) *Am. J. Pathol.*, **163**, 609–619.

Horner, R.D., Kamins, F.G., Feussner, J.R., Grambow, S.C. *et al.* (2003) *Neurology*, **61**, 742–749.

Hough, M.A., Grossmann, J.G., Antonyuk, S.V., Strange, R.W. *et al.* (2004) *Proc. Natl. Acad. Sci. USA*, **101**, 5976–5981.

Hough, M.A. and Hasnain, S.S. (2003) *Structure*, **11**, 937–946.

Howland, D.S., Liu, J., She, Y., Goad, B. *et al.* (2002) *Proc. Natl. Acad. Sci. USA*, **99**, 1604–1609.

Hutton, M., Lendon, C.L., Rizzu, P. *et al.* (1998) *Nature*, **393**, 702–705.

Ince, P.G., Shaw, P.J., Slade, J.Y., Jones, C. and Hudgson, P. (1996) *Acta Neuropathol. (Berlin)*, **92**, 395–403.

Ince, P., Stout, N., Shaw, P.J., Slade, J.Y. *et al.* (1993) *Neuropathol. Appl. Neurobiol.*, **19**, 291–299.

Ito, T., Niwa, J., Hishikawa, N., Ishigaki, S. *et al.* (2003) *J. Biol. Chem.*, **278**, 29106–29114.

Julien, J.P. (2001) *Cell*, **104**, 581–591.

Kaspar, B.K., Llado, J., Sherkat, N., Rothstein, J.D. and Gage, F.H. (2003) *Science*, **301**, 839–842.

Kawamata, T., Akiyama, H., Yamada, T. and McGeer, P.L. (1992) *Am. J. Pathol.*, **140**, 691–707.

Kokubo, Y., Kuzuhara, S., Narita, Y., Kikugawa, K. *et al.* (1999) *Arch. Neurol.*, **56**, 1506–1508.

LaMonte, B.H., Wallace, K.E., Holloway, B.A., Shelly, S.S. *et al.* (2002) *Neuron*, **34**, 715–727.

Lambrechts, D., Storkebaum, E., Morimoto, M., Del-Favero, J. *et al.* (2003) *Nat. Genet.*, **34**, 383–394.

Majoor-Krakauer, D., Willems, P.J. and Hofmann, A. (2003) *Clin. Genet.*, **63**, 83–101.

Niwa, J., Ishigaki, S., Hishikawa, N., Yamamoto, M. *et al.* (2002) *J. Biol. Chem.*, **277**, 36793–36798.

Oosthuyse, B., Moons, L., Storkebaum, E., Beck, H. *et al.* (2001) *Nat. Genet.*, **28**, 131–138.

Paschal, B.M. and Vallee, R.B. (1987) *Nature*, **330**, 181–183.

Pasinelli, P., Houseweart, M.K., Brown, R.H. Jr. and Cleveland, D.W. (2000) *Proc. Natl. Acad. Sci. USA*, **97**, 13901–13906.

Rae, T.D., Schmidt, P.J., Pufahl, R.A., Culotta, V.C. and O'Halloran, T.V. (1999) *Science*, **284**, 805–808.

Rakhit, R., Cunningham, P., Furtos-Matei, A., Dahan, S. *et al.* (2002) *J. Biol. Chem.*, **277**, 147551–47556.

Rakhit, R., Crow, J.P., Lepock,. J.R., Kondejewski, L.H. *et al.* (2004) *J. Biol. Chem.*, **279**, 15499–15504.

Raoul, C., Estevez, A.G., Nishimune, H., Cleveland, D.W. *et al.* (2002) *Neuron*, **35**, 1067–1083.

Ray, S.S. and Lansbury, P.T., Jr. (2004) *Proc. Natl. Acad. Sci. USA*, **101**, 5701–5702.

Ray; S.S., Nowak, R.J., Strokovich, K., Brown, R.H., Jr. *et al.* (2004) *Biochem.*, **43**, 4899–4905.

Rosen, D.R., Siddique, T., Patterson, D., Figlewicz, D.A. *et al.* (1993) *Nature*, **362**, 59–62.

Rosen, D.R., Bowling, A.C., Patterson, D., Usdin, T.B. *et al.* (1994) *Hum. Mol. Genet.*, **3**, 981–987.

Rothstein, J.D., Dykes-Hoberg, M., Pardo, C.A., Bristol, L.A. *et al.* (1996) *Neuron*, **16**, 675–686.

Rothstein, J.D., Kuncl, R., Chaudry, V., Clawson, L. *et al.* (1991) *Ann. Neurol.*, **30**, 224–225.

Rothstein, J.D., Tsai, G., Kuncl, R.W., Clawson, L. *et al.* (1990) *Ann. Neurol.*, **28**, 18–25.

Rothstein, J.D., Van Kammen, M., Levey, A.I., Martin, L.J. *et al.* (1995) *Ann. Neurol.*, **38**, 73–84.

Sacks, O. (1996) '*The Island of the Color-Blind*' and '*Cycad Island*', Picador, London.

Shah, J.V., Flanagan, L.A., Janmey, P.A. and Leterrier, J.F. (2000) *Biol. Cell.*, **11**, 3495–3508.

Shaw, P.J., Forrest, V., Ince, P.G., Richardson, J.P. and Wastell, H.J. (1995) *Neurodegeneration*, **4**, 209–216.

Shinder, G.A., Lacourse, M.C., Minotti, S. and Durham, H.D. (2001) *J. Biol.Chem.*, **276**, 12791–12796.

Siddique, G., Figlewitz, D.A., Pericak-Vance, M.A. *et al.* (1991) *New Eng. J. Med.*, **324**, 1381–1384.

Son, M., Fathallah-Shayk, H.M. and Elliott, J.L. (2001) *Ann. Neurol.*, **50**, 273.

Subramaniam, J.R., Lyons, W.E., Liu, J., Bartnikas, T.B. *et al.* (2002) *Nat. Neurosci.*, **5**, 301–307.

Tanaka, K., Watase, K., Manabe, T., Yamada, K. *et al.* (1997) *Science*, **276**, 1699–1702.

Trotti, D., Aoki, M., Pasinelli, P., Berger, U.V. *et al.* (2001) *J. Biol. Chem.*, **276**, 576–582.

Vukosavic, S., Stefanis, L., Jackson-Lewis, V., Guegan, C. *et al.* (2000) *J. Neurosci.*, **20**, 9119–9125.

Wang, L., Ho, C., Sun, D., Liem, R.K.H. and Brown, A. (2000) *Nat. Cell Biol.*, **2**, 137–141.

Wang, J., Slunt, H., Gonzales, V., Fromholt, D. *et al.* (2003) *Hum. Mol. Genet.*, **12**, 2753–2764.

Wilhelmsen, K.C., Lynch, T., Pavlou, E., Higgins, M. and Nygaard, T.G. (1994) *Am. J. Hum. Genet.*, **55**, 1159–1165.

Williamson, T.L., Bruijn, L.I., Zhu, Q., Anderson, K.L. *et al.* (1998) *Proc. Natl. Acad. Sci. USA*, **95**, 9631–9636.

Williamson, T.L., Corson, L.B., Huang, L., Burlingame, A. *et al.* (2000) *Science*, **288**, 399.

Xiong, Z.-Q. and McNamara, J.O. (2002) *Neuron*, **35**, 1011–1013.

9
Other Neurological Diseases

9.1 INTRODUCTION

In addition to the major neurodegenerative diseases which we have discussed in the previous chapters, there are of course a large number of others where the metal/oxidative stress connection probably also plays an important role. We discuss these below, in no particular order, beginning with aceruloplasminaemia, a disease which links iron with copper; Wilson's disease and Menkes disease, both caused by defective copper transporting ATPases; neuroferritinopathy, caused by a mutation in the ferritin light chain; the Hallervorden-Spatz syndrome (pantothenate kinase associated neurodegeneration); multiple sclerosis, an auto-immune disease resulting in demyelination in the central nervous system; HIV-associated dementia, a progressive encephalopathy observed in AIDS patients.

9.2 ACERULOPLASMINAEMIA

As was pointed out earlier (Chapter 1) ceruloplasmin is thought to play an important role as a ferroxidase, as Frieden demonstrated (Osaki et al., 1996), and together with the detailed nutritional studies by Cartwright on copper-deficient pigs (Lee et al., 1968), this suggested an important role for ceruloplasmin in iron metabolism – bringing together Mars and Venus (Crichton and Pierre, 2001).[1] That ceruloplasmin did indeed play an essential role in iron metabolism was established unequivocally in 1995 with the identification of patients with aceruloplasminaemia (Harris et al., 1995; Yoshida et al., 1995). Ceruloplasmin, as was pointed out earlier, is a member of the multicopper oxidase family of enzymes (**Figure 9.1**), which is synthesized in liver, the major source of serum ceruloplasmin, but also in other tissues, including spleen, lung, testis and brain. Within the CNS, ceruloplasmin is expressed in populations of glial cells associated with brain microvasculature surrounding dopaminergic melanin-containing neurons in the substantia nigra and within the inner cortex of the retina (Klomp and Gitlin, 1993). In astrocytes and Sertoli cells, ceruloplasmin is synthesized as a glycophosphatidylinositol (GPI)-anchored protein, suggestive of a role in oxidation and

---

[1] Mars, the powerful Roman god of war, and Venus, the goddess of love and beauty, were associated by the early alchemists respectively with the metals iron and copper.

Metal-based Neurodegeneration: From Molecular Mechanisms to Therapeutic Strategies   R. R. Crichton and R. J. Ward
© 2006 John Wiley & Sons, Ltd

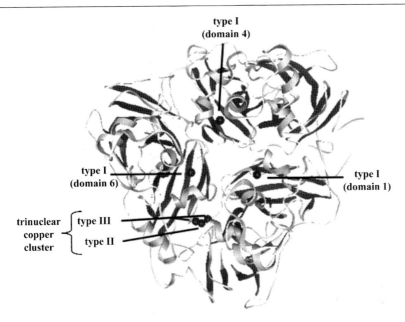

type I
(domain 4)

type I
(domain 6)   type I
                                                                   (domain 1)

trinuclear ⎡ type III
copper   ⎨
cluster   ⎣ type II

Figure 9.1: Structural model of human ceruloplasmin based on X-ray crystallographic data (Zaitseva et al., 1996). The type I, II and III coppers are indicated, as well as the site of the trinuclear copper cluster. From Hellman and Gatlin, reprinted, with permission, from the *Annual Review of Nutrition*, Volume 22, © 2002 by Annual Reviews, www.annualreviews.org.

mobilization of iron at the blood-brain and blood-testis barriers (reviewed in Hellman and Gitlin, 2002).

The first case of aceruloplasminaemia was reported in 1987 when Miyajima and colleagues reported on a 52 year old Japanese woman with diabetes, retinal degeneration and basal ganglia symptoms, associated with a total lack of serum ceruloplasmin (Miyajima et al., 1987). Since then, a number of mutations in the ceruloplasmin gene have been identified in affected patients and family members (reviewed in Hellman and Gitlin, 2002). Patients with aceruloplasminaemia usually present in their 40s or 50s with a classic triad of neurologic symptoms, including dementia, dysarthria and dystonia[2], a history of insulin-dependent diabetes, and retinal degeneration, all reflecting iron accumulation in most parenchymal tissues, including the basal ganglia in the brain (a 10-fold increase, with iron accumulation in both neurons and microglia). While serum ferritin is elevated, reflecting significant hepatic iron accumulation, liver function tests are normal.

In order to understand the disease mechanism in aceruloplasminaemia, we need to examine current thinking on the role of ceruloplasmin in the iron cycle (**Figure 9.2**). Within the reticuloendothelial system of macrophages, effete red blood cells are captured by phagocytosis, and the iron derived from haem oxygenase-dependent degradation of haem is returned to the plasma via the membrane transporter IREG1 (also known as ferroportin). Ceruloplasmin plays an essential role in determining the rate of iron efflux from the macrophages through its ferroxidase activity, oxidizing Fe^{2+} prior to its incorporation into apotransferrin.

---

[2] Dystonia is a movement disorder which is characterized by abnormal muscle tone.

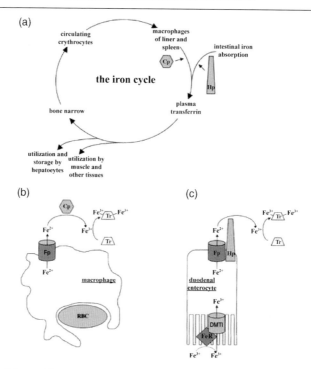

Figure 9.2: Role of the multicopper oxidases in the iron cycle. (**a**) The iron cycle depicting movement between storage and utilization sites. (**b**) In the reticuloendothelial system (macrophage) iron derived from haem is returned to the plasma via the membrane transporter ferroportin (Fp). Ceruloplasmin (Cp) plays an essential role in determining the rate of iron efflux via oxidation, which is required for binding to transferrin (Tf). (**c**) Iron absorption in the gut enterocyte requires the apical membrane reductase (FeR) and the divalent metal transporter-1 (DMT1) as well as the basolateral transporter Fp and the ceruloplasmin homologue hephaestin (Hp). From Hellman and Gitlin, reprinted, with permission, from the *Annual Review of Nutrition*, Volume 22, © 2002 by Annual Reviews www.annualreviews.org.

This is consistent with the clinical findings in aceruloplasminaemia, namely that iron accumulates in parenchymal tissues because ceruloplasmin is necessary for iron efflux, although this view had been considered to be controversial because of studies in cultured cells which suggested that ceruloplasmin promotes cellular iron uptake (Attieh et al., 1999). The unequivocal role of ceruloplasmin in cellular iron efflux has already been indicated by the early studies of the Utah group, who showed that administration of ceruloplasmin to copper-deficient pigs resulted in the rapid release of iron into the circulation, detectable in circulating transferrin (Lee et al., 1968; Roeser et al., 1970). This view is further reinforced by the finding that administration of ceruloplasmin to patients with aceruloplasminaemia results in a rapid increase in serum iron (Logan et al., 1994; Yonekawa et al., 1999), and that administration of a soluble form of the yeast homologue of ceruloplasmin restores iron homeostasis in aceruloplasminaemic mice (Harris et al., 2004).

The increase in brain iron observed in aceruloplasminaemia does not result from increased levels of plasma iron, since accumulation of brain iron is not found in other condition such as atransferrinaemia or haemochromatosis. Since ceruloplasmin does not cross the blood-brain barrier, this means that the ceruloplasmin which is synthesized and secreted by astrocytes must be directly involved in brain iron homeostasis. The mechanisms of neurodegeneration in aceruloplasminaemia are not well established. It is presumed that an iron cycle (**Figure 9.2a**) similar to, but separate from, that occurring in the systemic circulation, is functional in the brain. In the absence of ceruloplasmin, the excessive accumulation of iron within the central nervous system might result in either glial cell injury or direct oxidative damage to neurons. Consistent with this latter idea, affected patients have increased levels of lipid peroxidation and defective fatty acid oxidation (reviewed in Hellman and Gitlin, 2002). The role of iron accumulation in pathogenesis is supported by the finding that neurologic symptoms are improved by therapy with the iron chelator desferrioxamine (Miyajima et al., 1997).

9.3 WILSON'S AND MENKES DISEASES

In 1912, Samuel Alexander Kinnier Wilson, a young London registrar, described his observations on the disease to which he unwittingly gave his name – progressive lenticular degradation, a familial nervous disease associated with cirrhosis of the liver (Wilson, 1912). The demonstration of large amounts of copper in the brain and liver of affected individuals (Cummings, 1948) was quickly followed by the demonstration that ceruloplasmin was deficient in the serum of patients with the disease (Scheinberg and Gitlin, 1952), and a simple and effective treatment became available with the introduction of penicillamine as an oral copper chelator (Walshe, 1956).

Wilson's disease is a chronic disease of brain and liver with progressive neurological dysfunction, due to a disturbance of copper metabolism, with progressive accumulation of copper in the brain, liver, kidneys, and cornea. It is characterized by progressive degeneration of the basal ganglia of the brain, a brownish ring (Kayser-Fleischer ring) at the outer margin of the cornea caused by deposition of copper in the Descemet membrane, cirrhosis of the liver, splenomegaly, tremor, muscular rigidity, involuntary movements, spastic contractures, psychic disturbances, and progressive weakness and emaciation.

Wilson's disease is inherited as an autosomal recessive disorder with the affected gene located on chromosome 13. The gene locus encodes a copper-transporting P-type ATPase which is highly conserved in evolution and permits the efficient excretion of copper into the bile (reviewed in Gitlin, 2003). The hepatocytes play the key role in copper homeostasis, both as a storage site (mostly in metallothionein) and as the determinant which regulates biliary excretion, the only physiological route for copper excretion. This means that under steady state conditions the amount of copper excreted in the bile is directly proportional to the size of the hepatic copper pool, thus ensuring that hepatic copper overload occurs only rarely.

As we saw in Chapter 1, copper is transported across the hepatocyte basolateral membrane by the membrane transporter protein Ctr1 (**Figure 9.3**), transferring its copper to a family of copper chaperone proteins. The copper chaperone Atox1 is essential for transport of copper to the hepatocyte secretory pathway through its interaction with the Wilson's disease P-type ATPase, ATP7b (**Figure 9.4**). ATP7b is predominantly located in the trans-Golgi network and its function is to transfer copper into the secretory pathway both for excretion in the bile and for incorporation into ceruloplasmin. In Wilson's disease, lack of functional ATP7b results in secretion of the rapidly degraded apoceruloplasmin: a diagnostic hallmark of the disease is the decreased serum levels of ceruloplasmin. When the hepatocyte copper content increases, ATP7b cycles to a cytoplasmic compartment near the bile canicular membrane, where copper is accumulated in vesicles prior to its biliary excretion.

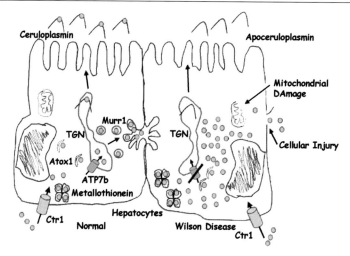

Figure 9.3: Illustration of the proteins and pathways critical for hepatocyte copper metabolism. The Wilson's disease ATPase, ATP7b, transports copper into the trans-Golgi network (TGN) and late secretory pathway. In Wilson's disease, inherited loss-of-function mutations in the gene encoding ATP7b result in cytosolic copper accumulation with associated cellular injury. Reprinted from *Gastroenterology*, Vol 125(6), Gitlin, Wilson's disease, pp 1868–1877, Copyright 2003, with permission from the American Gastroenterological Association.

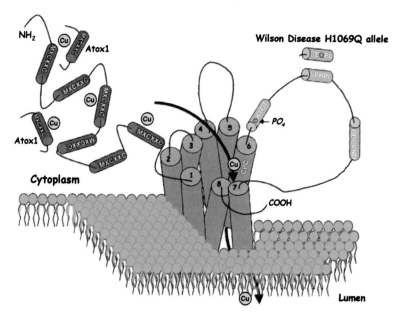

Figure 9.4: Structural model of the Wilson's disease copper-transporting ATPase, ATP7b, illustrating adenosine triphosphate (ATP)-dependent copper transport across the lipid bilayer. Highlighted are the MXCXXC copper-binding regions, the DKTGT-containing site of the aspartyl phosphate, the GDGVND ATP-binding site, and the CPC copper-binding region in the 6th transmembrane domain. The site of the most common mis-sense mutation (H1069Q) within the SEHPL sequence is also shown. Reprinted from *Gastroenterology*, Vol 125(6), Gitlin, Wilson's disease, Copyright 2003, with permission from the American Gastroenterological Association.

While the precise mechanisms of vesicular copper excretion at the canicular membrane is not known, it has recently been shown that the small, ubiquitously expressed protein Murr1 is required for this process (**Figure 9.3**). Murr1 is the product of the gene defective in canine copper toxicosis, an autosomal recessive disease characterized by massive lysosomal copper accumulation in the livers of affected dogs, and defective in biliary copper excretion (van de Sluis et al., 2002; Klomp et al., 2003). It was subsequently established that Murr1 interacts directly with ATP7b and that the interaction is mediated by the copper-binding amino terminus of ATP7b (Tao et al., 2003). Interestingly, it has recently been found that the inhibitor of apoptosis XIAP is involved in the control of intracellular copper homeostasis through regulation of Murr1 (Burstein et al., 2004).

ATP7b has many of the characteristic features of P-type ATPases, including the invariant aspartate residue which is phosphorylated in the course of ATP-dependent copper transport across the lipid bilayer (**Figure 9.4**). The six copper-binding MXCXXC motifs in the amino terminus of ATP7b are also the sites of Atox1 interaction. Copper transport involves transfer of the copper from these amino terminal sites to a high affinity copper site in the transmembrane channel and requires ATP binding and aspartate phosphorylation (Lutsenko and Petris, 2003). More than 200 distinct mutations have been found in the ATP7b gene in patients with Wilson's disease, most of them in transmembrane domains or other well defined motifs, such as the H1069Q mis-sense mutation within the highly conserved SEHPL motif in the cytoplasmic loop between the fifth and sixth transmembrane domains, which is the most common disease allele in Northern European populations. The analysis of patient mutations has established specific abnormalities in ATP7b copper transport, subcellular localization, copper-induced trafficking and interaction with Atox1. The loss of ATP7b function impairs incorporation of copper into ceruloplasmin and of biliary copper excretion, and results in copper-mediated oxidative damage, activation of cell death pathways, leakage of copper into the plasma and finally copper overload in most tissues (Sokol, 1996; Strand et al., 1998). However, the widespread copper accumulation is most probably due to loss of hepatic ATP7b function, since it is reversed after liver transplantation in affected patients (Schilsky, 2002).

In marked contrast (**Figure 9.5**) to the excessive accumulation of toxic copper in Wilson's disease, the disease described by John Menkes in 1962 is an X-chromosome-linked fatal neurodegenerative disorder of childhood characterized by massive copper deficiency (Menkes et al., 1962). The boys affected generally die in early childhood, usually in their first decade, with multiple abnormalities which can all be related to deficiencies in copper-containing enzymes. The lack of hair pigmentation is due to deficiency of tyrosinase, required for melanin synthesis. The connective tissue abnormalities, including aortic aneurisms, loose skin and fragile bones, result from decreased activity of lysyl oxidase, required for the maturation of collagen and elastase. The severe neurological defects are attributed to reduced activity of cytochrome c oxidase, the terminal enzyme of the mitochondrial respiratory chain (Kaler, 1994). And the characteristic kinky (or steely) hair (the disease is often referred to as kinky hair disease) is caused by the reduced degree of keratin cross-linking, a process catalysed by a copper oxidase (Gillespie, 1973). The link between copper and hair formation was first observed in copper-deficient sheep, which produce 'steely wool', and played an important part in establishing the 'copper link' in Menkes disease (Danks et al., 1972). Paradoxically for a disease characterized by copper deficiency, in Menkes patients some tissues, notably kidney and intestinal epithelial cells, accumulate copper. This reflects the fact that the defective protein is involved in the export of copper from intestinal and renal epithelial cells (reviewed in Mercer, 2001).

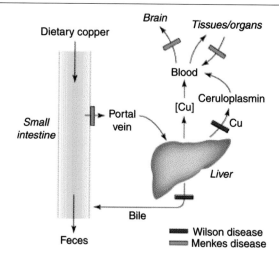

Figure 9.5: Pathways of copper in the body which are blocked in Menkes and Wilson's diseases. In Wilson's disease, copper incorporation into ceruloplasmin in the liver is blocked, as well as exportation of excess hepatic copper in the bile due to the mutations in ATP7b, resulting in copper accumulation in the liver. In Menkes disease the transport of copper across the intestinal tract is blocked, resulting in overall copper deficiency. The transport of copper to the brain is also blocked in Menkes disease, resulting in the severe neurological abnormalities characteristic of the disease. Reprinted from *Trends in Molecular Medicine*, Vol 7, Mercer, The molecular basis of copper-transport diseases, pp 64–69, Copyright 2001, with permission from Elsevier.

   Using the genetic strategy of positional cloning the affected gene in Menkes disease was isolated by three groups (Mercer et al., 1993; Chelly et al., 1993; Vulpe et al., 1993) and identified as a P-type ATPase (Vulpe et al., 1993). The Menkes protein is known as ATP7a and like the Wilson protein (**Figure 9.4**) the amino terminal region contains six copper-binding motifs, which also interact with copper chaperones, while the eight transmembrane domains form a channel through which copper is pumped, driven by the hydrolysis of ATP. ATP7a plays a vital role in systemic copper absorption in the gut and copper reabsorption in the kidney. The protein localizes to the trans-Golgi network, but when copper concentrations are increased, it relocalizes to the basolateral membrane in polarized kidney cells (Greenough et al., 2004), where, as previously shown in non-polarized cells (Petris et al., 1996), the metal binding sites in the amino terminal domain are required for copper-regulated trafficking of copper from the Golgi to the plasma membrane. Transport of copper to the brain is also blocked in Menkes disease (**Figure 9.5**). In very recent studies (Schlief et al., 2005), ATP7a has been shown to be abundantly expressed in the late Golgi of primary cultures of hippocampal neurons. Activation of glutamate receptors (specifically NMDA- but not AMPA/kainite-type receptors) results in the rapid and reversible trafficking of ATP7a to neuronal processes, independent of intracellular copper concentration, associated with rapid release of copper from hippocampal neurons. When hippocampal cultures from animals lacking a functional ATP7a were studied, no copper release was observed. These observations would appear to establish a mechanism whereby copper homeostasis and neuronal activation in the CNS are linked.
   Many mutations have been found in classical Menkes disease (Tümer et al., 1997), which would be predicted to prevent formation of any functional protein. Occipital horn syndrome is an X-linked connective tissue disorder with only mild neurological disease,

and it is likely here that the mutations (often splice site mutations) allow the production of small amounts of the normal protein (Moller et al., 2000) which, while sufficient to prevent neurological effects, cannot supply the requirements of lysyl oxidase for collagen maturation.

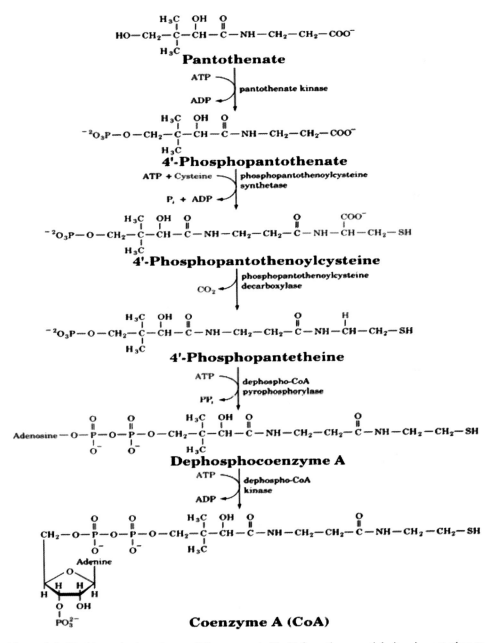

Figure 9.6: The biosynthetic pathway of Coenzyme A (CoA) from the essential vitamin pantothenate. CoA is vitally important for metabolism – acetyl-CoA is the link between the metabolism of amino acids, fats and sugars and the citric acid cycle. From Voet and Voet (1995).

9.4 HALLERVORDEN-SPATZ SYNDROME

The original description of Hallervorden-Spatz syndrome concerned 12 siblings, three of whom died in infancy: of the remaining nine, five showed clinically increasing dysarthria and progressive dementia, and all five died. At autopsy, brown discoloration of the globus pallidus and substantia nigra (Hallervorden and Spatz, 1922) was observed. The disease is relatively uncommon, is inherited as an autosomal recessive trait, and is characterized by progressive Parkinson-like rigidity and mental and emotional retardation. Onset is in late childhood, with death occurring usually within 10 years. The aetiology is unknown, but it can be considered as a form of iron storage disease, since the dark brown colour of both the globus pallidus and the substantia nigra is due to the accumulation of iron; routine iron staining shows the iron mostly in microglia and macrophages, but scattered neurons are also reactive. The disease presents not only in the classic forms (characterized by early onset and rapid progression), but also in an atypical form (later onset and slower progression). Many patients with classic Hallervorden-Spatz syndrome have mutations in the gene encoding pantothenate kinase 2 (PANK2), and in a study of 123 patients, all those with the classic form, and one third of those with the atypical form, had PANK2 mutations (Hayflick et al., 2003). Pantothenate kinase is the first enzyme in the biosynthesis of the key metabolic intermediate, coenzyme A, which plays a central role in intermediary metabolism, from its vitamin precursor, pantothenate (**Figure 9.6**). PANK2 is one of four human pantothenate kinase genes, and is the only one of the four predicted to be targeted to, and localized within, mitochondria (Johnson et al., 2004). It is proposed that the disease, for which the term pantothenate kinase-associated neurodegeneration (PKAN2) is proposed[3] (Gordon, 2002; Hayflick, 2003), may result in tissue-specific coenzyme A deficiency, resulting in the accumulation of cysteine in the basal ganglia, which may chelate iron and lead to its accumulation in these areas (Gordon, 2002; Hayflick, 2003). The cysteine-iron complex could also promote oxidative stress, resulting in neurodegenerative damage, as in other neurodegenerative diseases.

A characteristic diagnostic feature of Hallervorden-Spatz syndrome in T_2-weighted magnetic resonance image (MRI) scans is "the eye of the tiger" (**Figure 9.7a**), which shows diffuse bilateral low signal intensity of the globus pallidus (due to iron deposition) with a region of hyperintensity in the internal segment (high signal is thought to represent tissue oedema), due to axonal vacuolization (Hayflick et al., 2003).

9.5 NEUROFERRITINOPATHY

In 2001 a previously unknown, dominantly inherited late-onset basal ganglia disease, variably presenting with features similar to those of Huntington's disease or Parkinson's disease was reported (Curtis et al., 2001). This movement disorder, accompanied by behavioural disturbances and cognitive decline was found in a large family from Cumbria in north west England. Genetic analysis showed that the disease resulted from the insertion of an adenine residue at position 460-461 of the gene for the ferritin light chain, which was

---

[3] Controversy surrounds Julius Hallervorden's role in carrying out research on brains from metally sick patients subjected to "mercy killings" during World War II. Since the syndrome was originally discovered in 1922, and its name is still extensively used to describe this rare condition, we have left the name unchanged.

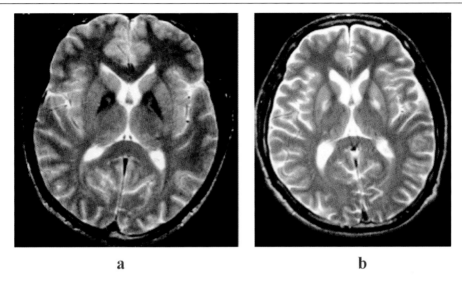

a   b

Figure 9.7: (**a**) Hallervorden-Spatz syndrome (PANK2), "the eye of the tiger" sign. This characteristic magnetic resonance imaging (MRI) picture is a T_2-weighted image which shows diffuse bilateral low signal intensity of the globus pallidus (due to iron deposition) with a region of hyperintensity in the internal segment, due to axonal vacuolization. From Healy et al. (2004). (**b**) Neuroferritino-pathy. The T_2-weighted image shows a high signal bilaterally in the globus pallidus. From Healy et al. (2004). Reprinted with permission from Elsevier (*The Lancet*, 2004, Vol 3, pp 652–662).

predicted to alter the carboxy terminal sequence of the protein. The same mutation has been found in a French family (Chinnery et al., 2003). An apparently similar ferritinopathy has been described accompanied by intranuclear and intracytoplasmic bodies found in glia and subsets of neurons in the CNS as well as in extraneural tissues (Vidal et al., 2003; 2004). More detailed analysis revealed that the main constituents of these bodies isolated from the striatum and cerebellar cortex were ubiquitinated ferritin light and heavy chains, which stained by the Perl's reagent for ferric iron (Vidal et al., 2004). Molecular genetic studies showed the presence of a 2-base pair insertion mutation in exon 4 of the ferritin light chain gene.

The T_2-weighted MRI images in neuroferritinopathy (**Figure 9.7b**) are quite character-istic, with symmetrical degeneration of the globus pallidus and putamen and low signal intensity in the internal capsule (Curtis et al., 2001). It has been proposed that ferritino-pathies may be diagnosed by a simple muscle or nerve biopsy, without the requirement of brain biopsy, autopsy or molecular genetic testing (Schroder, 2005).

9.6 MULTIPLE SCLEROSIS

The prototype inflammatory autoimmune disorder of the central nervous system, with a lifetime risk of one in four hundred, potentially the most common cause of neurological disability in young adults, multiple sclerosis is now one of the most common reasons for admission to a neurological ward. The brutal statistics, with 2.5 million affected individuals throughout the world, and an estimated annual expenditure in the UK alone of £1,200

(a)

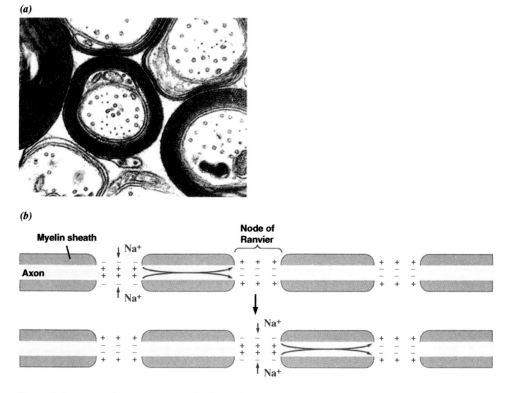

(b)

Figure 9.8: (**a**) An electron micrograph of myelinated nerve fibres in cross section. The myelin sheath surrounding the axon is the plasma membrane of an oligodendrocyte or a Schwann cell, which extrudes its cytoplasm from between the layers as it grows spirally around the axon. The resulting bilayer, which makes between 10 to 150 turns about the axon, is a good conductor of electricity because of its high lipid content (about 80%). (**b**) A schematic diagram of a myelinated axon in longitudinal cross section. The axonal membrane is in contact with the external medium at the nodes of Ranvier. A depolarization generated by an action potential at one node, hops down the myelinated axon (arrows) the the neighbouring node, where it induces a new action potential. This results in saltatory conduction. From Voet and Voet (1995).

million, conceal the individual personal anguish of young adults[4] who have seen their hopes raised by apparent remission, only to be shattered by subsequent relapse. Multiple sclerosis is an autoimmune disorder of the CNS characterized by inflammatory destruction of the myelin sheath of the axons of neurons. The axons of the long motor neurons are sheathed with myelin, a sort of "electrical insulating tape", which is wrapped around the axon (**Figure 9.8**), electrically isolating it from the surrounding medium. Nerve impulses in myelinated nerves travel much faster than in non-myelinated nerves[5] – up to $100\,\mathrm{m.s}^{-1}$

---

[4] Jacqueline du Pré was a brilliant young cellist, who acquired from her teacher William Pleeth the habit of putting a lot of body movement into her playing. She began suffering in July 1971 from a mystery ailment which affected her playing. Multiple sclerosis was diagnosed, and after a cruel series of remissions and relapses, she was never able to play the cello again, and died in 1987.

[5] As has been pointed out by more than one author, the difficulties of coordination in a giraffe, if motor neurons were not myelinated, hardly bears thinking about.

compared to a maximum of $10 \, \text{m.s}^{-1}$. This is because the myelinated axons have their Na^+ channels localized uniquely at the myelin-free nodes of Ranvier, compared to the rather sparse distribution in non-myelinated axons. The action potential of myelinated axons literally hops between the nodes of Ranvier, in a process termed saltatory conduction. Myelin is produced by specialized cells: oligodendrocytes in the central nervous system, and Schwann cells in the peripheral nervous system. The myelin sheaths, which are in fact the plasma membrane of the oligodendrocyte or Schwann cell, wrap themselves around the axons. The resulting bilayer, which makes between 10 to 150 turns around the axon, is a good electrical insulator because of its high lipid content. Each oligodendrocyte can myelinate up to 40 neighbouring axons. The oligodendrocyte is a principal target of attack in multiple sclerosis, and the consequences of demyelination for saltatory conduction explain many of the features of the disease. Partially demyelinated axons conduct nerve impulses more slowly. Demyelinated axons can discharge spontaneously and show increased mechanical sensitivity, accounting for flashes of light on eye movement and electrical sensations running down the spine or limbs on flexing the neck. Axons which have lost part of their myelin sheath are unable to sustain the fall in membrane capacitance induced by a rise in temperature, and conduction fails, leading to the appearance of symptoms after exercise or a hot bath. And crosstalk between demyelinated axons can result in paroxysmal symptoms.

Multiple sclerosis is caused by an interplay between genes and environment, but until now no clear genetic markers have been identified. The results of genome screening studies have strongly suggested that there is not a major genetic locus in MS (reviewed in Dyment et al., 2004). Many genes have been identified which seem to have an association with MS. The MHC[6] is unambiguously associated with MS (Olerup and Hillert, 1991; Sotgiu et al., 2002), and a number of HLA class I and II antigens have been shown to be associated with MS. So too have T-cell receptors, which bind directly to HLA antigens, and the cytotoxic T lymphocyte antigen 4, the expression of which is up regulated in the course of T cell activation, but the evidence that these genes or others which have been implicated have an effect on disease pathogenesis is not clear (Dyment et al., 2004).

Curiously, MS affects northern Europeans with a much greater frequency than other populations, and close relatives are at greater risk than second and third degree relatives (Compston and Coles, 2002). But population genetics do not explain the distribution of MS – the risk is higher for English-speaking people who migrate to South Africa as adults than as children, while the low frequency of MS in Africans increases significantly for first generation descendants raised in the UK. MS also affects twice as many women as it does men: this is in agreement with data for other autoimmune diseases. It is of course no coincidence that many of the genes suggested as being associated with MS are involved in immune function, either in recognition of self and non-self, or in later steps in the activation of T cells. The major pathological difference which distinguishes MC from other inflammatory diseases of the nervous system is the presence of large, multifocal, demyelinated plaques with reactive glial scar formation (Lassmann et al., 2001). The pathology of inflammation in MS lesions is consistent with a T-cell-mediated immune

---

[6] The Major Histocompatability Complex (MHC) encodes a series of membrane-bound proteins which are the antigen-presenting markers through which the immune system distinguishes body cells from invading antigens (Class I MHC proteins) and immune system cells from other cells (Class II MHC proteins). They are often referred to as HLA (human-leukocyte-associated) Class I and Class II antigens. They are among the most polymorphic genes known in higher vertebrates, such that two unrelated individuals are unlikely to have the same set of MHC genes.

reaction leading to the recruitment of blood-borne macrophages and activation of microglia (Lassmann et al., 2001). This is similar to experimental allergic encephalomyelitis (EAE), an animal model induced by immunization of animals with CNS tissue, myelin or myelin proteins. In particular, in MS and in EAE, the inflammatory process appears to be driven by T helper 1 (Th1) cell-mediated autoimmune response, with expression of Th1-related cytokines (Merril et al., 1992), chemokines and chemokine receptors (Sorensen et al., 1999).

For more than a century, multiple sclerosis was considered to be a disease process characterized by oligodendrocyte and myelin loss, and research was focused on the mechanisms of inflammation, often associated with redox-active metal ions, However, the development of more sophisticated molecular biological and neuroimaging techniques has revealed that tissue destruction, mostly axonal loss and neurodegeneration, is also a key element in the disease progression (reviewed in Minagar et al., 2004). Brain atrophy and loss of axonal integrity begins early in the disease process, often in patients with MS for less than 5 years, as determined by magnetic resonance imaging and spectroscopy. It may be that the initial neurodegeneration and axonal loss in MS patients are initially to some extent compensated by local responses from oligodendrocyte progenitor cells with some remyelination. However, these repair mechanisms eventually fail, resulting in generalized brain atrophy, progressive cognitive decline and permanent disability.

It has therefore been suggested that the pathogenic mechanisms involved in formation of MS lesions involve four progressive stages, namely inflammation, demyelination, followed by axonal injury, which becomes chronic in active plaques (Lassmann et al, 2001) (**Figure 9.9**). In the first phase, evidence indicates that T helper 1 (Th1) cells have a role in inducing inflammatory reactions in the central nervous system; by the release of proinflammatory cytokines they can activate macrophages, which are responsible for the majority of demyelination and axonal injury. In addition, T helper 2 (Th2) cells and Class-I cytotoxic T (Tc1) cells (which secrete a similar spectrum of cytokines to Th1 cells), might also modify the outcome of the lesions. The second phase involves demyelination in which oligodendrocytes and myelin sheaths are destroyed, possibly by different mechanisms in different individuals, resulting in distinctly different patterns of demyelination in active lesions. Demyelination could be induced by macrophages and/or their toxic products (pattern I), by specific demyelinating antibodies and complement (pattern II), by degenerative processes in distal processes, notably those of periaxonal oligodendrocytes (distal oligodendrogliopathy), followed by apoptosis (resulting in pattern III) or by a primary degeneration of oligodendrocytes followed by myelin destruction (resulting in pattern IV). Possible mediators of myelin and oligodendrocyte destruction include tumor necrosis factor α (TNF-α), reactive oxygen intermediates (ROI) which could be generated by redox active metals, antibodies against myelin oligodendrocyte glycoprotein (anti-MOG) or galactocerebroside (anti-GC). In the third phase, axonal injury follows acute destruction of myelin sheaths. In the active phase of demyelination, axonal injury is likely to be induced by macrophage toxins or by the direct effects of cytotoxic T cells. The chronic axonal injury observed in active plaques may be caused by a lack of growth factors supplied by glial cells, but could also involve inflammatory mediators produced by macrophages, that persist in most active chronic lesions. In any event, it now seems clear that multiple sclerosis, while in its initial stages associated with an inflammatory autoimmune response, probably associated with metal-mediated oxidative stress, progresses with involvement of the complete repertoire of the external pathway to full blown apoptosis.

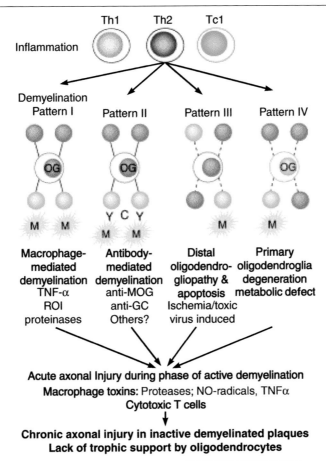

Th1   Th2   Tc1

Inflammation

Demyelination
Pattern I   Pattern II   Pattern III   Pattern IV

M   M   Y C Y   M   M
                M   M

Macrophage-   Antibody-   Distal   Primary
mediated   mediated   oligodendro-   oligodendroglia
demyelination demyelination   gliopathy &   degeneration
TNF-α   anti-MOG   apoptosis   metabolic defect
ROI   anti-GC   Ischemia/toxic
proteinases   Others?   virus induced

Acute axonal Injury during phase of active demyelination
Macrophage toxins: Proteases; NO-radicals, TNFα
Cytotoxic T cells

Chronic axonal injury in inactive demyelinated plaques
Lack of trophic support by oligodendrocytes

TRENDS in Molecular Medicine

Figure 9.9: Summary of pathogenic mechanisms involved in the formation of multiple sclerosis lesions. (i) Inflammation: T helper 1 (Th1) cells have a role in inducing inflammatory reactions in the central nervous system by releasing proinflammatory cytokines which activate macrophages; these latter are responsible for the majority of demyelination and axonal injury. In addition, T helper 2 (Th2) cells and Class-I cytotoxic T (Tc1) cells, might also be involved. (ii) Demyelination: myelin sheaths and oligodendrocytes (OG) can be destroyed, possibly by different mechanisms in different individuals. This results in distinctly different patterns of demyelination in active lesions. Demyelination may be induced by macrophages (M) and/or their toxic products (resulting in pattern I), by specific demyelinating antibodies and complement (C, resulting in pattern II), by degenerative changes in distal processes, in particular those of periaxonal oligodendrocytes (distal oligodendrogliopathy), followed by apoptosis (resulting in pattern III) or by a primary degeneration of oligodendrocytes followed by myelin destruction (resulting in pattern IV). Possible mediators of myelin and oligodendrocyte destruction include tumor necrosis factor α (TNF-α), reactive oxygen intermediates (ROI), antibodies against myelin oligodendrocyte glycoprotein (anti-MOG) or galactocerebroside (anti-GC). Axonal injury: axonal injury follows acute destruction of myelin sheaths. In the active phase of demyelination, axonal injury is likely to be induced by macrophage toxins or by the direct effects of cytotoxic T cells. The chronic axonal injury observed inactive plaques may be caused by a lack of trophic support by glial cells, such as oligodendrocytes, but could also involve inflammatory mediators, produced by macrophages, that persist in most active chronic lesions. Reprinted from *Trends in Molecular Medicine*, Vol 7, Lassman et al., Heterogeneity of multiple sclerosis pathogenesis: implications for diagnosis and therapy, pp 115–121, Copyright 2001, with permission from Elsevier.

9.7 HIV-ASSOCIATED DEMENTIA

Acquired immunodeficiency syndrome, resulting from infection by human immunodeficiency viruses (HIV), has caused devastation over the last two decades, with more than 60 million people infected and at present around 40 million living with the disease. The infection can cause a syndrome of cognitive, behavioural and motor dysfunction (Perry and Marotta, 1987), designated HIV-associated dementia (HAD), affecting about 20% of HIV patients (Adle-Biassette et al., 1999; Kolson and Gonzalez-Scarano, 2000). Since the introduction of highly active antiretroviral therapy (HAART), the incidence of HAD has decreased (Sacktor et al., 2001), whereas the prevalence rate is increasing as people with HIV survive longer. From a histopathological standpoint, HAD is characterized by infiltration of inflammatory cells into the CNS, increased microglial activity, pallor of myelin sheaths, abnormalities of dendritic processes and neuronal apoptosis (Gray et al., 1996). The curious thing about HAD is that the virus does not infect neurons directly, nor is it by itself neurotoxic.

Two interesting hypotheses have been advanced, based on the observations that the level of tumor necrosis factor-α (TNF-α), released by infected microglia and macrophages, plays a role in neuronal injury (reviewed in Saha and Pahan, 2003). The first attributes to TNF-α the role of inducer and mediator of neurodegeneration. The infected and activated microglia, macrophages and astrocytes secrete a veritable plethora of proinflammatory cytokines, including TNF-α. The latter may kill neurons directly through its receptor by activation of caspases, or by synergistically enhancing the toxicity of viral toxins, like gp120. Indirectly, TNF-α may kill neurons by NO-mediated peroxynitrite toxicity, and upregulation of the expression of gene products which are either directly neurotoxic (α-chemokines) or which may indirectly induce neuronal injury (ICAM and VCAM expression by astrocytes is increased which aids in HIV-1 trafficking across the BBB). In addition, TNF-α induces the production of excitotoxins, like glutamate from glial cells (Bezzi et al., 2001). Elevated levels of excitotoxins in the vicinity of neurons activate the NMDA receptor-operated channels, allowing an influx of Ca^{++} into the neurons, subsequent loss of cellular homeostasis, which may culminate in apoptosis (Foos and Wu, 2002).

In complete contrast to the arguments advanced above, a totally different role is envisaged in the second hypothesis, whereby TNF-α may ultimately play a neuroprotective role. This could involve protecting and maintaining Ca^{++} homeostasis in neurons (Cheng et al., 1994), activation of the transcription factor NFκB resulting in the upregulation of several pro-survival gene products (Mattson and Camandola, 2001), and production of neuroprotective chemokines, which may attenuate the toxicity of viral proteins like gp120 (Kaul and Lipton, 1999).

As indicated above, although the symptoms of HAD point clearly to neuronal dysfunction, neurons are not infected, but rather macrophages and microglia. Among the candidate inflammatory products from these infected cells, cytokines, chemokines, matrix metalloproteases, reactive oxygen or nitrogen species (Albright et al., 2003), we will most likely find the toxic players responsible for this dementia. Stromal cell-derived factor-1 (SDF-1) is a chemokine that is constitutively expressed in most tissues and displayed on the cell surface. Its numerous biological effects are mediated by a specific G protein-coupled receptor, CXCR4, and a number of cells inactivate SDF-1 by specific processing of its N-terminal domain. Recently it has been found that SDF-1 can be cleaved by a matrix metalloproteinase (MMP-2) produced by HIV-1-infected macrophages or microglia, to

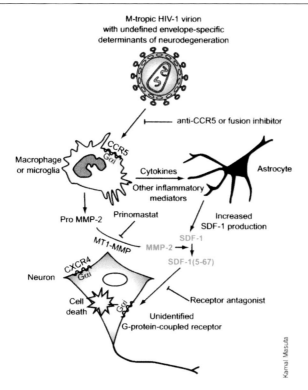

Figure 9.10: MMP-2 cleavage of SDF-1 at the 4-5 position generates a neurotoxin. Reprinted from Ransohoff, Snip, snip, kill, kill: truncated SDF-1, pp 1009–1011, *Nature Neuroscience*, Vol 6, Copyright 2003, with permission of Nature Publishing Group.

generate a potent neurotoxin (Zhang et al., 2003). **Figure 9.10** presents a mechanism for the MMP-2 cleavage of SDF-1 to generate a neurotoxin (Ransohoff, 2003). HIV infected macrophages secrete the matrix metalloproteinase-2 (MMP-2) in its inactive ProMMP-2 form, together with inflammatory cytokines. These cytokines act on nearby astrocytes, causing upregulation of secretion of SDF-1. The ProMMP-2 is converted to active MMP-2 by MT1-MMP, a matrix metalloprotease which is expressed abundantly by neurons. MMP-2 was converted to a highly neurotoxic protein after precise proteolytic processing by active MMP-2, which removed the N-terminal tetrapeptide. Implantation of cleaved SDF-1(5-67) into the basal ganglia of mice resulted in neuronal death and inflammation with ensuing neurobehavioural deficits that were abrogated by antibodies to SDF-1 and by an MMP inhibitor drug, prinomastat. This suggests that there may be *in vivo* pathways in which aberrant cleavage of a signalling protein by an HIV-1-induced metalloproteinase results in neuronal apoptosis, and neurodegeneration.

REFERENCES

Adle-Biassette, H., Levy, Y., Colombel, M., Poron, F. *et al.* (1999) *Neuropathol. Appl. Neurobiol.*, **21**, 218–227.
Albright, A.V., Soldan, S.S. and Gonzalez-Scarano, F. (2003) *J. Neurovirolog.*, **9**, 222–227.

Attieh, Z.K., Mukhopadhay, C.K., Seshadri, V., Tripoulas, N.A. and Fox, P.L. (1999) *J. Biol. Chem.*, **274**, 1116–1123.

Bezzi, P., Domercq, M., Brambilla, L., Galli, R. *et al.* (2001) *Nature Neurosci.*, **4**, 702–710.

Burstein, E., Ganesh, L., Dick, R.D., van de Sluis, B. *et al.* (2004) *EMBO J.*, **23**, 244–254.

Chelly, J., Turner, Z., Tonneson, T., Patterson, A. *et al.* (1993) *Nat. Genet.*, **3**, 14–19.

Cheng, B., Christakos, S. and Mattson, M.P. (1994) *Neuron*, **12**, 139–153.

Chinnery, P.F., Curtis, A.R., Fey, C., Coulthard, A. *et al.* (2003) *J. Med. Genet.*, **40**, e69.

Compston, A. and Coles, A. (2002) *Lancet*, **359**, 1221–1231.

Crichton, R.R. and Pierre, J.-L. (2001) *BioMetals*, **14**, 99–112.

Cummings, J.N. (1948) *Brain*, **71**, 410–417.

Curtis, A.R., Fey, C., Morris, C.M., Bindoff, L.A. *et al.* (2001) *Nat. Genet.*, **28**, 350–354.

Danks, D.M., Campbell, P.E., Walker-Smith, J., Stevens, B.J. *et al.* (1972) *Lancet*, **1**, 1100–1102.

Dyment, D.A., Ebers, G.C. and Sadovnik, A.D. (2004) *Lancet Neurol.*, **3**, 104–110.

Foos, T.M. and Wu, J.Y. (2002) *Neurochem. Res.*, **27**, 21–26.

Gillespie, J.M. (1973) *Aus. J. Derm.*, **14**, 127–131.

Gitlin, J.D. (2003) *Gastroenterology*, **125**, 1868–1877.

Gordon, N. (2002) *Eur. J. Pediatr. Neurol.*, **6**, 243–247.

Gray, F., Scaravilli, F. Everall, I., Chretien, F. *et al.* (1996) *Brain Pathol.*, **6**, 1–15.

Greenough, M., Pase, L., Voskoboinik, I., Petris, M.J. *et al.* (2004) *Am. J. Physiol. Cell Physiol.*, **287**, C1463–C1471.

Hallervorden, J. and Spatz, H. (1922) *Z. Ges. Neurol. Psychiat.*, **79**, 254–302.

Harris, Z.L., Davis-Kaplan, S.R., Gitlin, J.D. and Kaplan, J. (2004) *Blood*, **103**, 4672–4673.

Harris, Z.L., Takahashi, Y., Miyajima, H., Serizawa, M. *et al.* (1995) *Proc. Natl. Acad. Sci. USA*, **92**, 2539–2543.

Hayflick, S.J. (2003) *Curr. Opin. Pediatr.*, **15**, 572–577.

Hayflick, S.J., Westaway, S.K., Levinson, B., Zhou, B. *et al.* (2003) *N. Engl. J. Med.*, **348**, 33–40.

Healy, D., Abou-Sleiman, P., Wood, N. (2004) *Lancet Neurol.*, **3**, 652–662.

Hellman, N.E. and Gitlin, J.D. (2002) *Annu. Rev. Nutr.*, **22**, 439–458.

Johnson, M.A., Kuo, Y.M., Westaway, S.K., Parker, S.M. *et al.* (2004) *Ann. N. Y. Acad. Sci.*, **1012**, 282–298.

Kaler, S.G. (1994) *Adv. Pediatr.*, **41**, 262–303.

Kaul, M. and Lipton, S.A. (1999) *Proc. Natl. Acad. Sci. USA*, **96**, 8212–8216.

Klomp, A.E., van de Sluis, B., Klomp, L.W. and Wijmenga, C. (2003) *J. Hepatol.*, **39**, 703–709.

Klomp, L.W.J. and Gitlin, J.D. (1993) *Hum. Mol. Genet.*, **5**, 1989–1996.

Kolson, D.L. and Gonzalez-Scarano, F. (2000) *J. Clin. Invest.*, **106**, 11–13.

Lassmann, H., Brück, W. and Lucchinetti, C. (2001) *TRENDS Mol. Med.*, **7**, 115–121.

Lee, G.R., Nacht, S., Lukens, J.N. and Cartwright, G.E. (1968) *J. Clin. Invest.*, **47**, 2058–2069.

Logan, J.L., Harveyson, K.B., Wisdom, G.B., Hughes, A.E. and Archibald, G.P. (1994) *Quart. J. Med.*, **87**, 663–6670.

Lutsenko, S. and Petris, M.J. (2003) *J. Membr. Biol.*, **191**, 1–12.

Mattson, M.P. and Camandola, S. (2001) *J. Clin. Invest.*, **107**, 247–254.

Menkes, J.H.M., Alter, M. and Steigleder, G.K. (1962) *Pediatr.*, **29**, 764–769.

Mercer, J.F.B. (2001) *TRENDS Mol. Med.*, **7**, 64–69.

Mercer, J.F., Livingston, J., Hall, B., Paynter, J.A. *et al.* (1993) *Nat. Genet.*, **3**, 20–25.

Merril, J.E. (1992) *J. Immunother.*, **12**, 167–170.

Minagar, A., Toledo, E.G., Alexander, J.S. and Kelley, R.E. (2004) *J. Neuroimaging*, **14**, 5S–10S.

Miyajima, H., Nishimura, Y., Mizoguchi, K., Sakamoto, M. *et al.* (1987) *Neurology*, **37**, 761–765.

Miyajima, H., Takahashi, Y., Serizawa, M., Kaneko, E. and Gitlin, J.D. (1997) *Ann. Neurol.*, **41**, 404–447.

Moller, L.B., Tümer, Z., Lund, C., Petersen, C. *et al.* (2000) *Am. J. Hum. Genet.*, **66**, 1211–1220.

Olerup, O. and Hillert, J. (1991) *Tissue Antigens*, **38**, 1–15.

Osaki, S., Johnson, D.A. and Frieden, E. (1996) *J. Biol. Chem.*, **241**, 2746–2757.

Perry, S. and Marotta, R.F. (1987) *Alzheimer Dis. Assoc. Disord.*, **1**, 221–235.

Petris, M.J., Mercer, J.F., Culvenor, J.G., Lockhart, P. *et al.* (1996) *EMBO J.*, **15**, 6084–6095.

Ransohoff, R.M. (2003) *Nature Neurosci.*, **6**, 1009–1011.

Roeser, H.P., Lee, G.R., Nacht, S. and Cartwright, G.E. (1970) *J. Clin. Invest.*, **49**, 2408–2417.

Sacktor, N., Lyles, R.H., Skolasky, R., Kleeberger, C. *et al.* (2001) *Neurology*, **56**, 257–260.

Saha, R.N. and Pahan, K. (2003) *J. Neurochem.*, **86**, 1057–1071.

Scheinberg, I.H. and Gitlin, D. (1952) *Science*, **116**, 484–450.

Schilsky, M.L. (2002) *Pediatr. Transplant.*, **6**, 15–19.

Schlief, M.L., Craig, A.M. and Gitlin, J.D. (2005) *J. Neurosci.*, **25**, 239–246.

Schroder, J.M. (2005) *Acta Neuropathol. (Berl.)*, in press.

Sokol, R.J. (1996) *Semin. Liver Dis.*, **16**, 39–46.

Sorenson, T.L., Tani, M., Jensen, J., Pierce, V. *et al.* (1999) *J. Clin. Invest.*, **103**, 807–815.

Sotgiu, S., Rosati, G., Sana, A. *et al.* (2002) *Eur. J. Neurol.*, **9**, 1–13.

Strand, S., Hofmann, W.J., Grambihler, A., Hug, H. *et al.* (1998) *Nat. Med.*, **4**, 588–593.

Tao, T.Y., Liu, F., Klomp, L., Wijmenga, C. and Gitlin, J.D. (2003) *J. Biol. Chem.*, **278**, 41593–41596.

Tümer, Z., Lund, C., Tolshave, J., Vural, B. *et al.* (1997) *Am. J. Hum. Genet.*, **60**, 63–71.

van de Sluis, B., Rothuizen, J., Pearson, P.L., van Oost, B.A. and Wijmenga, C. (2002) *Hum. Mol. Genet.*, **11**, 165–173.

Vidal, R., Delisle, M.B., Rascol, O. and Ghetti, B. (2003) *J. Neurol. Sci.*, **207**, 110–111.

Vidal, R., Ghetti, B., Takao, M., Brefel-Courbon, C. *et al.* (2004) *J. Neuropathol. Exp. Neurol.*, **63**, 363–380.

Voet, D. and Voet, J.G. (1995) *Biochemistry*, 2nd edn., John Wiley & Sons, Chichester.

Vulpe, C., Levison, B., Whitney, S., Packman, S. and Gitschier, J. (1993) *Nat. Genet.*, **3**, 7–13.

Walshe, J.M. (1956) *Am. J. Med.*, **21**, 487–492.

Wilson, S.A.K. (1912) *Brain*, **34**, 295–507.

Yonekawa, M., Okabe, T., Asamoto, Y. and Ohta, M. (1999) *Eur. Neurol.*, **42**, 157–162.

Yoshida, K., Furihata, K., Takeda, S., Nakamura, A. *et al.* (1995) *Nature Genet.*, **9**, 267–272.

Zaitseva, L., Zaitsev, V., Card, G., Moshkov, K. *et al.* (1998) *J. Biol. Inorg. Biochem.*, **1**, 15–23.

Zhang, K., McQuibban, G.A., Silva, C., Butler, G.S. *et al.* (2003) *Nature Neurosci.*, **6**, 1064–1071.

10

Therapeutic Strategies to Combat the Onset and Progression of Neurodegenerative Diseases

One of the early events that occur in the metal-based neurodegenerative diseases is the mishandling of specific proteins in their degradation by the proteosomal mechanism. Prevention of such cellular dysfunction is likely to retard the development and progression of the neurological lesion. At the present time, the treatment of each of these neurological diseases relies almost exclusively on therapeutic agents that merely treat the pathology of each of the diseases rather than their aetiology.

10.1 PARKINSON'S DISEASE

It is essential that there is early recognition of the disease, since timely pharmaceutical intervention will retard its progression. Unfortunately physical symptoms of the disease do not occur until there is between 60–80% loss of dopaminergic neurons. Physical techniques for the early detection of the disease include echogenicity (to detect increased iron content in SN) and single photon emission computed tomography (SPECT) (to detect various aspects of dopamine metabolism, e.g. injection of the radiolabelled 18F-fluorodopa or 99 m TcTRODAT-1 to assay dopamine uptake or dopamine transporter, respectively). However, such procedures, at this present time, are research techniques rather than routinely available diagnostics. There are no biochemical or molecular biological assays that identify early changes in dopamine metabolism prior to the presentation of the clinical symptoms.

A multi-neuroprotective drug regime is appropriate for the treatment of PD because of the wide range of pathologies presented. Currently, molecules that either alter dopamine metabolism or inhibit cholinergic release are widely used, **Table 10.1**, although radical scavengers, iron chelators, nitric oxide synthase inhibitors, glutamatergic inhibitors and certain calcium channel antagonists may be important therapeutics in the future.

A well-balanced diet is important in maintaining a patient's general health and strength. An improvement in motor capacity was evident in PD patients who removed red meat from

Metal-based Neurodegeneration: From Molecular Mechanisms to Therapeutic Strategies R. R. Crichton and R. J. Ward
© 2006 John Wiley & Sons, Ltd

Table 10.1: Current drug strategies for the treatment of Parkinson's disease

DRUG	MECHANISM
L-DOPA-carbidopa (Sinemet)	Precursor of dopamine+ enzyme inhibitor
Amantadine (Symmetrel)	Dopamine reuptake inhibitor
Bromocriptine (Parlodel)	Dopamine agonist (receptor stimulation)
Pergolide (Permax)	Dopamine agonist (receptor stimulation)
Pramipexole (Mirapex)	Dopamine agonist (receptor stimulation)
Ropinirole (Requip)	Dopamine agonist (receptor stimulation)
Selegline (Eldepryl)	MAO-B inhibitor
Tolcapone (Tasmar)	COMT inhibitor
Diphenhydramine (Benadryl)	Antihistamine
Trihexphenidyl (Artane)	Anticholinergic activity
Benztropine (Cogentin)	Anticholinergic activity

Name of active compound shown together with brand name in parentheses.

their diet while being supplemented with riboflavin (Coimbra and Junqueira, 2003). However, this study was criticized on two criteria: (a) the lack of an independent assessor, and (b) there was no placebo group. Furthermore, the beneficial results may have related to an increased availability of their medication, i.e. L-DOPA, due to decreased dietary protein intake (Ferraz et al., 2004). Other epidemiological studies, which included a placebo group, did not demonstrate any correlation between life-style or food habits and PD (Baldereschi et al., 2003; Tsai et al., 2002). However, these studies gave no data on red meat consumption, (Hellenbrand et al., 1996) or iron intake, (Powers et al., 2003), both of which are risk factors for PD.

Regular physical exercise is beneficial to the PD patient and essential for maintaining and improving mobility, flexibility, balance and a range of motion. This will provide some protection against many of the secondary symptoms and side effects.

As already described in Chapter 3 the accumulation of α-synuclein in Lewy bodies is the hallmark feature of the disease. Strategies, aimed at preventing α-synuclein aggregation, as well as enhancing its degradation are of fundamental importance and need to be developed.

When brain dopamine levels decline in the SN, as a result of 60–80% loss of dopaminergic neurons, classical symptoms of the disease occur, e.g. tremor in hands, arms, legs, rigidity, stiffness of the limbs or trunk, bradykinesia (abnormal movements) or slowness of movement, impaired balance and co-ordination. The first line drug is levodopa (L-DOPA) which increases brain dopamine content. L-DOPA, **[Sinemet]**, a dopamine precursor, is transformed to dopamine in the brain. It is principally metabolized by dopa decarboxylase and catechol-O-methyl transferase (COMT) such that co-administration of

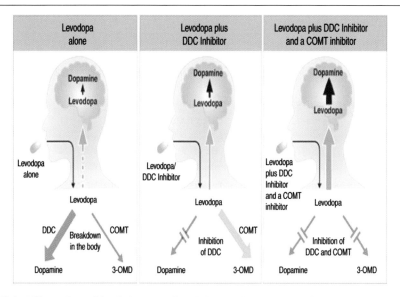

Figure 10.1: Effect of combined therapy of periphereal decarboxylase inhibitors and/or a COMT inhibitor with L-DOPA (levodopa).

peripheral inhibitors **[Tasmar]** will produce a 30–50% increase in L-DOPA half-life and a 25–100% increase in L-DOPA ensuring that more L-DOPA will reach the brain to be transformed to dopamine, **Figure 10.1**. Co-administration of L-DOPA with ascorbic acid may enhance its absorption, particularly in patients with poor GI absorption (Nagayama et al., 2004).

Recently, concern has been expressed that the use of L-DOPA might hasten the progression of the disease. In a randomized double blind controlled trial, 361 recently diagnosed Parkinsons' patients received COMT/L-DOPA, at varying doses, for a period of 40 weeks. The clinical data indicated that L-DOPA slowed disease progression as well as reducing the symptoms of the disease. In contrast, neuroimaging data showed that L-DOPA accelerated the loss of nigrostriatal dopamine nerve terminals or modified the dopamine transporter (Fahn et al., 2004). In recent years, the use of L-DOPA as a first line drug, particularly in young patients, has diminished because of its involvement in the generation of long-term motor complications and the possibility of neurotoxicity. Preliminary clinical studies have advocated that co-administration of nicotinic agonists with L-DOPA may have clinical advantages, in that the dose of L-DOPA can be reduced, but further clinical studies of PD patients are necessary.

Dopamine agonists **[Parlodel]**, **[Permax]**, **[Mirapex]** **[Requip]** were initially introduced to delay L-DOPA therapy. These drugs will retard the onset of dyskinesia but not motor fluctuations, while their co-administration with L-DOPA showed no added advantages (Ramaker and van Hilten, 1999; Ramaker and van Hilten, 2000). Apomorphine is a potent dopamine receptor agonist which needs to be administered subcutaneously because of its high first-pass metabolism by the liver (LeWitt, 2004). In small-scale pre-clinical studies it was shown that apomorphine was effective and safe for both inpatient and outpatient use (Frankel et al., 1990; Dewey et al., 2001). As yet this drug is not extensively used; the cost of such treatment, £10,000/year, may preclude its wide-spread clinical use (Clarke, 2002), although this may be offset by reductions in other expenses, such as residential care.

[Symmetrel] was initially investigated as an antiviral agent, but was also shown to decrease dopamine uptake, without causing appreciable changes in the release of the transmitter (Geldenhuys et al., 2004). [Symmetrel] may act synergistically with L-DOPA and is often used as a first line drug. In PD patients with advanced disease, its administration may reduce dyskinesias which is possibly due to the antagonism of specific glutamate receptors (Lange et al., 1997).

Selective dopamine blockers, such as clozaril and quetiapine, are effective in the treatment of psychosis and may be useful as an adjunctive to L-DOPA and dopamine agonists.

The use of these dopaminergic drugs is not without problems, side effects include nausea, sleepiness, dizziness, involuntary writhing movements and visual hallucinations. None of these drugs are effective long-term, as with time, the drugs will only be effective for a few hours, or become completely ineffective.

In the early sixties, anticholinergics were introduced to reduce tremor in Parkinson's disease patients which is caused by an imbalance between dopamine outputs and the intrinsic cholinergic innervation within the striatum. A review of randomized controlled trials of anticholinergic drugs, versus placebo or no treatment, in newly diagnosed or advanced PD patients, showed that benzhexol (mean dose 8–20 mg/day), bornaprine (8–8.25 mg/day) or benapryzine (200 mg/day) or orphenadrine and benztropine (no doses given for either) induced a significant improvement in motor function in comparison with baseline values (Katzenschlager et al., 2003). Currently the drug [Artane] is prescribed which has anticholinergic activity.

Metabotrophic glutamate receptors play a key role in striatal function and exert a profound modulatory role on the cholinergic inter-neuron excitability (Pisani et al., 2003). NMDA receptors trigger neurotoxicity, in part, mediated by increased synthesis and activation of nNOS. The excitatory amino acid antagonist riluzole is currently being assessed in clinical trials.

Excessive amounts of iron accumulate in the degenerating dopaminergic neurons of the substantia nigra and the noradrenergic neurons of the locus coeruleus. The source of this increase in iron is attributed to the degradation of the dopaminergic neurons containing iron-loaded neuromelanin as well as alterations in iron homeostasis. The role played by lactoferrin in contributing to this increasing iron burden in the SN remains unclear. Both MRI imaging and echogenicity will detect the augmented SN brain iron content (Gorell et al., 1995) and decreased putamenal and pallidial iron content with advanced disease (Ryvlin et al., 1995). Hence, its removal by iron chelators may reduce the inflammatory process, thereby, diminishing apoptosis and necrosis.

The use of desferrioxamine in the treatment of PD patients has not been advocated, since subcutaneous administration is required, and chelation therapy is not usually given to patients with reputed normal iron status. Therefore at this time there is an urgent requirement for the development of new orally bioactive chelating agents. The development of a new tridendate iron chelator, ICL670, for which clinical approval is currently being obtained for the treatment of thalassaemia patients, may be a potential therapeutic agent for PD patients. Extensive studies will be needed to ensure that iron is removed from specific brain areas and that the iron-chelated complex is not redistributed to other brain regions. Other molecules which have iron chelating properties as well as other beneficial effects include R-apomorphine, (Weinreb et al., 2003), VK-28, (5-[4-hydroxyethyl) piperazine-1-ylmethyl]-quiniline-8-ol) and the flavonoid polyphenols, e.g. (-)-epigallocatechin-3-gallate, in green tea (Mandel et al.,

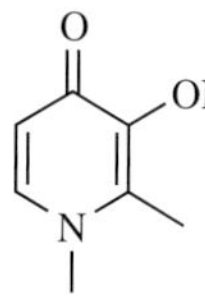

(3) Deferiprone (L1. CP20) 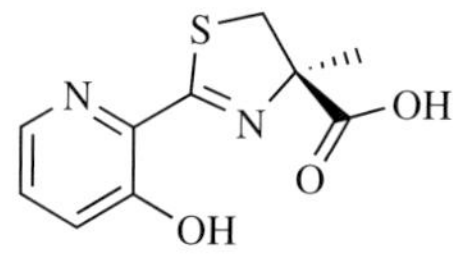   (4) Desferrithiocin

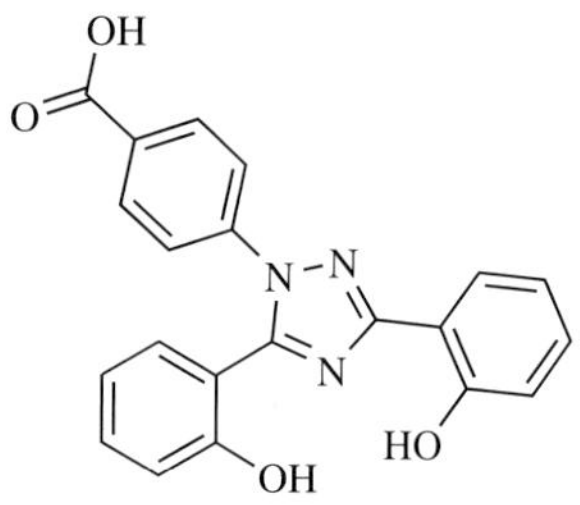

(5) ICL670A

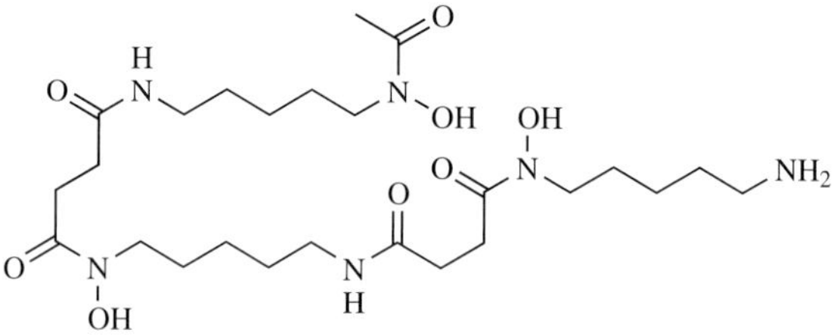

(9) Desferrioxamine (DFO)

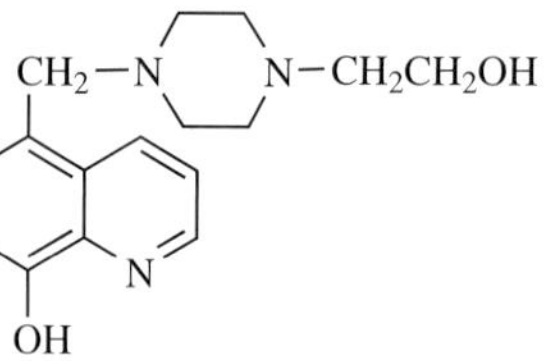

VK-28 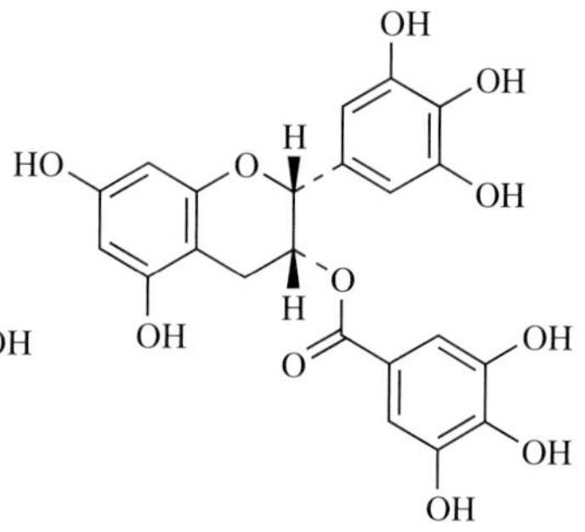   Epigallactocatechin-3 gallate

Figure 10.2: Iron chelators, past and future therapeutic agents for the removal of iron from neurodegenerative diseases where exceesive accumulation occurs. (**a**) bidendates, (**b**) tridendates, (**c**) hexadendates, (**d**) Epigallactocatechin-3-gallate (EGCG), (**e**) VK28.

2004), **Figure 10.2**. As yet, no clinical studies have commenced on the ability of these compounds to remove iron specifically from the SN in the brains of PD patients.

Oxidative stress has been put forward as one of the major causes of the nigral degeneration, such that its amelioration may retard the progression of the disease. An active inflammatory process will occur, with the induction of the transcription factor NFκB and of iNOS in brain glial cells (Ward and Ledeque, unpublished data). Increased CSF nitrite content was assayed in both untreated and treated PD patients in comparison with controls (Qureshi et al., 1995), while an increased NO signal in SN of PD patients was detectable by ESR in post-mortem samples (Shergill et al., 1996). Such increases in NO may have detrimental effects on a number of mitochondrial and cytosolic enzymes. Drugs which inhibit nNOS (7-nitroindazole) and iNOS (ginsenoside, one of the biological active ingredients of ginseng) (Chen et al., 2003) may help to prevent the destruction of dopaminergic neurons (Hantraye et al., 1996; Liberatore et al., 1999; Klivenyi et al., 2000).

Non-steroidal drugs, such as ibuprofen and aspirin, will primarily inhibit COX-1 (which is present in activated microglia) and COX-2, the rate limiting enzymes in prostaglandin synthesis and thereby inflammation. Whereas COX1 is constitutively expressed in most mammalian tissues, COX-2 is only expressed in certain tissues in response to inflammatory stimuli and is hence responsible for the elevated levels of prostaglandins found in inflammation (see Chapter 2). It therefore plays a role in the pathogenesis and selectivity of the PD neurodegenerative process. Both COX-2 and prostaglandin PGE_2 expression are upregulated within SN dopaminergic neurons of post-mortem PD specimens (Teismann et al., 2003). Furthermore, the release of PGE_2 from such affected neurons will promote the production of microglial-derived mediators, which in turn help in killing neurons. COX-2 inhibitors may be a useful adjunct therapy since they rapidly traverse the BBB. However, recent concern about their toxicity, via raised blood pressure and cardiovascular risks as well as changes in fatty acid synthesis, may preclude their use.

A range of cytoprotective enzymes are altered in the brains of PD patients. Our earlier studies failed to detect a reduction of α-tocopherol content in SN of PD (Dexter et al., 1992), thereby indicating that vitamin E supplementation may not yield any therapeutic advantage.

Glutathione content is depleted within the SN dopaminergic neurons, possibly due to increased γ-GT activity, and parallels the severity of the disease. Its replenishment might be of therapeutic advantage, either by increasing the synthesis of this tripeptide or by slowing its degradation. Administration of precursors of GSH metabolism, such as γ-glutamyl cysteine, or cysteine precursors, or GSH analogues, e.g. YM737, able to traverse the blood-brain barrier, may be of potential interest for further studies in PD (reviewed in Bharath et al., 2002).

The selegiline metabolite (a monoamine oxidase inhibitor), desmethylselegiline, reduces apoptosis by altering gene expression of SOD, Bcl-1, Bcl-xl, NOS and cJun, thereby preventing the progressive reduction of mitochondrial membrane potential in preapoptopic neurons (Ebadi and Sharma, 2003).

The increased activity of monoamine oxidase B in Parkinsonian brains will enhance oxidative metabolism of dopamine, **Figure 10.3**. such that the administration of a MAO B inhibitor, e.g. selegiline **[Eldepryl]**, will retard dopamine metabolism. A new melt tablet, Zydis selegiline, may exhibit less neurotoxicity. Second generation potent irreversible MAO B inhibitors, e.g. rasagiline (N-propargyl-1R-aminoindane), are now undergoing Stage III clinical trials (Youdim et al., 2005).

Techniques involving surgical intervention are currently being developed; experts believe that 1–10% of people with Parkinson's disease might be suitable for brain surgery. Fine needles, to which heat or radiofrequency is applied, are inserted into specific regions of the brain, e.g. the thalamus, the globus pallidus and subthalamic nucleus (subthalamotomy), to correct the movement disorders associated with PD. Such treatment has proved to be reasonably successful in the short term.

Intrastriatal transplants of fetal dopaminergic neurons may induce substantial and long lasting functional benefits in PD patients (Winkler et al., 2005), although all of the early studies were open label trials, i.e. small groups of patients received grafted embryonic human nigral neurons. However, recent double blind trials have questioned whether functional improvements reported were only marginal and that the primary end points were not achieved.

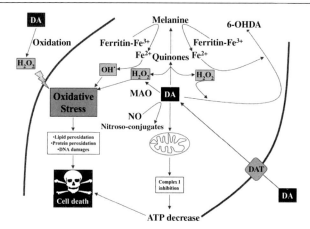

Figure 10.3: Role of monoamine oxidase in dopamine metabolism. Hypothetical mechanism of dopamine toxicity. Dopamine could induce catecholeminergic cell death by three main mechanisms, ROS generated by intra- or extracellular oxidation, hydrogen peroxide formed by the increased monamine oxidase activity, MAO, or direct inhibition of the respiratory chain. Reprinted from *Progress in Neurobiology*, Vol 65, Blum et al., Molecular pathways involved in the neurotoxicity of 6-OHDA, dopamine and MPTP: contribution to the apoptotic theory in Parkinson's disease, pp 135–172, Copyright 2001, with permission from Elsevier.

More recently, researchers have used the adeno-associated virus vector delivery system to insert the gene GAD into specific brain regions of PD patients. GAD is responsible for making GABA, which will be released by nerve cells thereby diminishing Parkinsonian-induced symptoms. In the first patient where this technique has been applied, an improvement of 20% was noted before administration of medication. It was predicted that an improvement of 60% might be possible when combined with low doses of anti-Parkinsonian drugs. Initially 12 PD patients with moderately advanced PD are being recruited into this study.

10.2 ALZHEIMER'S DISEASE

Unfortunately, a definitive diagnosis of Alzheimer's disease must await an autopsy, such that the search for sophisticated diagnostic tests will continue, e.g. brain scans, behavioural tests etc. Psychological testing generally focuses on memory, attention, abstract thinking, the ability to name objects, and other cognitive functions although the results of such tests do not easily distinguish between AD and other types of dementia.

The use of SPET (with carbon-labelled (R0-PK11195) to detect the peripheral benzodiazepine-binding site on activated microglia, has been used to identify inflammation in the entorhinal, tempoparietal and cingulated cortex of AD patients (Cagnin et al., 2001).

Drugs which reduce neurotransmitter degradation or diminish the inflammatory process may delay the symptoms and progression of the disease, **Table 10.2**. At present the therapy for AD is aimed at the pathological consequences of the disease, such as improving cognitive and behavioural symptoms, thereby improving the quality of life of these patients.

In later life, an active and socially integrated lifestyle protects against dementia and AD (Fratiglioni et al., 2004). An increased cortisol response to 'challenge' may be a risk factor associated with AD (Otte et al., 2005), although aging alone increases cortisol response, by almost 3 fold in women, when compared to men. Chronic stress is associated with hippocampal damage and impaired memory in humans. In a long term study, where detailed

Table 10.2: Current drug strategies for the treatment of Alzheimer's disease

Donepezil *(Aricept)*	Inhibits acetylcholinesterase
Rivastigmine (Exelon)	Inhibits acetylcholinesterase
Galantamine *(Reminyl)*	Inhibits acetylcholinesterase
	Enhances acetyl choline receptor

Name of active compound shown together with brand name in parentheses.

cognitive function information was collected from Catholic clergy during their retirement years, and whose brains were examined at post mortem to confirm AD, those considered to encounter high stress and anxiety during their later life span had twice the risk of developing AD (Wilson et al., 2004).

The fatty acid composition of neuronal cell membrane phospholipids reflects dietary intake. In animal models it has been shown that the ratio between omega-3 and omega-6 polyunsaturated fatty acids influences various aspects of serotoninergic and catecholaminergic neurotransmission as well as prostaglandin formation. Intervention trials in human subjects show that omega-3 fatty acids may have possible positive effects in the treatment of various psychiatric disorders (Haag, 2003).

β-secretase may be a candidate enzyme for directed inhibition to reduce Aβ. Since β-secretase needs a high cholesterol environment for its activity, lowering cholesterol concentration may reduce β-secretase activity (Passey, 2004), or alternatively binding it to an inhibitor drug to decrease its activity, **Figure 10.4**.

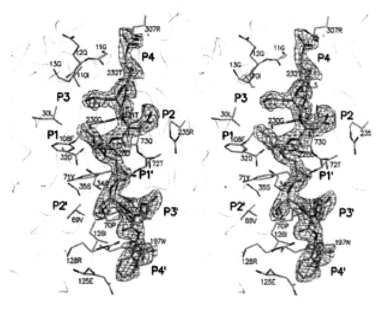

Figure 10.4: Stereoview of the electron density and subsite residues for OM00-3 bound to β-secretase; (from Hong et al., reprinted in part from *Biochemistry*, Vol 41, pp 10963–10969, Copyright 2002 American Chemical Society).

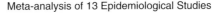

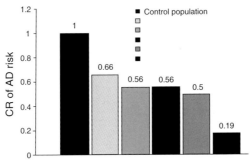

Figure 10.5: Epidemiological surveys of the use of anti-inflammatory therapy as a protective factor for AD (from Lema, 2002, reproduced with permission of Mark Lema). A meta analysis of 13 epidemiology surveys suggest that prolonged exposure to anti-inflammatory therapy confers a protective influence on the development of AD. Whether the variable was a diagnosis of arthritis or RA, or anti-inflammatory treatment with NSAI or both, the OR of a concomitant diagnosis of AD was less than 1.

Non-steroidal anti-inflammatory drugs (NSAIDs), such as aspirin, ibuprofen and indomethacin, may delay or prevent the onset of AD, **Figure 10.5**. For example, in a short term study (6 months), indomethacin (100–150 mg/day) provided slight but statistically significant improvement in a battery of cognitive tests in a group of aged individuals in contrast to the placebo group (Rogers et al., 1993) while a long term study of two years confirmed the protection of these drugs in preventing AD, which was calculated to be in excess of 50% (McGeer and McGeer, 2001). The main problem associated with long term administration of NSAIDs is the significant risk of stomach damage and gastrointestinal bleeding.

The recent introduction of an Alzheimer's disease vaccine, with the antibody $A\beta_{42}$ has not been successful due to brain inflammation caused by meningio-encephalitic presentation (Broytman and Malter, 2004). It is hoped that research will provide a better formulation and that it may be of use in people with a positive family AD history.

Abnormalities of a variety of neurotransmitter pathways, e.g. glutamatergic, adrenergic, serotonergic and dopamine, occur in AD. There is a selective loss of forebrain cholinergic neurons, such that drugs that enhance cholinergic activity in the synapses of the affected regions of the brain will be of therapeutic advantage. Anticholinesterase inhibitors, including tacrine, donepezil, **[Aricept]**, rivastigmine **[Exelon]** and galantamine **[Reminyl]**, induce modest memory and cognition improvements. However, a key body that guides Britain's NHS, the National Institute for Clinical Excellence (NICE), has concluded that such drugs are not appropriate for the treatment of AD, due to the expense of treatment, the lack of positive results from clinical studies and that the underlying progression of the disease continues.

NMDA receptor-mediated glutamate excitotoxicity plays a major role in $A\beta$-induced neuronal death. Early studies indicated that NMDA receptors might be a promising target for preventing the progression of AD. The NMDA antagonist memantine (1-amino adamantine derivative) was effective therapeutically, by inhibiting the neurotoxic functions of NMDA receptors (see Chapter 2) while physiological processes such as learning and memory were unaffected (Sonkusare et al., 2005). It has been approved for the treatment of moderate to severe AD patients in Europe.

Nicotinic receptors are markedly decreased in AD. Previous post-mortem observations that smokers' brains, in general, had more nicotinic receptors than non-smokers', led to the suggestion that smoking might be a protective factor for AD. Stimulation of nicotine receptors, via administration of nicotine and nicotine agonists e.g. ABT-418, improved acquisition and retention of verbal information and decreased errors in AD patients (Newhouse and Kelton, 2000).

The removal of iron, copper and zinc from specific brain regions may prevent brain $A\beta$ accumulation as well as disrupting preformed aggregates. Iron, zinc and copper induce $A\beta$ aggregation (see Chapter 4). In pre- and clinical trials, clioquinol, (an antibiotic and Zn/Cu chelator) induced a marked reduction of $A\beta$ deposition in APP transgenic mice after several months of treatment, and a reduction of $A\beta_{42}$ concentration in a placebo-controlled trial of AD patients with moderate to severe dementia. In addition, an increase in plasma zinc content and improvement in cognitive function, over a 24 week period, was recorded (Ritchie et al., 2003; Doraiswamy and Finefrock, 2004). Recently, clioquinol was withdrawn from use in Japan because of concerns of its association with myelo-optic neuropathy. There have been no reports of the use of specific iron chelating compounds in the treatment of AD which might reduce both inflammation and $A\beta$ formation.

Three mis-sense mutations in exon 17 of APP are reported to co-segregate in families with early onset of AD. These mutations may alter the structure of APP or may destabilize the stem of a putative IRE by inactivating this negative regulatory element (Zubenko et al., 1992).

The deposition of both plaques and tangles induces the inflammatory process, with the production of a variety of inflammatory cytokines, e.g. Il-1β TNF-α, iNOS, and induction of the transcription factor NFκB (Kaltschmidt et al., 1997), prostaglandins and free radicals, as well as infiltration of astrocytes and glial cells. IL-1β will further aggravate the immune/inflammatory response by promoting APP synthesis with the net result of more $A\beta$ production (Meda et al., 2001).

Non-steroidal anti-inflammatory drugs, NSAIDs, such as indomethacin, attenuate inflammatory reactions and protect against nerve cell death that results from the generation of free radicals. Many different NSAIDs have Alzheimer's-protective effects, including: ibuprofen (Motrin, Advil, Nuprin), naproxen (Naprosyn, Aleve, Anaprox), indomethacin (Indocin), meclofenamate (Meclomen) and possibly aspirin. NSAIDs will reduce the generation of free radicals from activated microglial cells. Some NSAIDs, ibuprofen, indomethacin, and sulindac sulphide, can lower toxic $A\beta$ levels by as much as 80%, independently of the inhibition of cyclooxygenase (COX) activity with a preferential increase of $A\beta_{38}$. The latter effect is possibly due to alterations in the activity of α- and β-secretase (Weggen et al., 2001). However, other studies where prostaglandin inhibitors have been used, i.e. diclofenac, which inhibits prostaglandin synthesis by interfering with the action of prostaglandin synthetase (Scharf et al., 1999), or prednisone (Aisen et al., 2000), showed no positive benefit in clinical studies of AD patients.

Chloroquine, the anti-malarial drug reduces the inflammatory stimuli by decreasing both tissue iron content and down-regulating NFκB activation in rat macrophages (Legssyer et al., 1999). However, a double blind parallel group multicentre trial of hydroxychloroquine for 18 months did not slow the rate of decline in minimal or mild AD (Van Gool et al., 2001) and showed no advantage, in comparison with placebo, with respect to quality of life and cognitive assessment. Antioxidants such as vitamins E and C might reduce the risk of Alzheimer's disease (Zandi et al., 2004) although no placebo-controlled clinical trails have been published.

In AD normal soluble cytoskeletal elements such as tau and neurofilaments are transformed into insoluble paired helical filaments. This is linked to the post-translational

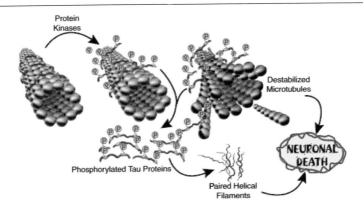

Figure 10.6: Hyperphosphorylated tau (from Calbiochem website, 2005, reprinted with permission from Merck Biosciences-Calbiochem).

change in Tau, primarily the hyperphosphorylation of Tau by a number of protein kinases, **Figure 10.6**, including cyclin-dependent kinase 5 (Cdk5) in conjunction with its neuron-specific activator p35. Inhibitors of Cdk5 may limit Tau phosphorylation. Hyperphosphorylation is ultimately linked with oxidative stress via the MAP kinase pathway and through activation of NFκB, **Figure 10.7**. Over-expression of interleukin-1 near amyloid plaques may promote the phosphorylation of tau protein, leading to the formation of neurofibrillary tangles (NFTs) and neuron death (Sheng et al., 2001). Tau phosphorylation inhibitors include cathepsin inhibitors, lithium, MAO kinase inhibitors and protein phosphatase 2A, but, as yet, there are no reported clinical studies of AD patients.

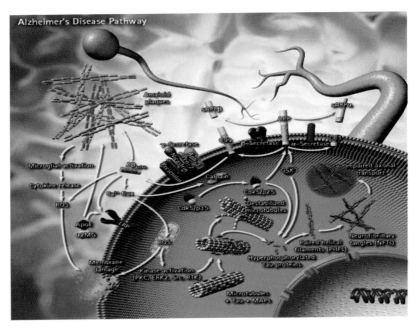

Figure 10.7: Formation of phosphorylated tau proteins. Phosphorylation is intimately tied to oxidative stress via MAP kinase pathway and via NFκB activation. Tau is a substrate for protein kinases including CaM kinase II, Cdk5 and MARK (from Calbiochem website, 2005, reprinted with permission from Merck Biosciences-Calbiochem).

An enzyme inhibitor that reduces cholesterol concentrations may be an appropriate treatment for AD. Inhibition of acyl-coenzyme A: cholesterol acyltransferase, an enzyme that controls storage of cholesterol, significantly reduced deposition of Aβ in a mouse model of AD. Preliminary studies of statins (cholesterol-lowering drugs) indicate that they may also play an important role in preventing or delaying Alzheimer's. Further studies are clearly warranted to ascertain the connection between cholesterol levels and the deposition of Aβ, although strict regard must be given to the known hepatotoxicity of statins.

Glycogen synthase kinase-3β, GSK-3β, a highly conserved ubiquitously expressed serine/threonine kinase protein kinase is involved in the signal transduction cascades of multiple cellular processes. High levels of GSK-3β are found in pre-tangles and in phosphorylated Tau-containing neurons. Beta-amyloid peptides activate GSK-3β indicating that this may be a key mechanism in AD pathogenesis. The development of GSK-3β inhibitors holds considerable promise for the reduction of Tau phosphorylation.

10.3 HUNTINGTON'S DISEASE AND OTHER POLYQ DISORDERS

Diseases caused by expanding CAG repeats coding for polyglutamine include; Spinal and Bulbar Muscular Atrophy (SBMA), the first to be discovered; Huntington's disease (HD), and one of the most actively studied; DentatoRubral and PallidoLuysian Atrophy (DRPLA), which is similar to HD; and several forms of Spino-Cerebellar Ataxia (SCA). Each is characterized by selective neuronal cell death in specific regions of the brain. While the exact areas affected in each disease differ, there is considerable overlap, including basal ganglia, brain stem nuclei, cerebellum, and spinal motor nuclei.

Huntington's disease (HD) is caused by polyglutamine (polyQ) expansion in the N terminus of the huntingtin protein (Chapter 5). The presence of polyQ stretches of ≥ 36 in huntingtin cause disease, whereas ≤ 35 do not. The longer the polyQ repeats, the earlier the onset, and the more severe the disease manifestations. Inclusions containing aggregates of huntingtin and ubiquitin are present in regions of the brain that degenerate, with a good correlation, between the length of the CAG repeat and the density of inclusions. The aggregates contain fibres and appear to have extensive β-sheet structure.

A recent review of double-blind, placebo-controlled trials of therapy for HD concluded that there is a tendency to concentrate on the motor aspects of the disorder, although the major problems are behavioural (Bonelli et al., 2004). Their recommendations are the drugs riluzole, olanzapine and amantidine for treatment of the movement disorders, selective serotonin reuptake inhibitors and mirtazapine for the treatment of depression, and atypical antipsychotic drugs for psychosis and behavioural problems.

Copolymer-1 has been granted a patent by the USA for protection from neurodegeneration and as an anti-inflammatory. Miraxion has completed one Phase III clinical trial for the treatment of Huntington's disease.

10.4 FRIEDREICH'S ATAXIA AND OTHER DISEASES LINKED TO NON-CODING TRIPLET REPEATS

Friedreich's ataxia, FRDA, the most common aut.somal recessive ataxia, is characterized by degeneration of large sensory neurons and spinocerebral tracts, cardiomyopathy and increased incidence of diabetes. It is caused by severely reduced levels of frataxin, a

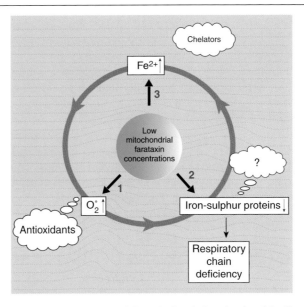

Figure 10.8: Consequences of decreased frataxin levels in mitochondria (from Durr, 2002).

mitochondrial protein necessary for iron incorporation into iron-sulphur clusters and haem biosynthesis, resulting in deficiency of iron-sulphur protein activity and increased mitochondrial iron overload, **Figure 10.8**. Its major neurological symptoms include muscle weakness, and ataxia, (loss of balance and co-ordination).

As our understanding of the function of frataxin (the consequences of its greatly decreased expression in FRDA patients and the availability of animal models of FRDA) increases, so we can hope to develop appropriate therapies. Since iron accumulation within the mitochondria was initially thought to play a major role in the pathogenesis of FRDA, it was suggested that iron chelation therapy could be useful. However, while most available chelators decrease intracellular iron, they do not remove mitochondrial iron, and may have important side effects (Delatycki et al., 2000). Furthermore, if the situation in man is similar to that in the animal models, the iron accumulation is a secondary event and not the pathological cause (Puccio et al., 2001). Nonetheless, the potential of iron chelators (notably analogues of 2-pyridylcarboxaldehde isonicotinoyl hydrazide) to target mitochondrial iron has been proposed (Richardson, 2003).

The hypothesis of oxidative stress in FRDA is supported by the similar clinical presentation caused by inherited deficiency of vitamin E (Ouahcki et al., 1995). Preliminary studies in an *in vitro* human heart homogenate model showed that, of known antioxidants, ascorbic acid is not protective, but idebenone, a short chain analogue of coenzyme Q10 (ubiquinone), does protect (Rustin et al., 2002). Idebenone is known to cross the blood-brain barrier (Nagy, 1999) and is available as a drug, Mnesis®. Encouraging results have been obtained in stabilizing or decreasing cardiac hypertrophy in FRDA patients with idebenone (Rötig et al., 2002; Dürr, 2002; Cooper and Schapira, 2003), but no positive effects on the neurological signs of FRDA have been observed. Co-administration with vitamin E could increase energy production in the cardiac and voluntary muscles of patients with FRDA.

Yet another possibility for therapy is to find pharmacological agents which will up regulate frataxin expression, even in the presence of the trinucleotide intron repeat.

Enhancement of FRDA gene expression in cell cultures by haemin and butyric acid has been demonstrated (Sarsero et al., 2003), as well as by the mitochondrial oxidative stress agent 3-nitropropionic acid (Turano et al., 2003).

But perhaps if, as is increasingly likely, the fundamental defect in FDA is in mitochondrial iron-sulphur cluster assembly, what we really require is some kind of surrogate iron-sulphur cluster assembly system with which to rescue mitochondria from their lack of iron-sulphur cluster formation consequent to their deficiency in frataxin.

Fragile X syndrome is the leading inherited form of mental retardation, caused by a defect in the fragile X mental retardation gene (FMR1), which is located near the end of the long arm of the X chromosome. It is caused by large methylated expansions of a CGG repeat in the FMR1 gene, leading to loss of expression of FMRP, an RNA-binding protein. FMRP is suggested to play a role in synaptic maturation and function.

10.5 PRION DISEASES

Prion diseases, often known as transmissible spongiform encephalopathies, are caused by conformational changes in a normal host glycoprotein, PrP^c, of unknown function, which is normally anchored in the plasma membrane. For reasons which remain unknown, PrP^c changes its protein folding to a form which has greatly increased β-sheet content, known as PrP^{Sc}, and it is this form which forms the aggregates which are typically found in intracellular inclusions in the various neurodegenerative diseases of animals and man.

The therapeutic focus (Mallucci and Collinge, 2005) can be directed at a number of levels. Intervention during the peripheral phase of prion propagation, before neuroinvasation has occurred, would allow the use of drugs that do not need to cross the blood-brain barrier. This would, however, necessitate early identification of infected individuals, which is not yet possible. Although tonsil biopsy can be used to diagnose variant CJD at an early stage (Hilton et al., 1998), it is not suitable for large scale screening, and a reliable diagnostic blood test for either PrP^{Sc} or another specific marker of the disease therefore remains a major research objective.

An alternative approach would be either to stabilize PrP^c itself, or to prevent PrP^c being transformed into PrP^{Sc} which should impede the formation of the mutant form. The potential for therapy based on drugs which would bind to PrP^c and stabilize its conformational state, thus preventing its transformation is clear, but unexploited. Similar approaches, using ligands which bind and maintain the stability of proteins in which mutations or altered conformation result in disease, have been successful for the central core of the tumour protein p53 (Foster et al., 1999) and the thyroid hormone transporter transthyretin, responsible for systemic amyliodosis (Klabunde et al., 2000).

10.6 AMYOTROPHIC LATERAL SCLEROSIS, ALS

Motor neurons are nerve cells which are located in the brain, brain stem and spinal cord and serve as controlling units and vital communication links between the nervous system and the voluntary muscles of the body. Messages from motor neurons in the brain (upper motor neurons) are transmitted to motor neurons in the spinal cord (lower motor neurons) and then forwarded to particular muscles. In ALS both the upper motor neurons and lower motor neurons degenerate and die, ceasing to send messages to the muscles, which gradually weaken and waste away (atrophy). The typical age of onset for ALS is between 50 and 60 years. Between 5–10% is inherited of which approximately 20% is due to an inherited defect in the Cu/Zn-superoxide dismutase, SOD-1. The cause of sporadic ALS remains unknown, although a multitude of both genes (**Table 8.1**) and pathways (**Figure 8.9**) have been identified which may be involved in the aetiology or contribute to the motor neuron degeneration. The clinical course is highly variable, although failure of the respiratory muscles is generally the fatal event and occurs within one to five years of disease onset. However, about 10% of ALS patients survive for 10 or more years.

Growth factors have long been considered as a therapy for motor neuron diseases, although human trials with neurotrophins, including insulin-like growth factor 1 (IGF-1) have shown no effect (Borasio et al., 1998) or only mild benefit (Lai et al., 1997). Similarly negative trials have been obtained with brain-derived growth factor (BDNF) (BDNF study Group, 1999) and ciliary neurotrophic factor (CNTF). Studies with the vascular endothelial growth factor (VEGF) in the SOD-1 mice model were successful in slowing the progression of the disease. However, the levels of VEGF are not reduced in ALS patients but were increased (Iizecka, 2004) or unaltered (Nygren et al. 2002) in post-mortem spinal cord samples or CSF, respectively.

For the future, IGF-1-producing virus injected into target muscles innervated by motor neurons in the cervical, thoracic and lumbar regions may be of promise (**Figure 10.9**). However, the poor understanding of the molecular basis for ALS has precluded the rational design of effective and safe treatments.

ALS patients have high levels of glutamate in the serum and spinal cord. Riluzole, a glutamate antagonist, is currently the only drug that has been approved for the treatment of

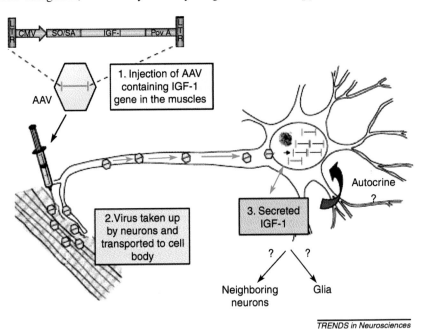

TRENDS in Neurosciences

Figure 10.9: Adeno-associated virus vector containing the IGF-1- producing gene is injected into target muscles innervated by motor neurons in the cervical, thoracic and lumbar regions to increase the synthesis of this neurotrophic growth factor in specific cells. Reprinted from *Trends in Neuroscience*, Vol 27, Boilée and Cleveland, Gene therapy for ALS delivers, pp 235–238, copyright 2004, with permission from Elsevier.

ALS. It provides only marginal therapeutic benefit, by decreasing the release of glutamate to prevent motor neuron damage, thereby delaying the decline in strength of limb muscles, but only prolongs survival by a few months (Lancomblez et al. 1996)

10.7 ACERULOPLASMINAEMIA

Aceruloplasminaemia is characterized by iron accumulation in the brain and in the visceral organs. The characteristic triad of retinal degeneration, diabetes mellitus (DM), and neurological disease is associated with movement disorders and ataxia. Aceruloplasminae-mia is an autosomal recessive disease of iron metabolism (Gitlin, 1998) associated with mutations in the ceruloplasmin gene, resulting in neurodegeneration of the retina and basal ganglia, and long-term accumulation of parenchymal iron similar to that in hereditary haemochromatosis resulting in diabetes, retinal degeneration and neurological symptoms. There is complete absence of serum ceruloplasmin which reflects specific mutations in the ceruloplasmin gene (Yoshida et al., 1995; Harris et al., 1995). However, in contrast to other iron overload symptoms, aceruloplasminaemia is unique in that the neurological manifesta-tions dominate the clinical picture, with all patients eventually succumbing to the effects of increased iron in the basal ganglia.

Early treatment with iron chelators can be useful in individuals with aceruloplasminaemia to diminish iron accumulation and to ameliorate symptoms. Treatment with desferrioxamine for 10 months in one patient was found to decrease brain iron stores, prevent progression of the neurological symptoms and decrease plasma lipid peroxidation (Miyajima et al., 1997). Chronic subcutaneous infusion of desferrioxamine was found to be remarkably effective in reducing hepatic iron overload in a female patient (Loreal et al., 2002).

10.8 MENKES DISEASE

Menkes disease is a neurodegenerative disease with X-linked recessive inheritance, in which defective intestinal absorption of copper results in copper deficiency in liver and brain. A milder form known as occipital horn syndrome is also found. The neurological disturbances, arterial degeneration and hair abnormalities can all be explained by a decreased activity of copper enzymes. The treatment accepted currently is parenteral administration of copper. When treatment is started in patients with classical Menkes disease above the age of 2 months, it does not improve the neurological degeneration. When the treatment is initiated in affected newborn babies, the neurological degeneration can be prevented in some, but not all, cases (Kodama et al., 1999). Moreover, early treatment cannot improve non-neurological problems, such as connective tissue laxity. Therefore, it seems that we should be searching for alternative therapies for Menkes disease and occipital horn syndrome.

10.9 WILSON'S DISEASE

Wilson's disease is an autosomal recessive inherited disorder of copper metabolism in which hepatic copper is neither excreted in the bile nor incorporated into ceruloplasmin and therefore accumulates to toxic levels in the liver. Although it was once considered fatal, identification of the Wilson's disease gene, the P-type ATPase, ATP7b, has resulted in better diagnosis. Initial treatment for symptomatic patients involves chelation therapy (Ala and Schilsky, 2004; Ferenci, 2004), aimed at mobilizing copper from the affected organs and promoting its excretion in the urine. The major chelating agent is d-penicillamine, which is quite effective but not without some side effects. Alternative chelating agents such as trientine and tetrathiomolybdate have also been successfully employed. Treatment of presymptomatic patients or maintenance therapy can also be accomplished with zinc. Zinc salts promote copper excretion by inducing the synthesis of metallothionein in the intestine, thereby blocking copper absorption from the gut, and have almost no side effects. They cannot be used as an initial treatment, but are very effective for maintenance therapy. In patients with acute liver failure, liver transplantation is the only hope for survival. Future cell-based and genetic therapies may provide a cure for this disorder.

10.10 MULTIPLE SCLEROSIS

Multiple sclerosis is a chronic progressive disease of the brain and spinal cord, where there is initially an inflammatory demyelinating process, which later develops into multiple sclerosis. Genetic and environmental factors, as well as stress, have been implicated in the aetiology of the disease, which by some unknown process have significant effects on the immune system. There is a significant hormonal influence, possibly oestriol, since the frequency of the disease declines during pregnancy.

A viral infection in genetically susceptible individuals, e.g. the cytomegalovirus and Epstein-Barr virus which have similar mimicry motifs, may modulate co-stimulatory signals thereby lowering the threshold for autoimmunity.

Pathologically the blood-brain barrier may become damaged, macrophages and T cells enter into the CNS, oligodentrocytes and myelin are destroyed, astrocytes and microglia undergo gliosis and axons become transected. Data from several biochemical and pharmacological studies indicate that free radicals participate in the pathogenesis of this disease. In the NWE region of Australia, the frequency of C282Y increased in MS cases because of its linkage disequilibrium with the ancestral DR15 susceptibility haplotype (Rubio et al., 2004). Although C282Y plays no independent role in predisposition to MS, this research highlights the fact that iron metabolism may play a role in the severity of MS.

The ultimate goal of drug therapies for MS is to reinforce immune tolerance to CNS antigens. Anti-inflammatory therapies show some promise although this may not retard the progression of the disease. Natalizumab, a humanized IgG4 monoclonal antibody has specificity for the α-chain of α4β1 integrin. Alpha4β1 integrin is expressed on activated monocytes and lymphocytes and mediates transendothelial migration and immune activation, particularly during CNF inflammation. Natalizumab blocks the interaction of α4β1 integrin with its ligands. In a six month randomized placebo controlled trial, monthly infusions of Natalizumab reduced both the neurological lesions and clinical relapses, although during the wash out period, both of these parameters returned to baseline values. It was concluded that Natalizumab altered the effector stage of the disease but not the immune process. Further clinical trails of this compound are close to completion, and if successful, may be marketed as a suitable therapy for MS. Interferon-β also has a modest clinical effect. Mitoxantrone, an anticycline-derived immunosuppressive drugs has been approved for the treatment of active MS. Its prolonged use is limited because of cariotoxic effects.

The use of cannabis to ameliorate some of the symptoms of MS has been the subject of considerable debate. There is evidence to suggest that muscle spasticity may be greatly reduced by using this drug, although the number of patients included in such trials was small. Since cannabis is a "schedule one drug" its use is associated with Misuse of Drugs Regulations and it is not possible to obtain it on prescription. A recently commenced clinical trial will recruit 660 patients with MS from the UK who have significant spasticity in some of their leg muscles and each patient will then be randomly allocated to one of three treatments: cannabis oil, tetrahydrocannabinol (a constituent of cannabis) or placebo capsules (containing only vegetable oil).

10.11 FUTURE DIRECTION FOR THERAPEUTIC AGENTS

Despite our increasing understanding of the biochemical pathways involved in the various neurodegenerative diseases, therapy is confined to the treatment of pathologies of each neurodegenerative diseases rather than their causes.

Metals play an important role in the neurodegeneration of many neurological diseases. Copper-containing proteins are associated with some of these diseases, Cu/Zn superoxide dismutase (amyotrophic lateral sclerosis), amyloid precursor protein (Alzheimer's disease), and prions (Creutzfeldt-Jakob disease) while iron is a prominent player in each of the neurodegenerative diseases, involved in the formation of aggregates, e.g. neuromelanin, as well as the exacerbation of inflammation.

Treatment strategies for PD in the future should include drugs which (a) restore mitochondrial function, specifically Complex 1, (b) delay or prevent the loss of dopaminergic neurons and (c) reduce oxidative stress. Up-regulation of cellular chaperones, such as Hsp70 and its co-chaperone Hps40, may ensure that protein folding and function are intact, and that there is normal processing by proteosomes. As already mentioned, the implantation of specific molecules into discrete brain regions, i.e. GAD, is beginning to show some success, although it should be emphasized that this technique is only treating the symptoms of the disease rather than its aetiology.

It is therefore anticipated that the development of "anti-amyloid" drugs that selectively target production of the highly amyloidogenic $A\beta_{42}$ species without inhibiting either COX activity or the vital physiological functions of γ-secretase will be of therapeutic importance for AD patients.

Good therapeutic targets for the treatment of AD would be alteration of β- and γ-secretase activity to limit the conversion of APP to $A\beta$. There has been progress in the development of secretase inhibitors, several target both PS1 and PS2. The use of antisense RNA to APP to reduce its expression and ultimately $A\beta$ aggregation, would appear to be a promising approach. As yet, iron chelators have not been administered to AD patients, which may reflect the lack of suitable molecules which will cross the BBB to chelate iron in specific brain regions. Naturally occurring compounds such as gingkolides may have some therapeutic application as in placebo-controlled trials similar therapeutic efficacy to that of tacrine and donepezil was found (Perry et al., 1999).

There is a growing body of opinion that indicates that insufficient neurotrophic support may play an important role in the pathology of several neurodegenerative diseases. Neurotrophic factors such as vascular endothelial growth factor, VEGF, brain-derived neurophic factor, BDNF, and insulin-like growth factor, IGF-1 and IGF-11, will influence the survival of neurons, and are currently being evaluated in clinical trials involving AD, PD and MS patients (Thoenen and Sendtner, 2002).

A greater understanding of the cellular function of many of these therapeutic targets will be needed since currently it is unknown whether additional cellular dysfunction and toxicity will ensue by the up-regulation and down-regulation of specific enzymes and molecules within the cell. Most importantly, such manipulations of cellular components will need to be focused and localized within precise brain regions. Currently there is considerable toxicity associated with many of the drugs used to treat the metal-based neurodegenerative diseases, which results in bad compliance and eventual withdrawal of some drugs.

REFERENCES

AD 2000 Collaborative Group (2004) *Lancet*, **363**, 2105–2115.
Aisen, P.S., Davis, K.L., Berg, J.D. Schafer, K. *et al.* (2000) *Neurology.*, **54**, 588–593.
Ala, A. and Shilsky, M.L. (2004) *Clin. Liver Dis.*, **8**, 787–805.
BDNF Study Group (1999) *Neurology*, **52**, 1427–1433.
Baldereschi, M., DiCarlo, A., Vanni, P., Ghetti, A. *et al.* (2003) *Acta. Neurol. Scand.*, **108**, 239–244.
Bharath, S., Hsu, M., Kaur, D., Rajagopalan, S. *et al.* (2002) *Biochem. Pharmacol.*, **64**, 1037–1048.
Blum, D., Torch, S., Lambeng, N., Nissou, M.-F. *et al.* (2001) *Prog. Neurobiol.*, **65**, 135–172.
Boilée, S. and Cleveland, D.W. (2004) *TRENDS Neurosci.*, **27**, 235–238.
Bonelli, R.M., Wenning, G.K. and Kafhammer, H.P. (2004) *Int. Clin. Psychopharmacol.*, **19**, 51–62.
Bonini, N.M. (2002) *Proc. Natl. Acad. Sci. USA*, **99**, 16407–16411.
Borasio, G.D. Robberecht, W., Leigh, P.N., Emile, J. *et al.* (1998) *Neurology*, **51**, 583–586.
Broytman, O. and Malter, J.S. (2004) *J. Neurosci. Res.*, **75**, 301–306.
Cagnin, A., Brooks, D.J., Kennedy, A.M. Gunn, R.N. *et al.* (2001) *Lancet*, **358**, 461–467.
Chen, X.C., Zhu, Y.G., Zhu, L.A., Huang, C. *et al.* (2003) *Eur. J. Pharmacol.*, **473**, 1–7.
Clarke, C.E. (2002) *J. Neurol. Neurosci. Psychiatr.*, **72**, i22–i27.
Coimbra, C.G. and Junqueira, V.B.C. (2003) *Braz. J. Med. Biol. Res.*, **36**, 1409–1417.
Cooper, J.M. and Schapira, A.H. (2003) *Biofactors*, **18**, 163–171.
Delatcycki, M.B., Williamson, M.B. and Forrest, S.M. (2000) *J. Med. Genet.*, **37**, 1–8.
Dewey, R.B., Hutton, J.T., LeWitt, P.A. and Factor, S.A. (2001) *Arch. Neurol.*, **58**, 1385–1392.
Dexter, D.T., Ward, R.J., Wells, F.J., Daniel, S.E. *et al.* (1992) *Ann. Neurol.*, **32**, 591–593.
Doraiswamy, P.M. and Finefrock, A.E. (2004) *Lancet Neurol.*, **3**, 431–434.
Dürr, A. (2002) *Lancet Neurol.*, **1**, 370–374.
Ebadi, M. and Sharma, S.K. (2003) *Antioxid. Redox Signal*, **5**, 319–335.
Fahn, S., Oakes, D., Shoulson, I., Kieburtz, K. *et al.* (2004) *New Eng. J. Med.*, **351**, 2498–2508.
Ferenci, P. (2004) *Metab. Brain Dis.*, **19**, 229–239.
Ferraz, H.B., Quagliato, E.A.B., Rieder, C.R.M. *et al.* (2004) *Braz. J. Med. Biol. Res.*, **36**, 1409–14117.
Foster, B.A., Coffey, H.A., Morin, M.J. and Rastinejad, F. (1999) *Science*, **286**, 2507–2510.
Frankel, J.P., Lees, A.J., Kempster, P.A. and Stern, G.M. (1990) *Neurol. Neurosurg. Psychiatry*, **53**, 96–101.
Fratiglioni, L., Paillard-Borg, S. and Winblad, B. (2004) *Lancet Neurol.*, **3**, 343–353.
Geldenhuys, W.G., Malan, S.F., Murugesan, T., Van der Schyf, *et al.* (2004) *Bioorg. Med. Chem.*, **12**, 1799–1806.
Gitlin, J.D. (1998) *Pediatr. Res.*, **44**, 271–276.
Gorell, J.M., Ordidge, R.J., Brown, G.G. Deniau, J.C. *et al.* (1995) *Neurology*, **45**, 1138–1143.
Haag, M. (2003) *Can. J. Psychiatry*, **48**, 195–203.
Hantraye, P., Brouillet, E., Ferrante, R., Palfi, S. *et al.* (1996) *Nat. Med.*, **2**, 1017–1021.
Harris, Z.L., Takahashi, Y., Miyajima, H., Serizawa, M. *et al.* (1995) *Proc. Natl. Acad. Sci. USA*, **92**, 2539–2543.

Hellenbrand, W., Seidler, A., Boeing, H., Robra, B.P. *et al.* (1996) *Neurology*, **47**, 636–643.

Hilton, D.A., Fathers, E., Edwards, P., Ironside, J.W. *et al.* (1998) *Lancet*, **352**, 703–704.

Hong, L., Turner III, R.T., Koelsch, G., Shin, D. *et al.* (2002) *Biochem.*, **41**, 10963–10967.

Iizecka, J. (2004) *Clin. Neurol. Neurosurg.*, **106**, 289–293.

Kaltschmidt, B., Uherek, M., Volk, B., Baeuerle, P.A. *et al.* (1997) *Proc. Natl. Acad. Sci. USA*, **94**, 2642–2647.

Katzenschlager, R., Sampaio, C., Costa, J. and Lees, A. (2003) *Cochrane Database Syst. Rev.* CD003735.

Klabunde, T., Petrassi, H.M., Oza, V.B., Raman, P. *et al.* (2000) *Nature Struct. Biol.*, **7**, 312–321.

Klivenyi, P., Andreassen, O.A., Ferrante, R.J., Lancelot, E. *et al.* (2000) *Neuroreport*, **11**, 1265–1268.

Kodama, H., Murata, Y. and Kobayashi, M. (1999) *Pediatr. Int.*, **41**, 423–429.

Lai, E.C. *et al.* (1997) *Neurology*, **49**, 1621–1630.

Lancomblez *et al.* (1996) *Lancet*, **347**, 1425–1431.

Lange, K.W., Kornhuber, J. and Riederer, P. (1997) *Neurosci. Biobehav. Rev.*, **21**, 393–400.

Legssyer R., Ward R.J., Crichton R.R. and Boelaert J. (1999) *Biochem. Pharmacol.*, **57**, 907–911.

Lema, M.J. (2002) *Cleve. Clin. J. Med.*, **69**, S 176–184.

LeWitt, P.A. (2004) *Neurology*, **23**, S8–S11.

Liberatore, G.T., Jackson-Lewis, V., Vukosavic, S., Mandir, A.S. *et al.* (1999) *Nat. Med.*, **5**, 2213–2216.

Loreal, O., Turlin, B., Pigeon, C., Moisan, A. *et al.* (2002) *J. Hepatol.*, **36**, 851–856.

McGeer, P.L. and McGeer, E.G. (2001) *Neurobiol Aging*, **22**, 799–809.

Malucci, G. and Collinge, J. (2005) *Nature Rev. Neurosci.*, **6**, 23–34.

Mandel, S., Weinreb, O., Amit, T. and Youdim, M.B. (2004) *J. Neurochem.*, **88**, 1555–1569.

Meda, L., Baron, P. and Scarlato, G. (2001) *Neurobiol. Aging.*, **22**, 885–893.

Miyajima, H., Takahashi, Y., Kamata, T., Shimizu, H. *et al.* (1997) *Ann. Neurol.*, **41**, 404–407.

Nagayama, H., Hamamoto, M., Ueda, M., Nito, C. *et al.* (2004) *Clin. Neuropharmacol.*, **27**, 270–273.

Nagy, Z. (1990) *Arch. Gerontol. Geriatr.*, **11**, 177–186.

Newhouse, P.A. and Kilton, M. (2000) *Pharm. Acta. Helv.*, **74**, 91–101.

Nygren, I., Larsson, A., Johannsson, A. and Askmark, H. (2002) *Neuroreport*, **13**, 2199–2201.

Otte, C., Hart, S., Neylan, T.C., Marmar, C.R. *et al.* (2005) *Psychoneuroendocronol.*, **30**, 80–91.

Ouahchi, K., Arita, M., Kayden, H. Hentati, F. *et al.* (1995) *Nat. Genet.*, **9**, 141–145.

Passey (2004) *Neurology*, **12**, 700-.

Perry, E.K., Pickering, A.T., Wang, W.W., Houghton, P.J. *et al.* (1999) *J. Pharm. Pharmacol.*, **51**, 527–534.

Pisani, A., Bonsi, P., Centonze, D., Gubellini, P. *et al.* (2003) *Neuropharmacol.*, **45**, 45–56.

Powers, K.M., Smith-Weller, T., Franklin, G.M. *et al.* (2003) *Neurology*, **60**, 1761–1766.

Puccio, H., Simon, D., Cossée, M., Criqui-Filipe, P. *et al.* (2001) *Nat. Genet.*, **27**, 181–186.

Qureshi, G.A., Baig, S., Bednar, I., Sodersten, P. *et al.* (1995) *Neuroreport*, **6**, 1642–1644.

Ramaker, C. and van Hilten, J. (1999) *Parkinson. Rel. Disord.*, **5**, 82.

Ramaker, C. and van Hilten, J. (2000) *The Cochrane Library*.

Richardson, D.R. (2003) *Expert Opin. Investig. Drugs*, **12**, 235–245.

Ritchie, C.W., Bush, A.L., Mackinnon, A., Macfarlane, S. *et al.* (2003) *Arch. Neurol.*, **60**, 1678–1679.

Rogers, J., Kirby, L.C. and Hempelman, S.R. (1993) *Neurology*, **48**, 626–632.

Rötig, A., Sidi, D., Munnich, A. and Rustin, P. (2002) *TRENDS Mol. Med.*, **8**, 221–224.

Rubio, J.P., Bahlo, M., Tubridy, N. Stankovich, J. *et al.* (2004) *Hum. Genet.*, **114**, 573–580.

Rustin, P., Rötig, A., Munnich, A. and Sidi, D. (2002) *Free Radic. Res.*, **36**, 467–469.

Ryvlin, P., Broussolle, E., Piollet, H., Viallet, F. *et al.* (1995) *Arch. Neurol.*, **52**, 583–588.

Scharf, S., Mander, A., Ugoni, A. Vajda, F., McGinness, J.M. *et al.* (1999) *Neurology*, **53**, 197–201.

Sarsero, J.P., Li, L., Wardan, H., Sitte, K. *et al.* (2003) *J. Gene Med.*, **5**, 72–81.

Sheng, J.G., Jones, R.A., Zhou, X.Q. *et al.* (2001) *Neurochem. Int.*, **39**, 341–348.

Shergill, J.K., Cammack, R., Cooper, C.E., Cooper, J.M. *et al.* (1996) *Biochem. Biophys. Res. Commun.*, **228**, 298–305.

Sonkusare, S.K., Kaul, C.L. and Ramarao, P. (2005) *Pharmacol. Res.*, **51**, 1–17.

Teismann, P., Vila, M., Choi, D.K., Tieu, K. *et al.* (2003) *Ann. N. Y. Acad. Sci.*, **991**, 272–277.

Thoenen, H. and Sendtner, M. (2002) *Nat. Neurosci.*, **5**, 1046–1050.

Tsai, C.H., Lo, S.K., See, L.C. *et al.* (2002) *Clin. Neurol. Neurosci.*, **104**, 328–333.

Turano, M., Tammaro, A., De Biase, I., Lo Casale, M.S. *et al.* (2003) *Neurosci. Lett.*, **350**, 184–186.

Van Gool, W.A., Weinstein, H.C., Scheltens, P.K., Walstra, G.J.M. (2001) *Lancet*, **358**, 455–460.

Ward, R.J., Lallemand, F. and De Witte, P. (2005) *Alcohol Res.*, **9**, 273–278.

Wilson, R.S., Evans, D.A., Bienias, J.L., Mendes de Leon, C.F. *et al.* (2004) *Neurology*, **63**, 941–.

Winkler, C., Kirik, D. and Bjorklund, A. (2005) *Trends Neurosci.*, **28**, 86–92.

Weggen, S., Eriksen, J.L., Das, P., Sagi, S.A. *et al.* (2001) *Nature*, **414**, 212–216.

Weinreb, O., Mandel, S. and Youdim, M.B. (2003) *Ann. N. Y. Acad. Sci.*, **993**, 351–361.

Youdim, M.B., Bar, A.O., Yogev-Falach, M., Weinreb, O. *et al.* (2005) *J. Neurosci. Res.*, **79**, 172–179.

Yoshida, K., Furihata, K., Takeda, S., Nakamura, A. *et al.* (1995) *Nat. Genet.*, 267–272.

Zandi, P.P., James, C.A., Ara, S. *et al.* (2004) *Arch. Neurol.*, **61**, 82–88.

Zubenko, G.S., Farr, J., Stiffler, J.S., Hughes, H.B. *et al.* (1992) *J. Neuopathol. Exp. Neurol.*, **51**, 459–463.

11

Animal Models of the Various Neurodegenerative Diseases

As we move into the 21st century, the use of transgenic mice, where the expression of specific genes can be modulated, has tremendously advanced our knowledge of the function and biological role of specific proteins. In addition, such animal models can be used to test potential symptomatic or disease-modifying therapies for specific neurodegenerative diseases. Careful interpretation of such results is required, before their extrapolation to the human situation, where a multitude of other factors may also contribute to the specific neurodegenerative disease. Other non-human primate models still need to be developed which will more closely parallel the genetic and neuro-anatomical make-up of man.

11.1 PARKINSON'S DISEASE ANIMAL MODELS

Alpha-synuclein is crucial for dopamine neuronal viability as a presynaptic regulator of dopamine release. Over-expression of WT α-synuclein in the mouse model decreases striatal dopamine as well tyrosine hydroxylase activity, induces motor performance impairment, but microscopy reveals no α-synuclein fibrils or loss of dopamine neurons (Giasson et al., 2002), **Table 11.1**. Increased levels of cytosolic α-synuclein were present in many brain regions of mice which expressed a mutant of α-synuclein, e.g. A30P (hA30P-SYN) (Kahle et al., 2000), or A53T-SYN (Giasson et al., 2002; van der Putten et al., 2000), which are visualized microscopically as diffuse soluble protein. In addition, the transgenic mouse A53T-SYN did show α-synuclein inclusions together with a loss of dopaminergic nerve terminals in the basal ganglia (a hallmark feature of PD) (Masliah et al., 2000). All of these mouse models expressing a mutant of α-synuclein showed motor performance impairment. The α-synuclein knock-out mouse has decreased striatal dopamine function (Abeliovich et al., 2000).

Gene delivery via associated viruses has two major advantages over transgenic mice, firstly the over-expression of the gene is site specific and secondly it can be induced in adult or aged animals. In one study, adeno-associated virus (AAV) delivery vector with A30P-SYN induced Lewy neuritis, fibrillar α-synuclein accumulation and a 53% loss in dopamine

Metal-based Neurodegeneration: From Molecular Mechanisms to Therapeutic Strategies   R. R. Crichton and R. J. Ward
© 2006 John Wiley & Sons, Ltd

Table 11.1: Transgenic models of Parkinson's disease

A. Mouse and rats

Transgenic

1) Wild type SYN	Intranuclear and cytoplasmic α-synuclein inclusions
	Transgene product in many brain regions including SN
2) Mutant human α-synuclein	
A30P (hA30P-SYN)	Diffuse cytosolic accumulation of α-synuclein
A53T-SYN	Diffuse cytosolic accumulation of α-synuclein
	Staining of motor neuron
	Motor performance decline
	Axonal damage and muscle atrophy
3) Parkin	
Knock out	Levels of dopamine are increased in the limbic brain areas
	Levels of dopamine transporter protein reduced.
4) Viral vectors	
i) Adeno–associated virus, AAV	
A30P-SYN	Lewy neuritis
	Fibrillar α-synuclein
	Loss of dopamine neurons
A53T-SYN	Transient alteration in dopaminergic phenotype
	Nigrostriatal axonal pathology
ii) Lentiviral system, LV	
Wild type SYN	Selective loss of dopamine neurons
A30P-SYN	Selective loss of dopamine neurons
A53T-SYN	Selective loss of dopamine neurons

B. Drosphilia melanogaster

Mutant α-synuclein

A30P	Filamentous intraneuronal inclusions resembling LBs.
	Dopaminergic neurons with LBs show age-dependent degeneration

neurons but no motor impairment (Klein et al., 2002). Transient alterations in rat dopaminergic phenotype and nigrostriatal axonal pathology were evident after AAV delivery vector with A53T-SYN (Kirik et al., 2002) while there was a selective loss of dopaminergic neurons after transfection of the rats with a lentiviral system, LV, with either human WT or one of the mutants, A53T-SYN or A30P-SYN (La Bianco et al., 2002).

The pathology in α-synuclein transgenic mice can be enhanced by the simultaneous expression of a human APP transgene (Masliah et al., 2000). There is an age-dependent loss of cholinergic neurons in the nucleus basalis and the caudoputamen which parallels the loss of cholinergic neurons in this brain region in AD patients. Between 3 and 20 months the accumulation of human α-synuclein in the neocortex was 1.6x higher in hSYN/APP mice compared with hSYN mice.

Expression of wild type, the mutant A30P-SYN or A53T-SYN in the fruit fly *Drosophila*, induced formation of filamentous intraneuronal inclusions resembling LB, which induced dopaminergic degeneration, **Figure 11.1**. Locomotor dysfunction was also reported (Feany and Bender, 2000).

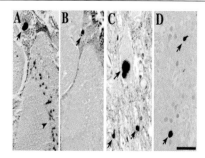

Figure 11.1: Alpha-synuclein Lewy-like body aggregates in flies and in Parkinson's disease patient tissue. (**a** and **b**) Brain sections through a 20-day-old fly expressing wild-type α-synuclein show Lewy-body-like aggregates in the cortex (arrow) and neutropil (arrowheads) which immunolabel for α-synuclein (**a**) and fly stress-induced HSP70 (**b**). (**c** and **d**) Tissue from substantia nigra of a patient with Parkinson's disease showing Lewy bodies and Lewy pathology which immunolabel for α-synuclein (**c**) and fly stress-induced HSP70 (**d**). Reprinted, with permission, from Bonini, *Proc Natl Acad Sci* 99, pp 16407–16411, Copyright 2002, National Academy of Sciences, USA.

The mouse mutant Quaking is a spontaneously occurring parkin knock-out mouse which shows a complete loss of parkin co-regulating gene in addition to parkin (Lockhart et al., 2004). Experimentally induced knock-out parkin mouse shows inhibition of both amphetamine-induced dopamine release and glutamate neurotransmission, in addition to motor and cognitive deficits (Itier et al., 2003). Adaptive changes in the nigrostriatal system occur in parkin mutant mouse where the increased dopamine levels in the limbic brain areas may be due to the decrease in dopamine transporter protein. Levels of GSH levels are increased in the striatum and fetal mesencephalic neurons which may indicate a protective mechanism to protect dopamine neurons. Levels of synphilin-1 and α-synuclein are unaltered in these mice (Goldberg et al., 2003). Over-expression of parkin generates aggresome-like inclusions in the ubiquitin/proteasome system in UPS-compromised cells (Ardley et al., 2004).

Chronic rotenone or paraquat administration to mice inhibits mitochondrial complex I (**Figure 11.2**) and induces degeneration of dopaminergic nerve cells in the SN resulting in hypokinesia and rigidity. Nerve cell death is preceded by the appearance of LB-like inclusions that are immunoreactive for both α-synuclein and ubiquitin (Betarbet, 2000).

The neurotoxins, MPTP and 6-OHDA, induce many of the pathological changes that occur in PD and are widely used as animal models of this disease. MPTP induces nigral degeneration in several species including rat, mouse, dog, cat and monkey (reviewed by Blum et al., 2001). Essentially, MPTP will cross the BBB to be converted by monamine oxidase B in glial cells to the active form, 1-methyl-4-phenylpyridinium, MPP^+, (**Figure 11.3**). MPP^+ will accumulate in dopaminergic cells prior to its entry into mitochondria, via an energy-dependent mechanism. MPP^+ will inhibit mitochondrial activity leading to decreases of ATP levels, thereby inducing cell death. MPTP induces changes in iron metabolism, up-regulating the expression of both transferrin and lactoferrin receptors, as well as increasing SN free iron content. Oxidative stress occurs which is associated with cellular changes of both GSH-GSSG ratio and cytoprotective enzymes. The loss of GSH may reflect the inactivation of glutathione peroxidase (Bharath et al., 2002). Primates treated with MPTP develop motor disturbances resembling those seen in idiopathic PD, including bradykinesia, rigidity and postural abnormalities.

6-Hydroxydopamine, 6-OHDA, a hydroxylated analogue of dopamine, is unable to cross the BBB, such that intracerebral administration is necessary to destroy nigral dopaminergic neurons in the striatum, the SN or the ascending medical forebrain bundle (reviewed by

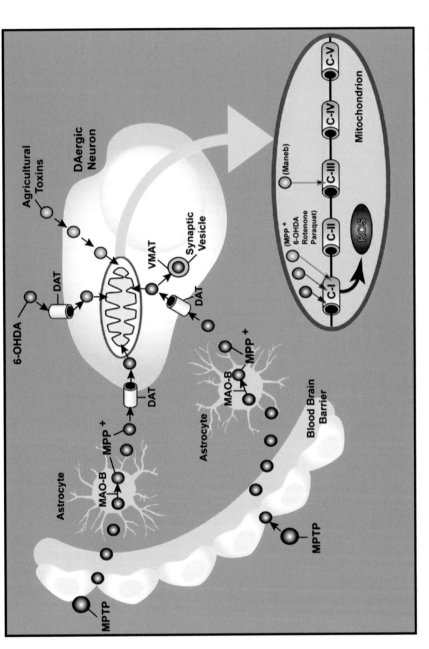

Figure 11.2: Schematic overview of molecular and intracellular pathways of dopaminergic neurotoxins in animal models of Parkinson's. MPTP crosses the BBB and is taken up by astrocytes, MPP$^+$ is formed, catalysed by MAO-B. MPP$^+$ is then transported into dopaminergic neurons via the dopamine transporter, DAT. Inside the mitochondria, 6-OHDA is taken up by DAT and accumulates in the mitochondria. Mitochondrial electron transfer chain 1–1V is represented in the box and shows the site of toxicity of the neurotoxins. Reprinted from *Cell Tissue Research*, Vol 318, 2004, pp 215–224, Classic toxin-induced animal models of Parkinson's disease, 6-OHDA and MPTP, Schober, A., with kind permission of Springer Science and Business Media.

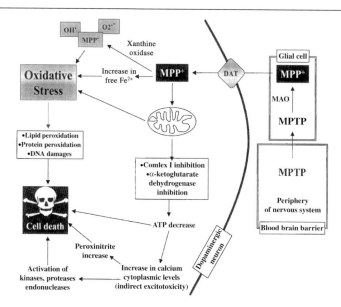

Figure 11.3: Hypothetical mechanism of MPTP toxicity. MPTP is injected peripherally, crosses the BBB and is transformed by glial MAO into the active compound MPP$^+$. Once inside the cells, MPP$^+$ will inhibit the respiratory chain and cause oxidative stress, both triggering cell death. Reprinted from *Progress in Neurobiology*, Vol 65, Blum et al., Molecular pathways involved in the neurotoxicity of 6-OHDA, dopamine and MPTP: contribution to the apoptotic theory in Parkinson's disease, pp 135–172, Copyright 2001, with permission from Elsevier.

Blum et al., 2001), **Figure 11.4**. The iron content of SN and striatum is increased, which will participate in Fenton chemistry to generate reactive oxygen species to exacerbate the lesion. The importance of iron in the exacerbation of this lesion can be verified by the facts that iron-deficient rats are resistant to 6-OHDA-induced damage (Shoham and Youdim 2000; Levenson et al., 2003), and iron chelating agents can prevent 6-OHDA-induced deleterious effects (Ben Shachar et al., 1991).

Both the MPTP and 6-OHDA animal models are extensively used to screen new molecules which may be of promise in delaying the progression of PD, **Figure 11.5**. For example, the MAO inhibitors clorgyline and pargyline can produce dose-dependent neuroprotection against the dopaminergic neurotoxicity of MPTP (Kurosaki et al., 2002), while 7-nitroindazole, an nNOS inhibitor, or pargyline, can protect against MPTP-induced depletion of tyrosine hydroxylase. Selective adenosine A2a receptor antagonists, such as the piperazine derivatives, [1,2,4] triazol [1,5-a][1,3,5]triazine derivative were effective in minimizing the 6-OHDA damage in the rat model (Vu et al., 2004).

The inflammatory processes induced by MPTP have been investigated in various knock-out mouse models. Both caspase-11 (Chapter 2) and nNOS knock-out mice were more resistant to MPTP-induced neurotoxicty than wild type, indicating that MPTP neurotoxicity is mediated via activation of the caspase-11 as well as NO-induced inhibition of various mitochondrial complexes and NO-induced dopamine depletion (Furuya et al., 2004; Ebadi and Sharma, 2003).

It has been difficult to engender an animal model which shows selective accumulation of iron in specific brain regions. In normal rats the blood-brain barrier will normally restrict iron uptake. However, the orally administered compound 3,5,5-trimethyl hexanoyl

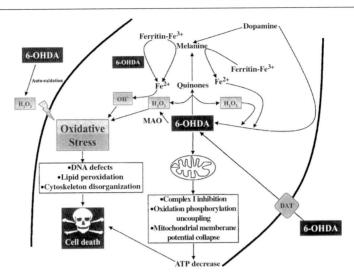

Figure 11.4: Hypothetical mechanism of 6-OHDA toxicity. This is induced by (a) reactive oxygen species generated by intra- or extracellular auto-oxidation, (b) hydrogen peroxide formation induced by MAO activity or (c) direct inhibition of the mitochondrial respiratory chain. Reprinted from *Progress in Neurobiology*, Vol 65, Blum et al., Molecular pathways involved in the neurotoxicity of 6-OHDA, dopamine and MPTP: contribution to the apoptotic theory in Parkinson's disease, pp 135–172, Copyright 2001, with permission from Elsevier.

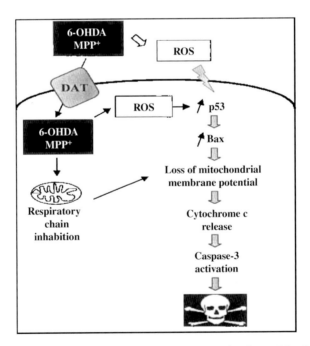

Figure 11.5: Hypothetical molecular pathways leading to apoptosis triggered by 6-OHDA and MPP$^+$ (from Blum et al., 2001). Reprinted from *Progress in Neurobiology*, Vol 65, Blum et al., Molecular pathways involved in the neurotoxicity of 6-OHDA, dopamine and MPTP: contribution to the apoptotic theory in Parkinson's disease, pp 135–172, Copyright 2001, with permission from Elsevier.

ferrocene, will rapidly traverse the BBB, its iron moiety being concealed between the two aromatic rings, releasing and increasing the iron content of various brain regions, including SN, cerebellum and cerebral cortex, by approximately 50%, after four weeks of administration. This animal model has been utilized to test the ability of a range of chelators to reduce brain iron content (Ward et al., 1995).

In our early study (Ward et al., 1995) intraperitoneal injection of either bidendates (e.g. deferripone), or the hexadendate, desferrioxamine, iron chelators (**Figure 10.2**) to ferrocene-loaded rats, reduced excess iron from a variety of brain regions, with no apparent adverse effect on brain iron metabolism. Dopamine metabolism was adversely affected by both groups of chelators in this study. Tridendates (e.g. desferrithiocein) were also efficient at removing iron from various brain regions in the ferrocene-loaded brain and most importantly did not interfere with dopamine metabolism (Dexter et al., 1999).

Both 6-OHDA and MPTP increase the iron content of the substantia nigra par compacta (SNPC) in rats and monkeys (Hall et al., 1992; Oestreicher et al., 1994, Temlett et al., 1994; Goto et al., 1996; Mochizuki et al., 1994) and in mice (Lan and Jiang, 1997a; Lan and Jiang, 1997b). Various factors are implicated in iron accumulation, which include up-regulation of DMT1 (Youdim et al., 2004; Wang et al., 2003a), down-regulation of transferrin receptors, loss of IRP-2 activity and iron release from ferritin (Mandel et al., 2003).

Many compounds have been evaluated in these two animal models for their iron chelating properties and anti-inflammatory action. In the MPTP model, desferal (Lan and Jiang, 1997a; Lan and Jiang, 1997b) and green tea catechin [(-)-epigallactocatechin-3-gallate) all show iron chelating properties and, as such, are potent neuroprotective agents against MPTP. DFO administration either by ICV pretreatment or IP prevented 6-OHDA-induced changes in dopaminagic neurons, (Youdim et al., 2004; Shachar et al., 2004). Another iron chelator, the lipophilic VK-28, (5-[4-hydroxyethyl) piperazine-1-ylmethyl]-quiniline-8-ol), **Figure 10.2**, traverses the blood-brain barrier to prevent 6-OHDA-induced MDA production, without altering dopamine metabolism.

IRP-1 knock-out mouse shows misregulation of iron metabolism in the kidney and brown fat, the two tissues in which the endogenous expression of IRP-1 exceeds that of IRP-2 (Meyron-Holtz et al., 2004). IRP-2 knock-out mice have dysregulated iron metabolism associated with cytosolic iron accumulation (possibly as ferritin) in neuronal axons, particularly striatum, which in normal circumstances has high IRP-2 content (la Vaute et al., 2001). Degradation of ferritin occurs in lysosomes, which could lead to increased release of free iron and oxidative damage. These animals exhibit movement disorders which include ataxia, tremor and bradykinesia. Mice that are homozygous for a targeted deletion of IRP-2 and heterozygous for a targeted deletion of IRP-1 (IRP+/-IRP2-/-) develop severe neurodegeneration, characterized by widespread axonopathy and vacuolization in several brain regions, including SN. Ultimately neuronal cell bodies degenerate in the SN activating microglia. Mice show gait and motor impairment when axonopathy is pronounced (Smith et al., 2004).

MnSOD knock-out mouse has reduced mitochondrial SOD activity, mSOD (by 50%), but no reduction of either CuZnSOD or glutathione peroxidase activities. Increased oxidative damage occurs in mitochondria, e.g. protein carbonyls and 8-hydroxydeoxyguanosine, which is associated with mitochondrial degeneration and extremely shortened life span, 2 weeks. CuZnSOD knock-out mice show perturbation of cellular antioxidant defence mechanisms but no evidence of neurodegeneration. Over-expression of CuZnSOD in mice increased enzyme levels 10 fold, in both myocytes and endothelial cells. An enhanced ability to combat a superoxide burst induced by experimental ischaemic damage was evident in these mice, therefore preventing functional damage, although there was no information on neurological function where excessive superoxide ions may be generated.

Both rodent and primate models have been utilized to investigate the use of different viral vector systems to deliver a gene to specific brain regions. Initially, dopamine synthesizing enzymes and GDNF were used but abandoned because of the unpredictable responses as well as uncertain consequences of their long term use. More latterly, AAV vectors expressing two isoforms of glutamic acid decarboxylase, GAD (which synthesize the major inhibitory neurotransmitter, GABA) have been infused into the subthalmic nucleus, and yielded encouraging results (reviewed in During et al., 2001).

11.2 ALZHEIMER'S DISEASE

Two histopathological hallmarks are crucial for the post-mortem diagnosis of AD, the extra cellular deposition of neuritic plaques, Aβ, and the intracellular aggregation of neurofibrillary tangles, NFT, composed of hyperphosphorylated cytoskeletal protein tau.

There has been considerable success in the development of such transgenic animals with these hallmark features of AD (**Table 11.2**). However, the reader should be reminded that

Table 11.2: Transgenic models of Alzheimer's disease

1. Mutant βAPP	
PDAPP	Diffuse and neuritic plaques and dystrophic neuritis/inflammation
Tg2576	Diffuse and neuritic plaques and dystrophic neuritis/inflammation
APP23	Diffuse and neuritic plaques and dystrophic neuritis/inflammation
CRND8	Diffuse and neuritic plaques and dystrophic neuritis/inflammation
2. Mutant PS1 and PS2	
PS1m146L	Selectively increase $A\beta_{42(43)}$, but no abnormal pathology
PS2n1411	Selectively increase $A\beta_{42(43)}$, but no abnormal pathology
Mutant PS1 + mutant βAPP	
PSAPP	Accelerated Aβ deposition
PS1M146L + Tg2576	Accelerated Aβ deposition
Mutant PS2 + mutant APP (Swe)	
PS2N1411 + APP (Swe) (K670N, M671L) (PS2APP)	Aβ deposition and inflammation
3. Tau-based transgenics	
JNPL3	NFT pathology
FTDP-17	Tau excluded from tau filiaments APP increased as well as $A\beta_{42}$ 5–7 fold
Tau + mutated APP	
JNPL3 + Tg2576	Aβ deposition and NFT pathology
4. Combined models of PD and AD	
hAPP + SYN	Locomotor deficits at 6 months linked to α-synuclein. Deficits in spatial learning and memory correlated with hAPP/β-amyloid expression. Age dependent loss of cholinergic neurons.

less than 5% of AD cases are caused by mutant proteins; the occurrence of AD is predominantly sporadic. Transgenic mice expressing single or multiple mutant proteins, PDAPP, Tg2576, APP23 and CRND8, develop diffuse neuritic plaques, dystrophic neuritis as well as inflammation but no NFT pathology. Tg2576 transgenic mice (mice which over-express the Swedish mutation in the human amyloid precursor protein 695) demonstrate a reduction in cell proliferation in the dentate gyrus of the hippocampus in comparison with non-transgenic litter mates. Isolation stress decreased hippocampal cell proliferation as well as accelerating the age-dependent deposition of $A\beta_{42}$, indicating that the magnitude of this impairment can be modulated by behavioural interventions (Dong et al., 2004).

BACE1 knock-out mice do not generate $A\beta$ and show no physical abnormalities even at 14 months (Luo et al., 2003). The presenilins, PS1 and PS2 are tightly linked to γ-secretase-mediated cleavage and probably constitute part of the γ-secretase complex. PS1 may have either inherent γ-secretase activity or act as a co-factor for γ-secretase Mice expressing mutant PS1, presenilin genes, selectively increase $A\beta_{42}$, but show no abnormal pathology (Duff et al., 1996). Crossing the mutant PS1 line (PS1m146L) with Tg2576, increases $A\beta$ deposition in the cerebral cortex and hippocampus in a shorter time period than the single transgenic Tg2576 mice. Interestingly, behavioural changes were apparent before $A\beta$ deposition (Holcomb et al., 1998). However, as these mice aged, non-fibrillar $A\beta$ deposits were detectable in regions not normally associated with AD (Gordon et al., 2002). Fibrillar $A\beta$ deposits were restricted to cortical and hippocampal regions and did not increase after 12 months. The transgenic mouse line PS2APP, which over-expresses mutant forms of human PS2 (N1411) and human βAPP (K670N, M671L), develops severe cerebral amyloidosis in the neo- and limbic cortices, including the hippocampal and amygdala (Grayson Richards et al., 2003). After 8 months the PS2APP mice show a range of cognitive defects (significant impairment in the acquisition of spatial learning, reduced platform site crossings, and increased float time) which was associated with $A\beta$ deposits and inflammation in two brain regions, the subiculum and frontolateral (motor and orbital) cortex. Cells obtained from PS1/PS2 double knock-out mice have no γ-secretase activity.

There are relatively few tau-based transgenics, e.g. JNPL3 (Lewis et al., 2000). The crossing of JNPL3 with Tg2576 mice results in the double transgenic mouse TAPP which exhibit both amyloid plaques and NFT pathology (Lewis et al., 2001), **Figure 11.6**. FTDP-17 tau double transgenic mice (expressing the Swedish mutation of APP and tau protein containing 3 mutations linked to chromosome 17, FTDP-17) showed increases in tau phosphorylation at serine S262 and S422 as well as sarkosyl insoluble polymers and wider tau filament in comparison with that of the single transgenic model (Perez et al., 2005). These results suggested that $A\beta$ could facilitate tau phosphorylation and tau aberrant aggregation.

Neuronal cells express a deubiquitylating enzyme, ubiquitin carboxy-terminal hydrolase-1, UCH L1 which associates and co-localizes with monoubiquitin and elongates ubiquitin in neurons (see Chapters 2 and 5). In the gad mouse, in which the function of UCH-L1 is lost (a deletion of a genomic fragment including exons 7 and 8 of UCH-L1), neurons contain a reduced level of monoubiquitin. Over-expression of UCH-L1 in mice increases ubiquitin levels (Osaka et al., 2003).

There is considerable evidence for abnormal metal homeostasis in AD. The presence of the 5'UTR in the APP transcript may indicate that APP is a metalloprotein. Iron chelation has been proposed as a possible therapeutic approach for the treatment of AD. Indeed, as already stated in Chapter 4, APP was selectively down regulated in response to iron chelation (Rogers et al., 2002). Chelation may also prevent the iron-induced inflammation as well as $A\beta$ aggregation. The therapeutic advantages of various chelators, such as clioquinol

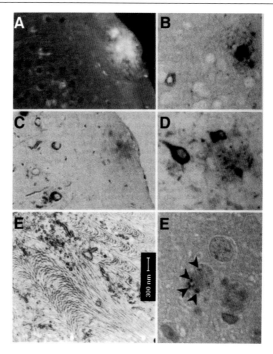

Figure 11.6: NFTs and amyloid plaques in TAPP mice. (**A** and **C**) Adjacent sections of entorhinal cortex viewed with thioflavin-S fluorescent microscopy (A) or Gallyas silver stain (C) show both amyloid plaques and NFTs in female TAPP mice. (**B** and **D**) Amyloid plaques are immunostained with a rabbit antibody to $A\beta42$ and double-immunostained with mouse antibodies to tau. In (B), a tangle-specific mAb ($A\beta39$) identifies a NFT (left) but no neurites in the plaque. In (D), double staining of a diffuse amyloid deposit in the frontal cortex shows local phospho-tau (PG5) immunoreactivity in neurons and neuronal cell processes associated with the plaque. (**E**) Ultrastructural studies of entorhinal NFTs reveal aggregates of criss-crossing straight filaments that are about 20 nm in diameter. (**F**) Granulovacuolar bodies (arrowheads) are detected in neurons in the amygdala, entorhinal cortex, and subiculum with phospho-tau antibodies (TG3). Mice were aged 9.5 to 10.5 months. Magnifications: (A) and (C), 200×; (B), (D), and (F), 400×. Reprinted with permission from Lewis et al., *SCIENCE* 293: 1487–1491. Copyright 2001 AAAS.

(copper chelator) desferioxamine (iron chelator) as well as polyphenols, e.g. EGCG and curcumin (a constituent of tumeric) (Baum and Ng, 2004), should be assessed in suitable animal models, for as yet there are no details of changes in iron metabolism in any of these transgenic AD animal models.

The genes for both amyloid precursor protein (APP) and Cu-Zn superoxide dismutase (SOD-1) reside on chromosome 21. Double-transgenic APP-SOD-1 mice show severe impairment in learning, working and long-term memory. In APP-SOD-1 mice, APP accumulated as membrane-bound high molecular weight species such that APP cleavage products do not increase and secreted APP levels were unchanged. However, severe morphological damage with lipofuscin accumulation and mitochondria abnormalities were identified in aged APP-SOD-1 (Harris-Cerruti et al., 2004).

Good therapeutic targets to ameliorate the production of $A\beta$, would be to decreases APP production or to inhibit either β- or γ-secretase. Binding of the phosphotyrosine binding domain of the neuronal protein X11a/mint-1 to the C-terminus of APP will inhibit its catabolism to $A\beta$, possibly by impairing its trafficking to sites of active γ-secretase complexes (King et al., 2004). In transgenic mice expressing mutant human APP, insertion of slow-release pellets of aceyl-coenzymeA:cholesterol acyltransferase, ACAT, inhibitors under the skin reduced the amyloid plaques after 2 months (Kovacs et al., 2004) Although these inhibitors are unsuitable for clinical use, the recent development of other ACAT inhibitors for cardiovascular disease (which are already in phase III clinical trials) may be appropriate for palliative treatment of AD. Progress in the development of γ-secretase inhibitors has been made with the identification of multiple classes of potent γ-secretase inhibitors which target both PS1 and PS2 (Vassar, 2004) However, further studies are needed to examine whether interference with the γ-secretase pathway may be potentially toxic to other cellular processes (Alves da Costa et al., 2004). The β-secretase inhibitors memapsin 2 and ibuprofen (possibly a β-secretase inhibitor) decreased levels of Aβ in brains of transgenic mice Tg2576 (Chang et al., 2004).

As already stated in Chapter 5 there is growing amount of evidence that cdk5 deregulation is involved in the pathogenesis of Alzheimer's disease. Transgenic mice over-expressing p25 show tau phosphorylation (Ahlijanian et al., 2000; Cruz et al., 2003). Bi-transgenic mice, that inducibly over-express human p25 under the control of the CamKII promoter, display progressive brain atrophy, significant neuronal loss and extensive astro-gliosis that strongly correlates with p25 expression (Cruz and Tsai 2004). Crossing mice expressing p25 under the control of the neuron-specific enolase promoter with mice containing a tau mutation (P301L-tau), (NSE-p24-P301L-tau) transgenic mice, resulted in enhanced formation of neurofibrillary tangles compared with the P301L-tau transgenic mice, confirming the role of cdk5 to initiate and affect tau pathology **(Figure 4.13)**.

Glial cells isolated from ApoE knock-out mice exhibit enhanced production of several pro-inflammatory markers in response to treatment with Aβ and other stimuli by comparison to wild type mice (LaDu et al., 2001). It was hypothesized that apoE receptors translate the presence of extra-cellular Aβ into cellular responses.

Nicotine administration to transgenic mice significantly reduced $Aβ_{42}$ plaques as compared to sucrose-administered controls (Nordberg et al., 2002). Direct nicotine injection into rat hippocampus elevated nerve growth factor (NGF) and enhanced the production and release of acetyl choline (Rattray, 2001).

11.3 HUNTINGTON'S DISEASE AND POLYQ

Mouse and rat models have been developed for the study of the polyQ-repeat diseases to reflect different aspects of these diseases (Beal and Ferrante, 2004). A transgenic HD mouse model expressing human huntingtin (Htt) exon 1 protein with ≈150 polyQs demonstrated that truncated mutant Htt was sufficient to cause an HD-like phenotype (Mangiarini et al., 1996). N-terminal fragments of mutant huntingtin form toxic protein aggregates in neurons, ultimately leading to neuronal dysfunction and death. There are three categories of mouse models – those which express full-length mutant human huntingtin, those that express a truncated form of the human protein and those with CAG repeats inserted into the murine gene (Beal and Ferrante, 2004). There is, however, no consensus as to which type of mouse model is the best model of human HD since there have been few clinical trials of treatments in humans on which to base comparisons.

Some investigators have chosen to study polyQ diseases in simpler organisms such as *Drosophila* (Marsh and Thompson, 2004) and *Caenorhabditis elegans* (Voisine and Hart, 2004). Studies in the *Drosophila* model have shown that a tandem repeat of the polyglutamine binding peptide (QBP1), previously identified from combinatorial peptide phage display libraries, significantly suppresses polyQ aggregation and neurodegeneration (Nagai et al., 2003).

A number of therapeutic strategies have been envisaged for the treatment of polyQ disorders, which have been tested in a number of organisms, as well as in cultured cells and brain slices. Since polyQ-dependent aggregation is clearly indicated as a cause of neurodegeneration, high-throughput cellular screening assays have been used to identify small-molecule inhibitors of polyQ aggregation. Promising candidate molecules can then be validated in mammalian cellular and animal models. Using such an approach, four primary chemical scaffolds have been identified as aggregation inhibitors, including a potent compound (IC50 = 10 nM) which had long-term inhibitory effects on polyQ aggregation in HD neurons (Zhang et al., 2005). This compound suppressed neurodegeneration *in vivo* in a *Drosophila* HD model, strongly supporting an essential role for polyQ aggregation in HD pathology. Aggregation can also be inhibited in a model neuronal cell line by modified single-stranded oligonucleotides (Parekh-Olmedo et al., 2004).

Another promising avenue of approach is presented by the observation that nuclear inclusions containing polyQ-expanded huntingtin recruit the transcriptional cofactor CREB(cAMP response element-binding protein)-binding protein (CBP) (Jiang et al., 2003). Histone acetylation/deacetylation is a master regulator of gene expression, and CBP is just one of several histone acetyl transferases whose transferase activities are inhibited by polyQ-huntingtin (Steffan et al., 2001). Indeed, reduced levels of acetylation of histones are found in cells expressing polyQ-huntingtin, and this effect can be reversed by inhibitors of histidine deacetylase (HDAC). Further, inhibitors of HDAC arrest polyQ-dependent neurodegeneration in *Drosophila* models of HD (Steffan et al., 2001), and more recently it has been shown that the HDAC inhibitors ameliorate neurological phenotypes in mouse models of HD (Hockly et al., 2003) and SBMA (Minamiyama et al., 2004).

AAV vector-mediated gene delivery of either brain-derived neurotrophic factor or glial cell line-derived neurotrophic factor was shown to be neuroprotective in a rat model of HD (Kells et al., 2004).

11.4 FRIEDREICH'S ATAXIA

Complete absence of frataxin in the mouse is embryonic lethal (hence the difficulty to create an animal model – in Friedreich's ataxia **some** frataxin is **always** produced, such that knock-out animal models cannot reproduce the human condition).

Several mouse models have been developed for Friedreich's ataxia. Complete inactivation of the FTR gene leads to embryonic lethality without iron accumulation (Cossée et al., 2000). In contrast, when mice, which had a 230 GAA repeat within the frataxin gene, were crossed with frataxin knock-out mice, viable double heterozygous mice were obtained which did not develop anomalies of motor coordination (Miranda et al., 2002). Subsequently, in view of the likelihood that mutations in the frataxin gene might not result in a diseased phenotype during the relatively short life-span of mice, mouse models were developed with tissue-targeted complete frataxin deficiency, which gave a rapidly progressive disease (Puccio et al., 2001). Viable animals developed cardiac hypertrophy, sensory neurone dysfunction and decreased activities of iron-sulphur proteins, notably in complexes I, II and II of the respiratory chain (Puccio et al., 2001). In a mouse model with isolated cardiac disease, iron-sulphur enzyme deficiency occurred at 4 weeks of age, prior to cardiomyopathy and significant accumulation of mitochondrial iron was observed at a terminal stage (Seznec et al., 2004). Using a similar gene-targeting approach, two mouse models for FRDA have been obtained which clearly show a slowly progressive neurological degeneration, with many of the prominent neurological features of FRDA (Simon et al., 2004). These animal models represent an excellent model for testing potential drugs. For example, ibedenone delays the onset of cardiac dysfunction without correcting the deficit in Fe-S enzymes in the mouse cardiac model of FRDA (Seznec et al., 2004).

11.4.1 Fragile X Mental Retardation Disease

Animal and *Drosophila* models of fragile X syndrome have been developed (Bakker and Oostra, 2003), the first in order to have an experimental tool closer to man in which potential therapeutic agents could be tested, the second to try to understand what exactly the role of FMRP is in neuronal development.

Since FMRP is an RNA binding protein, gene therapy in Fmr 1 knock-out mice using adenovirus vectors would seem to be a promising therapeutic approach (Ratazzi et al., 2004). It has been suggested that such knock-out mice have a defect in the expression of GABA receptors (D'Antuono et al., 2003), which could be a useful marker of restored FMRP function following gene transfer. The use of *Drosophila* as a model has shown that the fly homologue of FMRP plays an important role in regulating neuronal architecture and synaptic differentiation (Pan et al., 2004), and may be involved in direct interactions with components of the RNA interference pathway in this organism (Siomi et al., 2004).

Spinocerebral ataxias are a diverse group of rare, slowly progressive neurological diseases, which affect the cerebellum and its related pathways: they have few animal models and share no reliable biomarkers (Perlman, 2003).

11.5 PRION DISEASES

Prion diseases affect a large number of animal species, from the first to be recognized, scrapie in sheep, to man. The main common features are the presence of spongiform degenerative changes and the ability of transmission by inoculation into animals, including primates (Gajdusek et al., 1966) and rodents (Zlotnik and Rennie, 1965; Chandler, 1961). Indeed, many of the rodent models use the scrapie prion as infectious agent rather than one of the human variants of this class of diseases. There are, however, many animal models of the prion diseases. In the mouse alone, in addition to wild type mice infected directly with other animal prions, and knock outs for the mouse prion, transgenic mice expressing hamster, human, bovine, ovine and mouse prion proteins have all been developed (reviewed in Baron, 2002).

Some of these experimental models, particularly in hamsters and mice have served to demonstrate the major role of a post-translationally modified form of a host-encoded ubiquitously expressed neuronal protein, called the prion protein (PrP^c), which appears closely associated with, if not identical to, the infectious agent (Prusiner, 1982; Oesch et al., 1985) This abnormal form of the PrP^c (PrP^{Sc}), which accumulates in the infected tissues, is insoluble in non-denaturing detergents, and relatively resistant to proteinase K degradation.

Homozygous PrP^c knock-out mice showed no overt developmental or behavioural abnormalities (Büeler et al., 1992; Manson et al., 1994)[1], and when challenged intracerebrally with prions (Büeler et al., 1993; Weissmann et al., 1993) they not only lacked any clinical signs of scrapie, they did not appear to harbour any infectivity or protease resistant PrP, indicating that ablation of PrP^c abolished prion replication and propagation.

Mice which are heterozygous for PrP^c have remarkably mild symptoms of scrapie, despite high amounts of PrP^{Sc} and infectivity in their brains. In a model of forced release of prions into PrP^c-deficient host brain, neither clinical signs of scrapie disease nor pathological evidence of neuronal damage were observed, despite detectable levels of PrP^{Sc} and infectivity in the host brain (Brandner et al., 1996). The infected neurografts instead accumulated prions and underwent progressive neurodegeneration. That high levels of prion can accumulate without development of clinical signs of neurodegeneration is reinforced by the observation that no clinical signs develop in immunodeficient mice, which have been peripherally challenged by prions (Klein et al., 1997; Brown et al., 1997).

Another major finding in the experimental transmission of prion diseases, which has been followed up particularly in mice models is the 'species barrier', which limits, and in some cases prevents, the interspecies transmission of these diseases. When mice are inoculated with infected tissue from another species, variable but long incubation periods are observed at primary passage (Chandler, 1961), which can exceed the lifetime of the mouse (Dickinson et al., 1975). In marked contrast, the incubation period shortens considerably following inoculation of the brain of affected mice to other mice (Bruce, 1996). The 'species barrier' has been largely explained using transgenic mice. Three transgenic mouse lines were produced harbouring a Syrian hamster (Ha) prion protein (PrP) gene; all expressed the cellular HaPrP isoform in their brains. Inoculation of one of these mice lines, or of hamsters with Ha prions caused scrapie within 75 days; non-transgenic control mice failed to develop scrapie after greater than 500 days (Scott et al., 1989). Inoculation with mouse-derived prions resulted in the formation of exclusively mouse prions, and inoculation with hamster prions resulted in exclusive formation of hamster prions (Prusiner et al., 1990). The hamster PrP differs from the mouse PrP by only 16 of its 254 amino acid residues. Since these classic studies, several transgenic experiments have confirmed the relationship between the sequence of the prion protein and the specificity of transmission, although some studies have led to the suggestion that a species-specific protein factor is necessary for prion susceptibility (reviewed in Chien et al., 2004).

It has become clear that proteins can serve as genetic elements and that prions are more widespread in biology than previously thought. In particular the discovery of prions in yeast (Wickner, 1994) has furnished genetically and biochemically more tractable systems for studying prion behaviour and the mechanism of conformation-based inheritance and infection (Wickner et al., 2001; Serio and Lindquist, 2001). The yeast prion systems also show barriers to propagation analogous to that seen with mammalian prions. A model which integrates prion strains, species barriers and the physical principles that govern protein misfolding has been proposed recently (Chien et al., 2004).

Passive immunization with anti-prion antibodies can prevent peripheral prion replication and blocks disease progression in peripherally infected mice (Heppner et al., 2001; White et al., 2003). However, since antibodies do not readily cross the blood-brain barrier, no

---

[1] An apparent contradiction in which PrP knock-out mice suffered loss of Purkinje cells from 70 weeks of age (Sakaguchi et al., 1996) was shown to be due to ablation not of PrP, but to activation of *doppel*, a gene 16kD downstream from the PrP locus (Rossi et al., 2001).

protective effect was observed in intracerebrally infected mice. PrP^c knock-out mice are protected against prion disease, and the constitutive lack or acquired depletion of PrP^c is tolerated. The prospect of using an appropriately targeted viral vector system to deliver interfering RNA which could silence PrP^c is attractive, but would require effective CNS penetration.

Finally, preventing the accumulation of PrP^{Sc}, the disease-associated form of prion protein, in prion-infected cells would be an attractive option. A number of molecules such as polyanionic compounds, like pentosan polysulphate (PPS), the dye Congo red, amphotericin B, porphyrins and phenothiazine derivatives are active in cell cultures (reviewed in Mallucci and Collinge, 2005). However, they do not significantly prolong survival in mice with central nervous system prion infection, although intraventricular infusion of PPS prolonged the incubation time and decreased abnormal prion protein deposition and neurodegenerative changes in scrapie-infected mice (Doh-ura et al., 2004). In contrast, depleting endogenous neuronal PrP^c in mice with established neuroinvasive prion infection reversed early spongiform change and prevented neuronal loss and progression to clinical disease (Mallucci et al., 2003). This occurred despite the accumulation of extraneuronal PrP^{Sc} to levels seen in terminally ill wild type animals. Thus, the propagation of non-neuronal PrP^{Sc} is not pathogenic, but arresting the continued conversion of PrP^c to PrP^{Sc} within neurons during scrapie infection prevents prion neurotoxicity. Chemicals that affect the endocytosis, exocytosis intracellular trafficking and deradation of proteins, and in particular PrP may also be effective. Amphotericin is reported to delay prion disease in hamsters although it apparently has little effect in humans.

11.6 AMYOTROPHIC LATERAL SCLEROSIS, ALS

There are many animal models of motor neuron degeneration, which range from chronic aluminium toxicity in rodents to spinal muscular atrophy in cows. However, the majority of research into this disease has focused on mouse models of ALS. Although mutant SOD-1 is not present in sporadic ALS, there are striking similarities in both the pathology and clinical presentation between familial and sporadic ALS. As already stated, a small percentage of cases of ALS are caused by dominantly inherited mutations of SOD-1, such that the development of animal models based on such mutants might help to gain an insight into the mechanisms of the disease.

Although there are more than 100 mutations in human SOD-1, three have been well characterized in transgenic mouse models, namely G85R, G37R and G93A. The mutant protein is ubiquitously expressed and the transgenic animals are all characterized by ubiquitin-positive, intracellular aggregates in motor neurones and astrocytes (for further information see Bruijn et al., 2004). SOD-1-mediated toxicity in ALS is not due to a loss of SOD function (some mutant enzymes retain full dismutase activity), but due to some other toxic effect, as yet unknown. Transport along the extended axons is impaired in SOD-1 mutants that correlates with the development of the motor neuron disease.

Variable results have been obtained in animal models which over-express wild type SOD-1, either having no effect or accelerating the lesion. SOD-1 null mice do not develop motor neuron disease while removal of normal SOD-1 genes from mice that develop motor neuron disease as a result of expressing a SOD inactive mutant (SOD-1/G85R) did not affect onset or survival.

The evidence that mitochondria are important targets for damage in such SOD-1 mutants remains controversial. Vacuolated mitochondrial remnants have been identified in spinal motor neurons of mice with mutant SOD-1 but this was not confirmed in other rodent models (reviewed in Bruijn et al., 2004). The administration of either creatine (Klivenyi et al., 1999) (which may enhance energy storage capacity and inhibit opening of the mitochondrial transition pore), or of minocycline (Van Den Bosch et al., 2002; Zhu et al., 2002) (a derivative of tetracycline thought to inhibit activation of microglia as well as blocking cytochrome c mitochondrial release) will slow the progression of the disease by a few weeks in mouse models.

Neurofilaments are the most abundant structural proteins in many types of mature motor neurons and are possibly involved in some aspect of ALS. Multiple genetic manipulations involving either over-expression or deletion of various neurofilament subunits have confirmed their importance in the ALS model. Reduction of axonal neurofilaments, or an increase of assembled filaments or the neurofilament-M and H, retard the onset of SOD-1-mediated disease. Levels of neurofilaments are not altered in neurons isolated from transgenic mice expressing SOD-1 mutations in comparison with wild type (Williamson et al., 2000).

Excitotoxicity is a common occurrence in both sporadic and SOD-1 mutant; the SOD-1 mutant induces a focal loss of the astroglial EAAT2 (the glial glutamate transporter) within areas of the spinal cord containing motor neuron cell bodies. The drug Riluzole will reduce glutamate toxicity.

In initial hypotheses it was suggested that the mutant SOD-1-induced toxicity could be caused by (a) modifications of the binding sites for copper and zinc in the misfolded enzyme (Beckman et al., 1993) or (b) changes in SOD-1 substrate specificity, which results in abnormally increased production of hydroxyl radicals or peroxynitrite. In SOD-1 mutants, which lack the copper-coordinating histidine sites, progressive motor neuron disease still occurs (Wang et al., 2003a). Elimination of CCS, a specific copper chaperone, in mutant SOD-1 mice, G37R, G85R and G93A, significantly lowers copper loading in the mutant SOD-1, but did not affect onset or progression of motor neuron disease (Subramaniam et al., 2002).

Metallothioneins play an important role in regulating zinc availability; MT-1 and MT-2 are mainly glial while MT-III is neuronal. SOD-1G93A mice deficient in either MT-I, MT-2 or MT-III show enhanced disease onset although it is unclear whether this is caused by alterations in zinc binding to SOD-1.

In the mutant mouse, SOD-G93A, there is strong activation and proliferation of microglia in regions of motor neuron loss (Ince et al., 1996) with expression of pro-inflammatory mediators, TNF-α, IL-1β and COX-2, particularly during the initial development of the disease (Hensley et al., 2002). Minocycline, an antibiotic which blocks microglial activation, slows disease progression in such mice (Kriz et al., 2002), while celecoxib, an inhibitor of COX-2, prolongs survival by 25% (Drachman et al., 2002). However, deletion of iNOS in SOD-1 mutant mouse, did not alter their survival time (Son et al., 2001).

In the mouse SOD-1 mutant model, an early event in the mechanism of toxicity has been shown to be activation of caspase-1. Neuronal death, however, follows only after months of chronic caspase-1 activation, concomitantly with activation of the executioner caspase-3 as the final step in the toxic cascade (Pasinelli et al., 2000).

One of the puzzling facts of ALS is why the motor neurons are specifically targeted. Some work suggests that there is a novel Fas signalling pathway in these neurons which requires NO for cytotoxicity (Raoul et al., 2002). Fas-triggered apoptosis of these normal embryonic motor neurons requires transcriptional up-regulation of neuronal NOS (nNOS), which can be abolished by nNOS inhibitors. Motor neurons from transgenic mice expressing the SOD-1 mutant genes show increased susceptibility to activation of this pathway and were more sensitive to Fas- or NO-triggered cell death. Whether Fas activation is important in the survival of adult motor neurons in ALS remains to be established.

The spinal cord of Cu/Zn-SOD mouse mutant shows abnormalities in sphingolipid and cholesterol metabolism manifested by increased levels of sphingomyelin, ceramides and cholesterol esters. Pharmaceutical agents which prevent sphingolipid synthesis may protect motor neurons against oxidative and excitotoxic toxicity (Cutler et al., 2002).

Vascular endothelial growth factor has a crucial role in controlling the growth and permeability of blood vessels. Mice with reduced levels of VEGF develop adult-onset of motor neuron degeneration, comparable to that of human ALS (Storkebaum et al., 2004). Injection of a VEGF-expressing LV vector into various muscles of the SOD-1G93A mutant delayed both the onset and progression of ALS (Azzouz et al., 2004), while ICV delivery of recombinant VEGF to the SOD-1G93A rat model delayed onset of paralysis by 17 days as well as improving motor performance and prolonging survival time (Storkebaum et al., 2005) An opposite effect was observed, (i.e. lowering the age of onset of the disease as well shortening their life span) when levels of the growth factor were decreased in SOD-1G93A mice (reviewed in Bruijn et al., 2004). When hypoxia was induced in SOD-1G93A mice (thereby up-regulating VEGF in the spinal cord), their life span was unaffected. Further studies are required to ascertain whether VEGF has a direct or indirect function as a neurotrophic factor for motor neurons. The role of other neurotrophic factors in the development of ALS is unclear. In recent studies, where the AAV virus expressing GDNF or IGF-1 was injected into the hind-limb of SOD-1G93A mice, there was prolonged survival only in mice which received IGF-1 (Kaspar et al., 2003).

11.7 ACERULOPLASMINAEMIA

Disruption of the murine ceruloplasmin gene creates an animal model of aceruloplasminaemia (Harris et al., 1999) in which, although normal at birth, by one year of age all animals have elevated serum ferritin levels and 3 to 6 fold increases in liver and spleen iron. The animals show no differences from controls in cellular iron uptake, but a striking impairment in iron movement out of reticuloendothelial cells and hepatocytes. The divalent metal transporter 1 (DMT1), ferroportin 1 (FPN1), and hephaestin (HEPH) genes were not up-regulated in the duodenum from CP(-/-) mice nor was any increase of gene expression for DMT1 and transferrin receptors (TFR1 and TFR2) found in hepatocytes of CP(-/-) mice (Yamamoto et al., 2002). This result supports the hypothesis that CP mainly acts to release iron from cells in the liver, as does the demonstration that the copper homologue of ceruloplasmin, Fet3p, can restore iron homeostasis in aceruloplasminaemic mice (Harris et al., 2004).

11.8 MENKES DISEASE

Menkes disease, an X-linked recessive inherited disorder that is characterized by accumulation of dietary copper in the intestine, is characterized by copper deficiency in brain and liver, as a consequence of the defective copper absorption. Mottled or brindled mouse mutants (Mo(br/y)) (Mann et al., 1979), which suffer from lethal hypocupraemia, were known well before the Menkes protein was identified in 1993 as the P-type ATPase, ATP7a. These mice, which are hypopigmented, die around 15 days after birth, but can be saved by treatment with copper before the 10th day postnatal. They have a deletion of two amino acids in a highly conserved, but uncharacterized region of ATP7b (Grimes et al., 1997). A number of other murine mutants at the mottled locus are known, which resemble more closely mild Menkes disease and occipital horn syndrome (OHS). The brindled phenotype resembles severe Menkes disease, with severe copper deficiency and profound neurological problems, whereas the so-called blotchy mice, like the OHS patients, have a much milder phenotype, with predominantly connective tissue defects (La Fontaine et al., 1999). In the brindled mutant, large numbers of apoptotic cells were observed in the neocortex and in the hippocampus (Rossi et al., 2001). Not only were lower levels of copper and copper-dependent enzymes like cytochrome c oxidase found, but the expression of the anti-apoptotic potein Bcl-2 was dramatically decreased while cytochrome c release from mitochondria into the cytosol was significantly increased. The authors conclude that down-regulation of Bcl-2 might trigger mitochondrial damage leading to neurodegeneration due to copper depletion during brain development in (Mo(br/y)) mice.

11.9 WILSON'S DISEASE

In Wilson's disease, an autosomal recessive inherited disease of copper metabolism, hepatic copper is neither excreted in the bile nor incorporated into ceruloplasmin, and so it accumulates to toxic levels. The rat homologue of the Wilson's disease protein, the P-type ATPas7b, is abnormal in Long-Evans rats with a cinnamon-like coat colour (LEC), making this the animal model of choice. The LEC rat manifests elevated hepatic copper, defective incorporation of copper into ceruloplasmin, and reduced biliary excretion of copper in the bile (Cuthbert, 1995). This rat model is also characterized by development of hereditary hepatitis and hepatomas, which initially led to the conclusion that copper was a possible cause of hepatic cancer (Powell, 1994). It has been shown that the expression of alpha1-6 fucosyl transferase, which catalyses the transfer of fucose to complex glycoproteins, is up-regulated during hepatocarcinogenesis of LEC rats (Miyoshi et al., 1999).

Tetrathiomolybdate (TTM) has been used to remove Cu from the liver of LEC rats (Suzuki and Ogura, 2000). The effect of long term treatment with Zn on both total metallothionin (MT) and, in particular, oxidized MT (MTox) concentrations in LEC rat liver (Santon et al., 2004) demonstrated there were no statistically different MT concentrations between Zn-treated and untreated rats. However, the Zn treatment was very effective in reducing the percentage of oxidized MT (MTox). MTox is not able to bind metals, so it does not perform its "scavenger" action against Cu accumulation in LEC rats, thus suggesting that in LEC rats one of zinc's roles is to protect from oxidative stress. Zn-induced MT may also protect efficiently against DNA damage by free radicals.

11.10 MULTIPLE SCLEROSIS

A non-human-primate model of chronic multiple sclerosis, MS-experimental autoimmune encephalitis EAE, has been developed in the common marmoset (*Callithrix jacchus*) which is superior to laboratory mouse and rat models. Many of the EAE models in rodents present as a rapidly progressing monophasic disease with clinical and pathological findings that are more characteristic of acute disseminated encephalomyelitis than chronic relapsing MS. The EAE model in Biozzi/ABH mice immunized with spinal-cord homogenate is, however, a suitable model of EAE.

Clinical and neuropathological signs of MS are induced by inoculation of marmosets with CNS myelin from patients with MS or with myelin proteins, i.e. myelin basic protein, proteolipid protein or myelin-oligodendrocyte glycoprotein. These proteins are emulsified in a suitable solution, such as mineral oil, to induce an inflammatory focus. All animals will develop MS and represent all different stages of inflammatory demyelination. Lesions III and IV are associated with oligodendrocyte degeneration rather than immune attack. Axonal pathology is prominent in early lesion stages in the marmoset model, with the presence of APP and non-phosphorylated neurofilaments identifiable by antibody staining. It remains questionable whether autoimmune reactions to CNS myelin are the cause of MS or whether the release of myelin antigens induced by some pathogenic events causes the oligodendrocytes to degenerate.

Both human and murine monoclonal antibodies could promote remyelination in the SJL/J mice after Theiler's virus induced inflammatory demyelination (Pirko et al., 2004).

REFERENCES

Abeliovich, A., Schmitz, Y., Farinas, I. *et al.* (2000) *Neuron*, **25**, 239–252.
Ahlijanian, M.K. *et al.* (2000) *Proc. Natl. Acad. Sci. USA*, **97**, 2910–2915.
Alves da Costa, C., Ayral, E., Hernandez, J.-F. *et al.* (2004) *J. Neurochem.*, **90**, 800–.
D'Antuono, M., Merlo, D. and Avoli, M. (2003) *Neuroscience*, **119**, 9–13.
Ardley, H.C., Scott, G.B., Rose, S.A., Tan, N. *et al.* (2004) *J. Neurochem.*, **90**, 379–391.
Azzouz, M., Ralph, G.S., Storkebaum, E., Walmsley, L.E. *et al.* (2004) *Nature*, **429**, 413–417.
Bakker, C.E. and Oostra, B.A. (2003) *Cytogenet. Genome Res.*, **100**, 111–123.
Baron, T. (2002) *TRENDS Mol. Med.*, **8**, 495–500.
Baum, L. and Ng, A. (2004) *J. Alzheimer's Dis.*, **6**, 367–377.
Beal, M.F. and Ferrante, R.J. (2004) *Nature Rev. Neurosci.*, **5**, 373–384.
Beckman, J.S., Carson, M., Smith, C.D., Koppenol, W.H. (1993) *Nature*, **364**, 584.
Ben Shachar, D., Eshel, G., Finberg, J.P. and Youdim, M.B. (1991) *J. Neurochem.*, **56**, 1441–1444.
Betarbet, R. (2000) *Nat. Neurosci.*, **3**, 1301–1306.
Bharath, S., Hsu, M., Kaur, D., Rajagopalan, S. *et al.* (2002) *Biochem. Pharmacol.*, **64**, 1037–1048.
Blum, D., Torch, S., Lambeng, N., Nissou, M.-F. *et al.* (2001) *Prog. Neurobiol.*, **65**, 135–172.
Bonini, N.M. (2002) *Proc. Natl. Acad. Sci. USA*, **99**, 16407–16411.
Brandner, S., Isenmann, S., Raeber, A., Fischer, M. *et al.* (1996) *Nature*, **379**, 339–343.
Brown, K.L., Stewart, K., Bruce, M.E. and Fraser, H. (1997) *J. Gen. Virol.*, **78**, 2707–2710.
Bruce, M. (1966) in *Methods in Molecular Medicine: Prion Diseases* (Baker, H. et al., eds.) pp. 223–236, Humana Press.
Bruijn, L.I., Miller, T.M. and Cleveland, D.W. (2004) *Annu. Rev. Neurosci.*, **27**, 723–749.
Büeler, H.R., Fischer, M., Lang, Y. *et al.* (1992) *Nature*, **356**, 577–582.
Büeler, H.R., Aguzzi, A., Sailer, A. *et al.* (1993) *Cell*, **73**, 1339–1347.
Chandler, R.L. (1961) *Lancet*, **1**, 1378–1379.
Chang, W-P., Koelsch, G., Wong, S. *et al.* (2004) *J. Neurochem.*, **89**, 1409-.
Chien, P., Weissman, J.S. and DePace, A.H. (2004) *Annu. Rev. Biochem*, **73**, 617–656.
Cossée, M., Puccio, H., Gansmuller, A. *et al.* (2000) *Hum. Mol. Genet*, **9**, 1219–1226.
Cruz, J.C., Tsen, H.-C., Goldman, J.A., Shih, H. and Tsai, L.-H. (2003) *Neuron*, **40**, 471–483.
Cruz, J.C. and Tsai, L.-H. (2004) *Trends Mol. Med.*, **10**, 452–458.
Cuthbert, J.A. (1995) *J. Investig. Med.*, **43**, 323–336.

Cutler, R.G., Pederson, W.A., Camandola, S., Rothstein, J.D. *et al.* (2002) *Ann. Neurol.*, **42**, 448–457.

Dexter, D.T., Ward, R.J., Florence, A., Jenner, P. *et al.* (1999) *Biochem. Pharmacol.*, **58**, 151–155.

Dickinson, A.G, Fraser, H. and Outram, G.W. (1975) *Nature*, **256**, 732–733.

Doh-ura, K., Ishikawa, K., Murakami-Kubo, I., Sasaki, K. *et al.* (2004) *J. Virol.*, **78**, 4999–5006.

Dong, H., Goico, B., Martin, M., Csernansky, C.A. *et al.* (2004) *Neurosci.*, **127**, 601–609.

Drachman, D.B., Frank, K., Dykes-Hoberg, M. *et al.* (2002) *Ann. Neurol.*, **52**, 771–778.

Duff, K., Eckman, C., Zehr, C. *et al.* (1996) *Nature*, **383**, 710–713.

During, M.J., Kaplitt, M.G., Stern, M.B. and Eidelberg, D. (2001) *Hum. Gene Ther.*, **12**, 1589–1591.

Ebadi, M. and Sharma, S.K. (2003) *Antioxid. Redox Signal.*, **5**, 319–335.

Feany, M.B. and Bender, W.W. (2000) *Nature*, **404**, 394–398.

Furuya, T., Hayakawa, H., Yamada, M., Yoshimi, K. *et al.* (2004) *J. Neurosci.*, **24**, 1865–1872.

Gajdusek, D.C., Gibbs, C.J. and Alpers, M. (1966) *Nature*, **209**, 794–796.

Giasson, B.I., Duda, J.E. Quinn, S.M. *et al.* (2002) *Neuron*, **34**, 521–533.

Goldberg, M., Fleming, S.M., Palacino, J.J., Cepeda, C. *et al.* (2003) *J. Biol. Chem.*, **278**, 43628–43635.

Gordon, M.N., Holcomb, L.A., Jantzen, P.T. *et al.* (2002) *Exp. Neurol.*, **173**, 183–195.

Goto, K., Mochizuki, H., Imai, H., Aiyama, H. *et al.* (1996) *Brain Res.*, **724**, 125–128.

Grayson Richards, J., Higgins, G.A., Ouagazzal, A.-M. *et al.* (2003) *J. Neurosci.*, **23**, 8989–9003.

Grimes, A., Hearn, C.J., Lockhart, P., Newgreen, D.F. *et al.* (1997) *Hum. Mol. Genet.*, **6**, 1037–1042.

Hall, S., Rutledge, J.N. and Schallert, T. (1992) *J. Neurol. Sci.*, **113**, 198–208.

Harris-Cerruti, C., Kamsler, A., Kaplan, B., Lamb, B. *et al.* (2004) *Eur. J. Neurosci.*, **19**, 1174–1190.

Harris, Z.L., Davis-Kaplan, S.R., Gitlin, J.D., Kaplan, J. (2004) *Blood.*, **103**, 4672–4673.

Harris, Z.L., Durley, A.P., Man, T.K., Gitlin, J.D. (1999) *Proc. Natl. Acad. Sci. USA*, **96**, 10812–10817.

Hensley, K., Floyd, R.A., Gordon, B. *et al.* (2002) *J. Neurochem.*, **82**, 365–374.

Heppner, F.L., Musahl, C., Arrighi, I., Klein, M.A. *et al.* (2001) *Science*, **294**, 178–182.

Hockly, E., Richon, V.M., Woodman, B., Smith, D.L. *et al.* (2003) *Proc. Natl Acad. Sci. USA*, **100**, 2041–2046.

Holcomb, L., Gordon, M.N., McGowan, E. *et al.* (1998) *Nat. Med.*, **4**, 97–100.

Ince, P.G., Shaw, P.J., Slade, J.Y. *et al.* (1996) *Acta Neuropath. (Berlin)*, **92**, 395–403.

Itier, J.M., Ibanez, P., Mena, M.A., Abbas, N. *et al.* (2003). *Hum. Mol. Genet.*, **12**, 2277–2291.

Jiang, H., Nucifora, F.C., Ross, C.A. and DeFranco, D.B. (2003) *Hum. Mol. Genet.*, **12**, 1–12.

Kahle, PH. *et al.* (2000) *J. Neurosci.*, **20**, 6365–6373.

Kaspar, B.K., Llado, J., Sherkat, N. *et al.* (2003) *Science*, **301**, 839–842.

Kells, A.P., Fong, D.M., Dragunow, M., During, M.J. *et al.* (2004) *Mol. Ther.*, **9**, 682–688.

King, G.D., Cherian, K. and Turner, R.S. (2004) *J. Neurochem.*, **88**, 971–982.

Kirik, D., Rosenblad, C., Burger, C. *et al.* (2002) *J. Neurosci.*, **22**, 2780–2791.

Klein, M.A., Frigg, R., Flechsig, E., Raeber, A.J. *et al.* (1997) *Nature*, **390**, 687–690.

Klein, R.L., King, M.A., Hamby, M.E. and Meyer, E.M. (2002) *Hum. Gene. Ther.*, **13**, 605–612.

Klivenyi, P., Ferrante, R.J., Matthews, R.T. *et al.* (1999) *Nat. Med.*, **5**, 347–350.

Kovacs *et al.* (2004) *Neuron*, **44**, 227–238.

Kriz, J., Nguyen, M.D. and Jukien, J.P. (2002) *Neurobiol*, **10**, 268–278.

Kurosaki, R., Muramatsu, Y., Michimata, M., Kato, H. *et al.* (2002) *Neurol. Res.*, **24**, 655–662.

La Bianco, C., Ridet, J.L., Schneider, B.L. *et al.* (2002) *Proc. Natl. Acad. Sci. USA*, **99**, 10813–10818.

LaDu, M.J., Shah, J.A., Reardon, C.A. *et al.* (2001) *Neurochem. Int.*, **39**, 427–434.

La Fontaine, S., Firth, S.D., Lockhart, P.J., Brooks, H. *et al.* (1999) *Hum. Mol. Genet.*, **8**, 1069–1075.

Lan, J. and Jiang, D.H. (1997a) *J. Neural. Transm. (Budapest)*, **104**, 469–481.

Lan, J. and Jiang, D.H. (1997b) *J. Neural. Transm.*, **104**, 649–660.

LaVaute, T., Smith, S., Cooperman, S. *et al.* (2001) *Nat. Genet.*, **27**, 209–214.

Levenson, C.W., Perkov, B. and Matteson, A. (2003) *J. Amer. Aging. Assoc.*, in press.

Lewis, J., McGowan, E., Rockwood, J., Melrose, H. *et al.* (2000) *Nat. Genet.*, **25**, 402–405.

Lewis, J., Dickson, D.W., Lin, W.L., Chisholm, L. *et al.* (2001) *Science*, **293**, 1487–1491.

Lockhart, P.J., O'Farrell, C.A., Farrer, M.J. (2004) *Mov. Disorder.*, **19**, 101–104.

Luo, Y., Bolon, B., Damore, M.A., Fitzpatrick, D. *et al.* (2003) *Neurobiol. Dis.*, **14**, 81–88.

Mallucci, G. and Collinge, J. (2005) *Nature Rev. Neurosci.*, **6**, 23–34.

Mallucci, G., Dickinson, A., Linehan, J., Klohn, P.C. *et al.* (2003) *Science*, **302**, 871–874.

Mandel, S., Grunblatt, E., Levites, Y., Maor, G. *et al.* (2003) *Adv. Neurol.*, **91**, 123–132.

Mangiarini, L., Sathasivam, K., Seller, M., Cozens, B. *et al.* (1996) *Cell*, **87**, 493–506.

Mann, J.R., Camakaris, J., Danks, D.M. and Walliczek, E.G. (1979) *Biochem. J.*, **180**, 605–612.

Manson, J.C., Clarke, A.R., Hooper, M.I., Aitchison, L. *et al.* (1994) *Mol. Neurobiol.*, **8**, 121–127.

Marsh, J.L. and Thompson, L.M. (2004) *Bioessays*, **26**, 485–496.

Masliah, E. *et al.* (2000) *Science*, **287**, 1265–1269.

Meyron-Holtz, E.G., Ghosh, M.C., Iwai, K. *et al.* (2004) *EMBO J.*, **23**, 386–395.

Minamiyama, M., Katsuno, M., Adachi, H., Waza, M. *et al.* (2003) *Hum. Mol. Genet.*, **13**, 1183–1192.

Miranda, C.J., Santos, M.M., Ohshima, K., Smith, J. *et al.* (2002) *FEBS Lett.*, **512**, 291–297.

Miyoshi, E., Noda, K., Yamaguchi Y., Inoue S. *et al.* (1999) *Biochim. Biophys. Acta*, **1473**, 9–20.

Mochizuki H., Imai, H., Endo., K., Yokomizi, K. *et al.* (1994) *Neurosci. Lett.*, **168**, 251–253.

Nagai, Y., Fujikake, N., Ohno, K., Higashiyama, H. *et al.* (2003) *Hum. Mol. Genet.*, **12**, 1253–1259.

Nordberg, A., Hellstrom-Lindahl, E., Lee, M., Johnson, M. *et al.* (2002) *J. Neurochem.*, **81**, 655–658.

Oesch, B., Westaway, D., Walchli, M., McKinley, M.P. *et al.* (1985) *Cell*, **40**, 735–746.

Oestreicher, E., Sengstock, G.J., Riederer, P., Olanow, C.W. *et al.* (1994) *Brain Res.*, **660**, 8–18.

Osaka, H., Wang, Y.-L., Takada, K. *et al.* (2003) *Hum. Mol. Genet.*, **16**, 1945–1958.

Pan, L., Zhang, Y.Q., Woodruff, E. and Broadie, K. (2004) *Curr. Biol.*, **14**, 1863–1870.

Parekh-Olmedo, H., Wang, J., Gusella, J.F. and Kmiec, E.B. (2004) *J. Mol. Neurosci.*, **24**, 257–267.

Pasinelli, P., Houseweart, M.K., Brown, R.H. *et al.* (2000) *Proc. Natl. Acad. Sci. USA*, **97**, 13901–13906.

Perlman, S.L. (2003) *Expert Opin. Pharmacother.*, **12**, 235–245.

Perez, M., Ribe, E., Rubio, A., Lim, F. *et al.* (2005) *Neurosci.*, **130**, 339–347.

Pirko, I., Ciric, B., Gamez, J., Bieber, A.J. *et al.* (2004) *FASEB J.*, **18**, 1577–1579.

Powell, C.J. (1994) *Hum. Exp. Toxicol.*, **13**, 910–912.

Prusiner, S.B. (1982) *Science*, **216**, 136–144.

Prusiner, S.B., Scott, M., Foster, D., Pan, K.M. *et al.* (1990) *Cell*, **63**, 673–686.

Puccio, H., Simon, D., Cossée, M., Criqui-Filipe, P. *et al.* (2001) *Nat. Genet.*, **27**, 181–186.

Raoul, C., Estevez, A.G., Nishimune, H. *et al.* (2002) *Neuron*, **35**, 1067–1083.

Ratazzi M.C., La Fauci, G. and Brown, W.T. (2004) *Ment. Retard. Dev. Disabil. Res. Rev.*, **10**, 75–81.

Rattray, M. (2001) *Biol. Psych.*, **49**, 185–193.

Rogers, J.T., Randall, J.D., Cahill, C.M., Eder, P.S. *et al.* (2002) *J. Biol. Chem.*, **277**, 45518–45528.

Rossi, L., De Martino, A., Marchese, E., Piccirilli, S. *et al.* (2001) *Neuroscience*, **103**, 181–188.

Santon, A., Albergoni, V., Santovito, G., Sturniolo, G.C. *et al.* (2004) *Eur. J. Histochem.*, **48**, 317–320.

Schober, A. (2004) *Cell Tissue Res.*, **318**, 215–224.

Scott, M., Foster, D., Mirenda, C., Serban, D. *et al.* (1989) *Cell*, **59**, 847–857.

Serio, T.R. and Lindquist, S.L. (2001) *Adv. Prot. Chem.*, **57**, 335–366.

Seznec, H., Simon, D., Monassier, L., Criqui-Filipe, P. *et al.* (2004) *Hum. Mol. Genet.*, **13**, 1017–1024.

Shachar, D.B., Kahana, N., Kampel, V., Warshawsky, A. *et al.* (2004) *Neuropharmacol.*, **46**, 254–263.

Shoham, S. and Youdim, M.B.H. (2000) *Cell Mol. Biol.*, **46**, 743–760.

Simon, D., Seznec, H., Gansmuller, A., Carelle, N., *et al.* (2004) *J. Neurosci.*, **24**, 1987–1995.

Siomi, H., Ishizuka, A. and Siomi, M.C. (2004) *Ment. Retard. Dev. Disabil. Res. Rev.*, **10**, 68–74.

Smith, S.R., Cooperman, S., Lavaute, T. *et al.* (2004) *Ann. N. Y. Acad. Sci.*, **1012**, 65–83.

Son, M., Fathallah-Shaykh, H.M. and Elliott, J.L. (2001) *Ann. Neurol.*, **50**, 273.

Steffan, J.S., Bodai, L., Pallos, J. and Poelman, M. (2001) *Nature*, **413**, 693–694.

Storkebaum, E., Lambrechts, D. and Carmeliet, P. (2004) *Bioessays*, **26**, 943–954.

Storkebaum, E., Lambrechts, D., Dewerchin, M., Moreno-Murciano, M.P. *et al.* (2005) *Nat. Neurosci.*, **8**, 85–92.

Subramaniam, J.R., Lyons, W.E., Liu, J. *et al.* (2002) *Nat. Neurosci.*, **5**, 301–307.

Suzuki, K.T. and Ogura, Y. (2000) *Yakugaku Zasshi*, **120**, 899–908.

Temlett, J.A., Landsberg, J.P., Watt, F. and Grime, G.W. (1994) *J. Neurochem.*, **62**, 134–146.

Van Den Bosch, L., Tilkin, P., Lemmens, G. *et al.* (2002) *Neuro. Report*, **13**, 1067–1070.

van der Putten *et al.* (2000) *J. Neurosci.*, **20**, 6021–6029.

Vassar, R. (2004) *J. Mol. Neurosci.*, **23**, 105–114.

Voisine, C. and Hart, A.C. (2004) *Methods Mol. Biol.*, **277**, 141–160.

Vu, C.B., Peng, B., Kumaravel, G., Smits, G. *et al.* (2004) *J. Med. Chem.*, **47**, 4291–4299.

Wang, J., Slunt, H., Gonzales, V., Fromholt, D. *et al.* (2003a) *Hum. Mol. Genet.*, **12**, 2753–2764.

Wang, X.S., Ong, W.Y. and Connor, J.R. (2003b) *Neurosci.*, **120**, 21–29.

Ward, R.J., Dexter, D., Florence, A. *et al.* (1995) *Biochem. Pharmacol.*, **49**, 1821–1826.

Weissmann, C., Büeler, H.R., Fischer, M. and Aguet, M. (1993) *Intervirology*, **35**, 164–175.

White, A.R., Enever, P., Tayebi, M., Mushens, R. *et al.* (2003) *Nature*, **422**, 80–83.

Wickner, R.B. (1994) *Science*, **264**, 566–569.

Wickner, R.B., Taylor, K.L., Edskes, H.K., Maddelein, M.L. *et al.* (2001) *Adv. Prot. Chem.*, **57**, 313–334.

Williamson, T.L., Corson, L.B., Huang, L. *et al.* (2000) *Science*, **288**, 399.

Yamamoto, K., Yoshida, K., Miyagoe, Y., Ishikawa, A. *et al.* (2002) *Biochim. Biophys. Acta*, **1588**, 195–202.

Youdim, M.B.H., Stehenson, G. and Ben Shachar, D. (2004) *Ann. N. Y. Acad. Sci.*, **1012**, 306–325.

Zhang, X., Smith, D.L., Meriin, A.B., Engemann, S. *et al.* (2005) *Proc. Natl Acad. Sci. USA*, **102**, 892–897.

Zhu, S., Stravrovskaya, I.G., Drozda, M. *et al.* (2002) *Nature*, **417**, 74–78.

Zlotnik, I. and Rennie, J.C. (1965) *J. Comp. Pathol.*, **75**, 147–157.

12

Concluding Remarks

The premise at the outset of this endeavour was to establish a clear path leading from (i) metal-based oxidative stress in brain, through (ii) the production of potentially toxic and harmful reactive molecules resulting from the peroxidation of unsaturated lipids, which in turn (iii) can then cause oxidative damage to proteins; (iv) these damaged, misfolded and aggregated proteins accumulate because (v) they fail to be removed by the cytosolic waste disposal service, involving labelling by ubiquitination and degradation by the proteasome; (vi) as a consequence, these protein aggregates, which frequently are rich in β-pleated sheets and in β-turns, are then found in inclusion bodies (which can be intranuclear, cytoplasmic or extracellular); these are the hallmark of these different neurodegenerative diseases (**Figure 12.1**). We will, in these concluding remarks, summarize the growing body of evidence which supports this hypothesis, and try to paint an optimistic picture of where the future may lie, in terms of improved and earlier diagnosis as well as therapeutic strategies.

We have pointed out earlier that the frequency of many (but not all) of these neurological disorders increases with age, and that metal ions such as copper, iron and zinc, accumulate in the brain with ageing and also with a number of neurodegenerative diseases. It is also clear that copper and iron can readily engage in Fenton chemistry with concomitant free radical production. There is an extensive body of evidence to show that in many neurodegenerative diseases oxidative stress plays an important role (for a recent review see Barnham et al., 2004). The generation of reactive oxygen and nitrogen species (ROS and RNS) including hydrogen peroxide, nitric oxide, peroxynitrite, and the highly reactive hydroxyl radical, combined with the high oxygen consumption and low antioxidant defence capacity of brain makes it particularly vulnerable to oxidative insult. These ROS and RNS can directly attack the four bases of DNA, the cellular proteins and their lipids. Starting with attack on the double bond of the unsaturated fatty acids in brain lipids, very reactive lipid peroxy radical are formed, which spawn a vast army of reactive breakdown products, including 4-hydroxy-2,3-nonenol and acrolein. In their turn, these molecules form covalent bonds with lysine, cysteine and histidine residues in proteins, which may result in crosslinking. It is likely that other covalent modifications may also be involved, including that recently described for prion protein with advanced glycosylation end products (Choi et al., 2004). What role these covalent modifications have in subsequent protein aggregation is not clear.

Metal-based Neurodegeneration: From Molecular Mechanisms to Therapeutic Strategies   R. R. Crichton and R. J. Ward
© 2006 John Wiley & Sons, Ltd

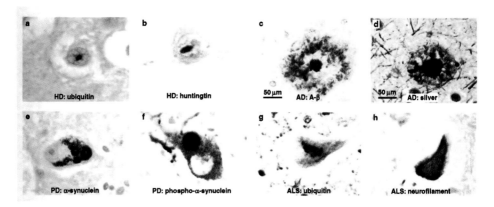

Figure 12.1: Characteristic neurodegenerative disease neuropathological lesions involve deposition of abnormal proteins, which can be intranuclear, cytoplasmic or extracelular. All are labelled with antibodies (except **d**) as indicated. (**a**) and (**b**) HD, intranuclear inclusion labelled for ubiquitin and huntingtin (cerebral cortex). (**c**) and (**d**) AD, neuritic plaque labelled with Aβ (cerebral cortex) and silver stained. (**e**) and (**f**) PD, Lewy bodies labelled for α-synuclein (fine granular brown label in this and next panel represent neuromelanin) and phosphorylated α-synuclein (substantia nigra). (**g**) and (**h**) ALS, cytoplasmic skein of neurofilaments labelled with ubiquitin and with neurofilament (medulla oblongata). From Ross and Poirier (2004), reproduced by permission of Nature Publishing Group.

However, it has become increasingly clear that many neurodegenerative diseases, including Alzheimer's disease (AD), Parkinson's disease (PD), Huntington's disease (HD), amyotrophic lateral sclerosis and prion diseases, have in common striking similarities. The selective neuronal vulnerability accompanied by degeneration in specific brain regions is accompanied by the deposition of abnormal aggregated proteins within inclusion bodies (**Table 12.1** and **Figure 12.1**). The protein aggregates often contain, in addition to the deposited disease proteins (**Table 12.1**), ubiquitin, a marker of misfolded proteins and signal for degradation by the proteasome. These aggregates usually consist of fibres, containing misfolded proteins with a β-sheet conformation commonly termed amyloid.

Amyloid fibrils are filamentous structures about 10 nm in width and from 0.1 to 10 μm long. A major distinguishing feature is the presence of cross-β structures. This structural motif consists of ribbon-like β-sheets, with the β-sheets running roughly at right angles to the long axis of the fibrils and the hydrogen bonds between them parallel to the long axis, and is found widely in the neuropathological lesions that characterize many of these diseases (reviewed in Ross and Poirier, 2004). The core structure of Aβ, α-synuclein and poly-glutamine aggregates found in AD, PD and HD all seem to involve compact β-sheet interspersed with β-turns (**Figure 12.2**). Further evidence that this may be a common structure of neurodegenerative disease-related amyloid comes from the observation that conformation-specific antibodies which bind to the amyloid fibril state of Aβ peptide, but not to its soluble monomeric form, will also bind to amyloid fibrils derived from other proteins of unrelated sequence (O'Nuallain and Wetzel, 2002). They do not, however, bind to non-native globular protein. Regarding the detailed structure of amyloid, and how it is assembled, there seem to be considerable similarities among the structures of different kinds of disease-related amyloid.

What, we may ask, are the causes of protein aggregation, and what initiates the aggregation process in all of these different diseases? Many of the neurodegenerative

Table 12.1: Neurodegenerative diseases: proteins and pathology

Disease	Etiology	Regions most affected	Characteristic pathology	Disease proteins deposited
Huntington's disease	Huntingtin (dominant)	Striatum, other basal ganglia, cortex, other regions	Intranuclear inclusions and cytoplasmic aggregates	Huntingtin with polyglutamine expansion
Other polyglutamine diseases (DRPLA, SCA1–3, etc., SBMA)	Atrophin-1, ataxin-1–3, etc.; androgen receptor (AR) (dominant)	Basal ganglia, brain stem cerebellum, and spinal cord	Intranuclear inclusions	Atrophin-1, ataxins or AR
Alzheimer's disease (AD)	Sporadic (ApoE risk factor)	Cortex, hippocampus, basal forebrain, brain stem	Neuritic plaques and neurofibrillary tangles	Aβ peptide (from APP) and hyperphosphorylated tau
	Amyloid precursor protein (APP) (dominant)	Same as sporadic	Same as sporadic	Same as sporadic
	Presenilin 1, 2 (dominant)	Same as sporadic	Same as sporadic	Same as sporadic
Fronto-temporal dementia with Parkinsonism	Tau mutations (dominant)	Frontal and temporal cortex, hippocampus	Pick bodies	Hyperphosphorylated tau protein
Parkinson's disease (PD)	Sporadic	Substantia nigra, cortex, locus ceruleus, raphe, etc.	Lewy bodies and Lewy neurites	α-Synuclein
	α-Synuclein (dominant)	Similar to sporadic, but more widespread	Similar to sporadic	α-Synuclein
	Parkin (also DJ-1, PINK1) recessive (some dominant)	Substantia nigra	Lewy bodies absent (or much less frequent)	α-Synuclein (when present)
Amyotrophic lateral sclerosis (ALS)	Sporadic	Spinal motor neurons and motor cortex	Bonina bodies and axonal spheroids	Unknown (neurofilaments)
	Superoxide dismutase-1 (dominant)	Same as sporadic	Same	Unknown
Prion diseases (kuru, CJD, GSS disease, fatal familial insomnia, new variant CJD)	Sporadic, genetic and infectious	Cortex, thalamus, brain stem, cerebellum, other areas	Spongiform degeneration, amyloid, other aggregates	Prion protein

ApoE, apolipoprotein E; APP, amyloid precursor protein; CJD, Creutzfeldt-Jakob disease; DRPLA, dento-rubral and pallido-Luysian atrophy; GSS, Gerstmann-Dtraussler-Scheinker; SBMA, apinal and bulbar muscular atrophy; SCA, spino-cerebellar ataxia. From Ross and Poirier (2004), reproduced by permission of Nature Publishing Group.

(a)

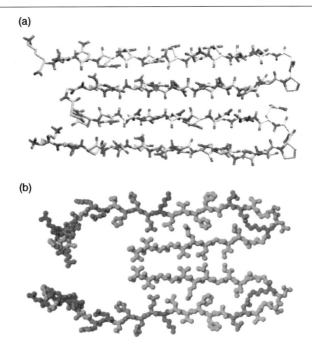

(b)

Figure 12.2: β-Sheet, β-turn models for expanded polyglutamine and Aβ amyloid suggest commonalities in amyloid structure in different neurodegenerative diseases. (**a**) Sketch of expanded polyglutamine with β-turns constrained by proline-glycine insertions every nine glutamines, thought to be similar to the structure of expanded pure polyglutamine. (**b**) Model for an Aβ(1-40) fibril with β-sheets formed by residues 12 to 24 and 30 to 40. From Ross and Poirier (2004), reproduced with permission of Nature Publishing Group.

disease proteins have an unfolded native structure, which may facilitate their transition to the beta-sheet-rich structures which have the ability to form insoluble neurotoxic amyloid deposits that accumulate in the brain. Covalent modification of the kind described above may also facilitate both aggregation and its initiation. Phosphorylation may also be involved, as has been proposed in the case of α-synuclein in PD, of ataxin-1 in models of spinocerebral ataxia, and even hyperphosphorylation of tau in neurofibrillary tangles in AD.

Proteolytic cleavage may also be involved, notably in the subtle interplay of α-, β- and γ-secretases in the cleavage of the amyloid precursor protein, to give the beta amyloid peptides, some of them non-amyloidogenic, others much more so (Esler and Wolfe, 2001). Proteolysis may also be involved in HD, where short N-terminal fragments containing the expanded polyglutamine repeat are substantially more toxic than longer huntingtin, and in PD as well.

We may also question whether the intracellular inclusion bodies illustrated for a few neurodegenerative conditions in **Figure 12.1** are the culprits responsible for the disease, or rather, the last despairing cry for help of a cell which finds its machinery for removing misfolded proteins totally overwhelmed. There is a cruel irony in the fact that some of the disease proteins, like parkin, are directly involved in the ubiquitin/proteasome pathway, (where it functions as a ubiquitin protein ligase). Further, recent studies suggest that IRP2, the iron responsive protein which, at least in the mouse, dominates the regulation of iron homeostasis, is itself degraded by the proteasome in conditions of iron excess (Meyron-Holz et al., 2004). On the other hand, there is little doubt, for example in the polyglutamine diseases like Huntington's, that the size of the polyglutamine repeat determines the severity and the age of onset of the disease, strongly implying that the diseased protein is itself involved in the neuropathology.

12.1 THERAPEUTIC STRATEGIES

Since, at the moment of writing these concluding remarks, we have just launched a new COST (European Cooperation in the field of Scientific and Technical Research) Chemistry Action D34 "Molecular Targeting and Drug Design in Neurological and Bacterial Diseases", it seems appropriate to conclude these remarks with some thoughts on therapeutic strategies. If we assume that the origin of many neurological disorders ultimately results from protein misfolding and aggregation (**Figure 12.3**) caused by metal-based oxidative stress, which leads to exposure of hydrophobic regions, inability of chaperones to direct misfolded proteins to their cellular locations, and progressive chaperone/proteasome overload, we can readily identify a number of areas where we could try to intervene (while still lacking the crucial answer to the question 'why **this** particular brain region, why **this** particular protein or peptide?').

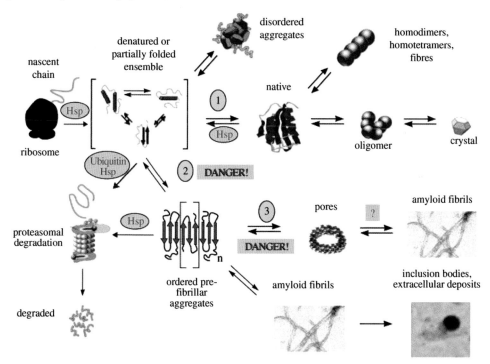

Figure 12.3 The possible fates of newly synthesized polypeptide chains, which may assemble into native structures, but (1) may also return to partly folded states. These will either be refolded by chaperones, or cleared by the ubiquitin/proteasome machinery. If the equilibrium (2) shifts to increased formation of β-sheet structures, which can subsequently (3) form amyloid pores and amyloid fibrils, the future of the cell may be compromised, with the formation of intracellular inclusion bodies or extracellular deposits. Reprinted from *Biochemica et Biophysica ACTA (BBA) – Molecular Basis of Disease*, Vol 1739, Stefani, Protein misfolding and aggregation: new examples in medicine and biology of the dark side of the protein world, pp 5–25, Copyright 2004, with permission from Elsevier.

The first therapeutic target is to retard metal accumulation in specific brain regions. And that is precisely the nature of the problem, namely getting metal chelators to reach the appropriate target regions in the brain, where they will complex the metal and diffuse back out as the metal chelate, without either interfering with the iron- and copper-dependent enzymes which play such an essential role in brain, or causing a redistribution of brain iron such that previously non-toxic iron changes its toxic potential by being moved to a different brain compartment. We showed some years ago, in iron-loaded rats, that while chelators were able to cross the blood-brain barrier, and reduce the levels of iron in specific brain regions, some of them also interfered with the metabolism of the neurotransmitter, dopamine (Dexter et al., 1999). Increasing efforts are being made to target chelators, or to use the more sophisticated recent jargon, metal-protein attenuating compounds (MPACs)[1], to cross the blood-brain barrier. Recent examples include incorporating chelators in nanoparticles (Cui et al., 2005) and the use of lipophilic brain-permeable molecules and polyphenols (reviewed in Zecca et al., 2004). Some success has been reported with the copper chelator clioquinol (5-chloro-7-iodo-8-hydroxyquinoline) in a phase 2 clinical trial in Alzheimer's disease (Ritchie et al., 2003).

A second site for therapeutic action could be to reduce the extent of oxidative stress by the use of appropriate antioxidants. A number of studies have shown beneficial effects of antioxidants in cell culture studies (reviewed in Moosmann and Behl, 2002). We obtain many antioxidants in our diet and various claims have been made for a variety of antioxidant supplements, including vitamin C, ubiquinone and derivatives, lipoic acid, β-carotene, creatine, melatonin, curcumin and the phenolics and flavonoids present in red wine (which may also act as metal chelators, notably of iron). While most of these studies have used cell cultures, there has been only a limited clinical evaluation of antioxidants. Alpha-tocopherol (vitamin E) was found to have no beneficial effects in PD, whereas positive effects were noted in an AD study, with an increase in median survival time, but no improvement in cognitive function (reviewed in Barnham et al., 2004).

The generation of ROS is known to initiate excitotoxicity, which is modulated through the over-activation of glutamate receptors. Memantine, which targets the NMDA receptor, has received FDA approval for use in moderately severe to severe AD, and amantadine, another NMDA receptor inhibitor, has also been used in the treatment of AD. Riluzole, which is used to treat ALS, is also thought to inhibit glutamate release.

Other strategies could be envisaged based on the formation of abnormal conformations of disease target proteins notably increased content of β-structure. Small molecules could be developed which target the protein misfolding pathways. The dye Congo red binds to proteins with β-sheet structure. Infusion of Congo red into a transgenic mouse model of Huntington's disease, well after the onset of symptoms, promotes the clearance of expanded repeats *in vivo* and exerts marked protective effects on survival, weight loss and motor function (Sanchez et al., 2003). Chemical chaperones could be developed to block protein aggregation. The disaccharide trehalose, widely used in biotechnological applications to stabilize protein structure, has had some success in a mouse model of HD (Tanaka et al., 2004), and automated small molecule screens have been developed to identify polyglutamine aggregation inhibitors. Similar approaches to identify small molecules which could inhibition aggregation of Aβ, α-synuclein and prions are being developed (reviewed in Ross and Poirier, 2004).

---

[1] A good example of not calling a spade a spade, but rather a heavy, flat-bladed, long-handled tool used for digging by pressing the metal blade into the ground with the foot.

And, in the case of diseases involving proteolytic cleavage, like AD, targeting the proteolytic enzymes themselves, both γ-secretase and β-secretase presents a considerable possibility for the development of powerful small molecule inhibitors (John et al., 2003).

Yet another strategy might be to enhance cellular defense mechanisms involved in protecting against misfolded proteins. Drugs like geldanamycin are known which can modulate and enhance chaperone levels in scrapie-infected mouse neuroblastoma cells (Winklhofer et al., 2001), and it may also be possible to find drugs which stimulate the activity of the ubiquitin-proteasome system itself. The enhancement of the activity of ubiquitin-conjugating enzymes has been demonstrated in Arabadopsis by a ubiquitin-conjugating enzyme variant (Yanagawa et al., 2004).

The neuropathology and motor dysfunction observed in a conditional mouse model of HD can be reversed when expression of the mutated huntingtin fragment is blocked, demonstrating that a continuous influx of the mutant protein is required to maintain inclusions and symptoms, and raising the possibility that if the production of the mutant polyglutamine huntingtin can be stopped, HD may be reversible (Yamamoto et al., 2000).

The recent discovery of RNA interference (RNAi) holds considerable promise as a means of silencing disease genes. RNAi, small duplexes of RNA complementary to specific target genes suppress protein expression by inhibiting translation or by degrading the targeted messenger RNA (mRNA). In important preclinical studies for disease therapies, inhibitory RNA has been introduced into cells by two main methods (**Figure 12.4**).

In the first, a duplex of short oligonucleotides, generally perfectly complementary to one another, is used with a reagent that facilitates entry of the duplex into cells. The duplex becomes incorporated into a complex of cytoplasmic proteins already present in the cell, known as the RNA-induced silencing complex (RISC), which directs the duplex to the appropriate target transcript mRNA, initiating its degradation. Only one strand of the duplex, the strand which is complementary to the targeted transcript, becomes incorporated into RISC, where it binds the complementary nucleotide sequence in the targeted mRNA. RISC then cleaves the mRNA at this point, leading to its destruction. The gene is now effectively silenced, since without its corresponding mRNA, no protein can be synthesized.

In the second, inhibitory RNAs can be introduced into cells through expression vectors – either plasmids or viruses, which have been engineered to express small interfering siRNA. Some systems express two independent RNAs, one a sense strand, the other antisense, which can form a duplex once expressed. The antisense strand from this duplex becomes incorporated into the RISC and causes suppression of the targeted gene.

The possible therapeutic applications of RNAi for neurological diseases are broad. However, the dominantly inherited neurodegenerative diseases are a particularly attractive group of candidates. These include Huntington's disease and related polyglutamine disorders, amyotrophic lateral sclerosis and familial Alzheimer's disease. While encouraging results have been reported in the suppression of dominant disease genes *in vitro*, in some cases even allele-specific silencing has been achieved, silencing the disease-causing allele while maintaining the expression of the normal allele (reviewed in Davidson and Paulson, 2004). The challenge now is to target the delivery vectors for the RNAi to the appropriate brain region. However, we should insist that these studies are still a long way from reaching realization in human disease, with the codicil of course that we are still extrapolating from an animal model to man.

Nonetheless, the hope is now great, there is optimism in the air, that we will make progress in the treatment of many of these debilitating neurological disorders. Indeed, as we advance in our understanding of the pathways by which the disease pathogenesis progresses,

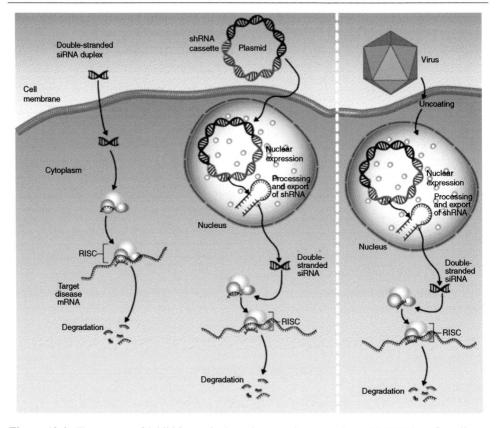

Figure 12.4: Three ways of inhibiting polyglutamine-protein expression with RNAi. Left: cells are transfected with preformed siRNA duplexes, generally in combination with a transfection reagent. The transfected siRNA becomes incorporated into the RISC following its entry into the cell, leading to degradation of target disease gene mRNA. Middle: transfected plasmid vectors must reach the nucleus for transcription of shRNA. The shRNA is a short hairpin, which consists of a sense sequence about 21 bases long followed by a six to eight base non-complementary loop and another 21-base sequence complementary (i.e. antisense) to the sense sequence. The shRNA is processed and exported to the cytoplasm where it is incorporated into the RISC for directed gene silencing. Right: viral vectors encoding siRNA or shRNA bind to the target cell via a receptor, followed by receptor-mediated endocytosis. Uncoating of the viral protein coat (adeno-associated viruses) or fusion of the viral envelope with cellular membranes (lentivirus) releases viral genomes and allows trafficking to the nucleus. From Davidson and Paulson (2004).

we can expect that this should lead to rational therapeutics. And that will make the lives of the millions of sufferers that much better, and, lest we forget them, it will make the task of their long-suffering carers that much easier.

REFERENCES

Barnham, K.J., Matsers, C.L. and Bush, A.I. (2004) *Nat. Rev. Drug Discov.*, **3**, 205–214.
Choi, Y.G., Kim, J.I., Jeon, Y.C., Park, S.J. *et al.* (2004) *J. Biol. Chem.*, **279**, 30402–30409.

Cui, Z., Lockman, P.R., Atwood, C.S., Hsu, C.H. *et al.* (2005) *Eur. J. Pharm. Biopharm.*, **59**, 263–272.

Davidson, B.L. and Paulson, H.L. (2004) *Lancet Neurol.*, **3**, 145–149.

Dexter, D.T., Ward, R.J., Florence, A., Jenner, P. and Crichton, R.R. (1999) *Biochem. Pharmacol.*, **58**, 151–155.

Esler, W.P. and Wolfe, M.S. (2001) *Science*, **293**, 1449–1454.

John, V., Beck, J.P., Bienkowski, M.J., Sinha, S. and Heinrikson, R.L. (2003) *J. Med. Chem.*, **46**, 4625–4630.

Meyron-Holz, E.G., Ghosh, M.C., Iwai, K., La Vaute, T. *et al.* (2004) *EMBO J.*, **23**, 386–395.

Moosmann, M. and Behl, C. (2002) *Exp. Opin. Invest. Drugs*, **11**, 1407–1435.

O'Nuallain, B. and Wetzel, R. (2002) *Proc. Natl. Acad. Sci. USA*, **99**, 1485–1490.

Ritchie, C.W., Bush, A.I., Mackinnon, A., Macfarlane, S. *et al.* (2003) *Arch. Neurol.*, **60**, 1685–1691.

Ross, C.A. and Poirier, M.A. (2004) *Nature Med.*, **10**, S10–17.

Sanchez, I., Mahlke, C. and Yuan, J. (2003) *Nature*, **421**, 373–379.

Stefani, M. (2004) *Biochim. Biophys. Acta*, **1739**, 5–25.

Tanaka, M., Machida, Y., Niu, S., Ikeda, T. *et al.* (2004) *Nature Med.*, **10**, 148–154.

Yamamoto, A., Lucas, J.J. and Hen, R. (2000) *Cell*, **101**, 57–66.

Yanagawa, Y., Sullivan, J.A., Komatsu, S., Gusmaroli, G. *et al.* (2004) *Genes Dev.*, **18**, 2172–2181.

Winklhofer, K.F., Reintjes, A., Hoener, M.C., Voellmy, R. and Tatzelt, J. (2001) *J. Biol. Chem.*, **276**, 45160–45167.

Zecca, L., Youdim, M.B.H., Riederer, P., Connor, J.R. and Crichton, R.R. (2004) *Nature Rev. Neurosci.*, **5**, 863–873.

Index

JACK THE RIPPER

The Theories and the Facts

JACK THE RIPPER

RIPPER

The Theories
and the Facts

COLIN KENDELL

ERLEY

For Emma, Dan, Tasha, Oli and Liz

First published 2010

Amberley Publishing Plc
Cirencester Road, Chalford,
Stroud, Gloucestershire, GL6 8PE

www.amberleybooks.com

Copyright © Colin Kendell, 2010

The right of Colin Kendell to be identified as the Author
of this work has been asserted in accordance with the
Copyrights, Designs and Patents Act 1988.

British Library Cataloguing in Publication Data.
A catalogue record for this book is available from the British Library.

ISBN 978 1 4456 0084 0

Typesetting and Origination by Amberley Publishing.
Printed in Great Britain.

Contents

CHAPTER 1

Mary Ann Nichols

At 1.40 a.m. on Friday, 31 August 1888, a forty-two-year-old prostitute named Mary Ann Nichols was in a common lodging house at 18 Thrawl Street in Spitalfields, Whitechapel. Nichols, known as Polly from her nickname Pretty Polly, often stayed at that particular address. She was drunk that night, as she often was, and probably because she had spent all her day's earnings in one of the local public houses, she was unable to pay her night's rent when the lodging house deputy asked her for it. After a short argument, the deputy ordered her out – and so began the story of the world's greatest crime mystery, the Jack the Ripper murders.

Polly's final words to the deputy are still remembered today, over a century after she walked out into the street on that August night. "Don't let my doss, I'll soon be back – see what a jolly bonnet I've got now."

Her intention was obviously to earn the money that she needed from the street and she hoped that her black, velvet-trimmed bonnet would help her to attract a client. It would not have been new – women like Polly could only afford second-hand clothes – but she had only just acquired it and was clearly pleased with it. The rest of her attire – an old russet-coloured ulster jacket with metal buttons, coarse brown linsey dress and cut down men's boots – would have been far less attractive.

Polly was the estranged wife of William Nichols, a printer. Their marriage had broken up some years earlier, largely because of her fondness for drink, and she had followed a wandering, dissolute existence ever since. Probably it had suited her. Earlier that year she had been given employment as a maid by Mr Samuel Cowdry, a Chief Clerk of the Works for the Metropolitan Police building department, who lived in Wandsworth. It would have been a more comfortable life than she had known for some time and she would have had a regular if small income, but she absconded after only a few weeks. Taking with her some articles of clothing belonging to the Cowdry family, which she later sold, she made her way to Spitalfields. There she could at least come and go, and drink, as she liked. She could not do that in the house of the strictly teetotal Mr and Mrs Cowdry.

Polly did find a client – probably more than one – after she left the doss-house. At half past two that morning she was seen by Ellen Holland, another of the regulars at 18 Thrawl Street, who later described her as "very drunk". Seeing her state, Ellen suggested that they should go back to Thrawl Street together but Polly refused. According to what she told her friend she was still without her doss money because, having earned it twice since she left the lodging house, she had spent it in the nearby Frying Pan public house. Apparently confident that she could earn it for a third time she wandered off, saying that she would soon be back at Thrawl Street.

According to Ellen Holland, Polly went in the direction of Buck's Row, a street south of the main Whitechapel High Street and running more or less parallel with it. It was in Buck's Row, about half a mile from where she left her friend, that Polly was found dead. At twenty to four that morning Charles Cross, a Bethnal Green carman, stopped on his way to work to look at an object lying by the gates of a stable yard. When he went closer to it he realised that it was a woman, dead or unconscious.

As he stood looking at the body and no doubt wondering what he should do, Cross heard somebody approaching. This was Robert Paul who, by coincidence, was also a carman from Bethnal Green on his way to work. Cross called him over and showed him the body. He believed that the woman was dead but Paul touched the body and thought he could detect breathing. After a quick discussion the two men decided to go on to their places of work and report the matter to the first policeman they met. This happened to be PC Jonas Mizen, who went back to Buck's Row and found another officer, PC John Neil, standing over the body. Shining his bull's-eye lantern on it, Neil saw that the throat had been deeply cut.

Knowing that other constables were in the area, Neil called for assistance and was heard by PC John Thain, who joined him in Buck's Row. While Neil stayed with the body, Thain went to fetch Dr Rees Ralph Llewellyn from his house at 152 Whitechapel Road. Mizen went to Bethnal Green police station to ask for assistance and for the police ambulance to be sent. Dr Llewellyn soon arrived and pronounced the woman dead. The body was removed when the police ambulance – little more than a coffin on wheels pushed like a hand-cart – was brought from Bethnal Green.

Inspector John Spratling, with other officers, had also come from the Bethnal Green station, and he accompanied the ambulance to the mortuary attached to the Old Montague Street workhouse. At the mortuary the body was stripped and it was only then that it was realised that the stomach had been cut deeply in several places, exposing the intestines. Seeing this, Spratling called Dr Llewellyn's attention to it. Llewellyn carried out an instant post-mortem and was of the opinion that the stomach wounds were severe enough to cause death. He also thought that they had been inflicted before the throat was cut.

Inspector Joseph Helson, examining the victim's clothing, found the mark of the Lambeth Workhouse on her petticoat. Nichols had been an inmate there before she went to work for Samuel Cowdry and following up this clue, the police were able to identify her and inform her relations. Formal identification of the body was made by Ellen Holland, who told the police of her meeting with Nichols shortly before she was murdered.

PC Neil was certain that the body had not been there when he passed through Bucks Row earlier that morning. That had been at ten past three – so it seemed clear that the murder had taken place at some time between then and 3.40, when Cross and Paul came upon the body. They had felt the hands and face and found them to be cold but Neil had touched her arm as he shone his lantern over her and thought he felt some warmth in it. If so, she had probably been dead for about fifteen minutes.

At that time in late August, with the summer of 1888 having been particularly hot, the night would probably have been a warm one, but Nichols would have lost a lot of blood from her various injuries, speeding the process by which she grew cold after death. If Cross and Paul were correct in what they said, she would have been dead for long enough for the exposed parts of her body to have become cold but other parts would have remained warm. Fifteen minutes would therefore be a fair estimate.

The obvious conclusion is that the murderer approached Nichols as a client, either in Bucks Row or as she wandered in that direction, after she had left Ellen Holland. One of them would probably have suggested the stable gateway as a suitable place to conduct their business and when they had reached it, the man killed her. If Dr Llewellyn was right, he did so by slashing her stomach. Her under clothing was not cut or bloodstained so she might have pulled it aside for the client's convenience.

The only alternative would be that she was unconscious when her assailant began his work, giving him free access to her body. Dr Llewellyn said –

"There was a bruise running along the lower
part of the jaw on the right side of the
face. That might have been caused by a blow
from a fist or pressure from a thumb."

As the police would have known, however, the bruise could also have been the result of some disagreement with a previous client or another woman. The possibility that Nichols had been made helpless or unconscious may have been thought more likely when the next murder took place. In that instance, evidence suggested strongly that the victim had been partially strangled.

Dr Llewellyn's belief that Nichols was already dead when her throat was cut was supported by the way in which the wound was inflicted. As he said in his report –

"On the left side of the neck, about one inch below the jaw, there was an incision about four inches in length, and ran from a point immediately below the ear. On the same side, but an inch below, and commencing at about one inch in front of it, was a circular incision, which terminated at about three inches below the right jaw. That incision completely severed all the tissues down to the vertebrae. The large vessels of the neck on both sides were severed. The incision was about eight inches in length."

There were, then, two cuts in the neck, suggesting that Nichols was helpless enough for the murderer to have been able to make a second attempt when the first was unsuccessful. The severity of the second cut, reaching right down to the spinal column, also supports that view. A wound like that could never have been inflicted while the victim was capable of any sort of struggle.

The belief that Jack the Ripper was left-handed seems to have begun with the murder of Nichols. Spratling noted that her throat had been cut from left to right and said that the abdominal injuries had been inflicted "supposedly by a left handed person". He may, however, have been echoing Llewellyn's words as the doctor said that "The injuries were from left to right and *might* (my italics) have been caused by a left-handed person."

In suggesting that the bruise on the right side of the face could have been made by pressure from a thumb, Llewellyn raised the possibility that the murderer forced his victim's head back with his right hand and cut her throat with a knife held in the left. That would certainly have been more likely to have been done if the murderer was left-handed, and would have been easier to accomplish if Nichols had been dead or unconscious at the time.

The question then arises of *why* the murderer would have cut her throat if Dr Llewellyn was correct in his opinion – strongly supported by the evidence – that she was already dead when that wound was inflicted. One explanation might be that in the darkness, the murderer was not certain that she was dead and was afraid that she might survive for long enough to tell somebody what had happened and to describe him. Another possibility is that it was done to complete some sort of ritual, as some theorists believe.

Llewellyn's opinion about the order in which the wounds were inflicted may have cast some doubt on the idea that the murder of Nichols was just another street crime – and a remark that he made about the crime scene certainly did. He was surprised by the small amount of blood on the ground where the body lay, estimating it was no more than enough to fill two large wine glasses or half a pint at the most. Inspector Helson emphasised this later that morning when he told *The Times* that "viewing the spot where the body was found, it was difficult to believe that the woman received her death wounds there."

At the inquest, Helson said that he was sure that she had been killed where she was found, but by then he would no doubt have discussed the matter and had possibly accepted an explanation of the lack of blood which some modern experts still adhere to. This was that it had been absorbed by her clothing and hair, which is too facile an answer. As the late author Stephen Knight pointed out, if that had been a valid reason, there would have been no speculation that she had not been murdered at that spot.

11

Another author, Melvyn Fairclough, shared Knight's belief that Nichols was killed at some other place and brought to Buck's Row in a coach. He suggested that she was carried from the vehicle by two men, one of them supporting her shoulders, and the other holding her legs, by the knees. This, he said, would have caused the blood to run down her back as the upper part of her body would have been tilted backwards. This seems quite possible, particularly if Dr Llewellyn was correct in saying that the throat had been cut *after* the other wounds had been inflicted. The loss of blood from the other wounds would have reduced the flow from the throat and if, as Fairclough suggested, Nichols was carried in a semi-upright position to where she was found, the blood might well have clung to the body as it thickened, and run down the back. This would account for the fact that there was blood soaking into the back of her coat and dress, down as far as her waist.

There are two alternatives to Fairclough's explanation, neither of which are completely compatible with the facts. One is that, as some authors believe, Nichols and other victims had their throats cut from behind, giving the murderer the advantage of surprise and preventing them from putting up any sort of struggle. If that had happened to Nichols, however, there would have been blood on the front of her clothing and probably on the ground, away from her body, but none was found. The other possibility is that she was somehow rendered unconscious or wrestled to the ground and her throat cut as she lay there, killing her instantly, with the blood from the wound spreading out under her body and head, soaking into her coat and hair. This is equally unlikely. Dr Llewellyn said that he could detect no signs of a struggle on the body, but more importantly, there was a marked difference in the evidence at the crime scene than at that of the murder of the third Ripper victim, Elizabeth Stride.

Because her assailant was interrupted by the arrival on the scene of another person, Stride was the only victim whose body was not mutilated. The only wound that she suffered was the deep cut across her throat which killed her. It severed the carotid artery, causing a sudden, violent release of blood which, following a slight slope in the ground where she lay, ran away from her body. A witness estimated that there were about four pints of it – about eight times the amount that Dr Llewellyn saw by the body of Nichols. Quite obviously there was not the same sudden outpouring which occurred when Stride was murdered, although again, the carotid artery was severed. This was probably one of the factors that had made Llewellyn suspect the wounds to Nichols's stomach had been the cause of her death, and her throat had been cut – perhaps for some ritual purpose – after they had been inflicted. Blood would still have flowed from the carotid artery but not to the extent that it would have done if she had been alive when it was severed.

Llewellyn was a doctor of some experience and having seen the victims of violent murders before, he was probably accurate in his assessment of the amount of blood at the crime scene. He made no suggestion that Nichols had been killed at some other place but his opinions pointed to that conclusion and, together with the theories of Knight and Fairclough, they must raise the the possibility that Nichols was taken to Buck's Row, already dead and mutilated, in some sort of vehicle, lifted out in such a way that the blood from her throat ran back over her shoulders and down the neck of her coat. When she was placed on the ground, a slight gradient made the blood that was still spilling from her throat flow round her head and into her hair as it lay on the cobbles.

Dr Llewellyn's comment on the lack of blood at the crime scene, his opinion on the order in which Nichols received her wounds and the wounds themselves, all pointed to an unusual murder. The appointment of the Scotland Yard detective Inspector Frederick George Abberline as co-ordinator if not the actual head of the investigation, may indicate that this was quickly realised in the police hierarchy. Some theorists who believe in a cover-up conspiracy, however, have made a fairly good case for their belief that Abberline's brief was really to ensure that the real truth about Jack the Ripper never emerged. His activities in another well-known case a few months later support that view.

Until Scotland Yard took an interest, officers like Spratling and Helson would probably not have seen the murder as anything more than a particularly unpleasant version of the type of street crime that had been occurring in that area. Earlier that month another prostitute, Martha Tabram, had been found dead, having been repeatedly stabbed with a bayonet-like instrument, and other gruesome murders had taken place in the area. These crimes and the general conditions in Whitechapel had put considerable pressure on the local police. Dr Llewellyn's opinions would have been respected, but it's unlikely that they would have resulted in any different approach to the murder.

Nichols had been murdered in the early hours of a Friday morning, and if the crime had been committed today, modern investigators would have wondered if the killer was a person who worked at night, such as a shift-worker or a watchman. At that time, however, the working day began much earlier, as is shown by the fact that Cross and Paul were on their way to work when they discovered the body at 3.40 a.m., so the time of the murder gives no real clue. It would almost certainly have been assumed that the murderer had been a man, probably one who had approached the victim posing as a would-be client, as it would have needed stronger hands than most women possess to inflict a cut to the throat as deep as the one that the victim received.

In modern investigation the psychological profiling of murderers has become an accepted practice but the Ripper's first murder gives very little scope for such an approach. In his book, *Whoever Fights Monsters*, the American expert Robert Ressler, who pioneered psychological profiling as an FBI agent, talks of the "Great Divide" between organised and disorganised murderers. He explains one particular difference in a way that gives us a good indication of how profiling works –

> "I say that the organised offender hides the
> bodies of his victims; in our research
> interviews, and in analysis of crime scenes, we
> found this to be true more than three quarters
> of the time. That's enough to make the
> generalisation hold up pretty well, but not
> enough to make it an absolute condition for our
> characterisation. All the 'rules' of profiling
> are like that."

This goes a long way to explaining why Ressler insists that profiling is an art, not a science. It has no infallible rules which would make it possible for anyone to practise it. In the hands of those who have mastered the art, however, it has had remarkable results.

It would be difficult now to build up an accurate profile of Jack the Ripper because the data is incomplete. With no clear photographs of the crimes scenes we can only rely on the statements of witnesses and the reports of the detectives and police surgeons who were involved in the investigation. In the case of Polly Nichols, the inquest documents were destroyed by fire during the Second World War. Evidence such as Dr Llewellyn's post mortem report survives only through newspaper reports of the proceedings, which may not be completely accurate. There are, in any case, very few definite facts concerning the murder.

As doubt exists as to whether or not she was killed in Buck's Row, the fact that PC Neil failed to see her when he passed the spot on his beat at 3.10 a.m. does not necessarily mean that she was alive at that time. All that can be said for certain is that she died at some time between 2.30, when Ellen Holland spoke to her, and 3.40, when Charles Cross discovered her body, with Constable Neil's belief that he felt warmth in her arm suggesting that she was killed at about 3.25. The murderer could have been one of many men on their way to work that in the morning.

Looking at that murder alone – and assuming, as the police probably did, that Nichols was murdered where she was found in Buck's Row – the killing would probably go down as a disorganised one. The victim would have been a random one, with the murderer making it impossible for himself to hide the body, although such a thing would probably not have occurred to him. If he had met Nichols, approached her as a client and walked with her to what he saw as a suitable place to kill her, it would be said that he had "controlled" his victim, but only in the most elementary and obvious way. It would certainly not have indicated any great intelligence or planning on his part.

If she was *not* killed in Buck's Row, however, a great amount of organisation would have gone into the crime. Again, there would have been no effort to conceal the body but there may have been an attempt at "staging" – that is, arranging the evidence at the crime scene to confuse the investigators. If Nichols was murdered at some other place, the very act of leaving her in Buck's Row was "staging", because it was almost certain that it would be assumed that she was murdered there. She could not, of course, have been killed at any great distance from where she was found, as the evidence of Ellen Holland proves, but the killer might have come from some distance. If so, the use of a vehicle would have enabled him to kill and escape quickly, and would also have created the impression that he lived near the crime scene. If that was his intention, the murderer made one mistake because the lack of blood mentioned by Dr Llewellyn raised some doubt as to whether she was actually murdered in Buck's Row. Whether or not this indicated a lack of medical knowledge is difficult to say but it seems that Jack the Ripper started his career in a way typical of a serial murderer. He began nervously – as can be seen when the killing of Nichols is compared with later murders.

As Robert Ressler puts it when he talks of the "predictable pattern" of serial murderers,

> "They begin cautiously, frightened of their
> crimes. Then the pace picks up, and they
> progress to become effective and efficient
> killing machines. Eventually, they become
> cavalier and careless, convinced that they
> cannot be caught by any mortal."

Later murders suggest that Jack the Ripper followed that pattern. The mutilation of Nichols – pointing to an introverted, woman-hating type of person – was slight in comparison with that of subsequent victims, but the process had begun. Having many times imagined himself killing and mutilating his victims, the murderer had now actually done so, and what Ressler calls the gap between fantasy and reality had been bridged. It was not long before there was confirmation of that, as it was only eight days later that Jack the Ripper killed his second victim.

CHAPTER 2

Annie Chapman

The second victim of Jack the Ripper was Annie Chapman, known in Whitechapel as "Dark Annie". She was murdered on 8 September 1888, and her fate was decided in a strangely similar way to that of Mary Ann Nichols, who had been killed eight days earlier. The report by Inspector Joseph Chandler, the police officer who was called to the scene of her murder, tells the story.

> "The woman has been identified by Timothy
> Donovan, deputy at Crossingham's lodging
> house at 35 Dorset Street, Spitalfields,
> who states that he has known her about
> 16 months as a prostitute, and for the past
> 4 months she had lodged at above house.
> At 1.45 a.m. 8th instant she was in the
> kitchen, the worse for liquor and eating
> potatoes. He (Donovan) sent to her for
> the money for her bed, which she said she
> had not got and asked him to trust her, which
> he declined to do. She then left, stating
> that she would not be long gone."

So, like Polly Nichols, Annie Chapman was ordered out because she had no money, and even left with the same intention of earning her night's rent from the street. As she went out, she is said to have told John Evans, the watchman at Crossingham's, "I won't be long, Brummy. See that Tim keeps the bed for me."

Annie, aged forty-five, was a widow. Her husband John Chapman, a coachman at Windsor, died in 1886 but they had lived apart for several years before then. The break-up occurred because like Polly Nichols, Annie become too fond of drink. She had been more fortunate than many of the Whitechapel prostitutes because until he died, John Chapman had given her an allowance of ten shillings (50p) a week.

There is no evidence of where she went after she finally left Crossingham's, which was at around 2 a.m. At about ten to six that morning John Davis, a carman, went into the backyard of the house in which he lived at No. 29 Hanbury Street, in Spitalfields, and found her there, dead and horribly mutilated. Her stomach had been cut open and the intestines taken out and placed over her shoulder. Doctors carrying out the post mortem examination found that the uterus was missing, presumably having been removed and taken away by the murderer.

Davis, shocked by what he had seen, went along the street to No. 23a, where Joseph and Thomas Bayley had a business making packing cases. Two of their employees, James Green and James Kent had already arrived for work and Davis persuaded them to return to the yard of No. 29 with him. When they had done so and looked at the body, Davis went with some other men to the nearby Commercial Street police station. They reported the murder to Inspector Chandler, the duty inspector. Chandler immediately went to Hanbury Street with Davis and the others, and having viewed the body, he sent for assistance from Commercial Street and for the divisional police surgeon Dr George Bagster Phillips to come to Hanbury Street.

Dr Phillips arrived at about 6.20 a.m., and pronounced the victim dead. He was then of the opinion that she had been dead for at least two hours. That would have meant that she was murdered at 4.20 a.m. at the latest, but soon there was conflicting evidence. A man named John Richardson told the police that he had been in the yard at 4.45 that morning and he was certain that the body was not there at that time.

Richardson's mother, Mrs Amelia Richardson, lived at 29 Hanbury Street where she and another occupant made wooden goods which they sold at the nearby Spitalfields Market. They kept their stock in a cellar under the back stairs of the house. Since it had been broken into a few weeks earlier, Richardson had made a habit of calling in on his way to work to make sure that another robbery had not taken place. He told the police that on that particular morning he sat down on the steps and trimmed some loose leather from the sole of his shoe with his knife. If Chapman's body had been in the yard at that time – and according to Dr Phillips she would then have been dead for over half an hour – her head would have been practically at his feet and he would certainly have seen her.

Dr Phillips had been a police surgeon for twenty-two years and his estimate of the time of death would have been regarded as accurate. Richardson's evidence may therefore have raised doubts, as in the case of Polly Nichols, that the victim had actually been murdered in the place where she had been found. There was another reminder of the murder of Nichols in Inspector Chandler's report, as it showed that there had been only a small amount of blood by the body. He said,

> "I...found a woman lying on her back, dead,
> left arm resting on the left breast, legs
> drawn up, abducted, small intestines and
> flap of abdomen lying on right side above
> right shoulder, attached by a cord with
> the rest of the intestines inside the body;
> two flaps of skin from the lower part of the
> abdomen lying in a large quantity of blood
> above the left shoulder; throat cut deeply
> from left and back in a jagged manner right
> around the throat. I at once sent for Dr
> Phillips, divisional surgeon, and to the
> station for the ambulance and assistance.
> The doctor pronounced life extinct and stated
> the woman had been dead at least two hours...
> *On examining the yard I found on the back wall*
> *of the house (at the head of the body) and about*
> *18 inches from the ground about six patches of*
> *blood varying in size from a sixpenny piece to a*
> *point and on the wooden paling on left of the*
> *body near head patches and smears of blood about*
> *14 inches from the ground.*" (My italics)

In his evidence at the inquest, Dr Phillips said very much the same thing –

"On the wooden paling...smears of blood
corresponding to where the head of the
deceased lay, were to be seen. These
were about 14 inches from the ground,
*and immediately above the part where the
blood lay that had flowed from the neck.*"
(My italics)

There was, then, blood which had apparently flowed from the victim's
throat, but not as much as would have been expected. In a report in *The
Times*, 10 September 1888, it was stated that

"Although, as in the case of Mary Ann Nichols,
a very small quantity of blood was found on
the ground (leading to the supposition that
the murder was committed elsewhere) its
absence is accounted for by the quantity
the clothes would absorb."

This report must almost certainly have been based on information from
the police, who were therefore sticking to the explanation put forward
in the case of Nichols, that the victim's clothing had soaked up much of
her blood – which was at the very least a remarkable coincidence.

The discrepancy between the evidence of Richardson and Dr Phillips
seemed to be explained by two other witnesses at the inquest, but their
evidence was not quite compatible. Albert Cadosche, a carpenter who lived at
27 Hanbury Street, told the coroner that he went into his back yard – which
adjoined the one in which Chapman was found – at 5.15 on the morning of
the murder. He said that from that yard he heard a voice say 'No!'. He went
back into the house but returned to the yard a few minutes later and heard
what sounded like something falling against the fence. He left for work at
5.30, and was certain of the time because the nearby Spitalfields Church
clock showed 5.32 as he passed. Several authors have quoted Cadosche as
saying that it was a woman's voice that he heard from the adjoining yard but
newspaper reports of the inquest say only that it was "a voice". Whether or
not it was a woman, however, the immediate conclusion was that Cardosche
had heard Chapman being murdered, with her body brushing against the
fence, by which she was later found, as she fell.

When he gave evidence at the inquest, Dr Phillips was probably aware that the testimony of other witnesses would question his estimate of the time of death. He said that he had thought Chapman to have been dead for at least two hours when he saw her in the yard, but with the coldness of the morning and the loss of blood that she had sustained, death might have appeared to have taken place earlier than it actually had. That qualification accommodated Cadosche's evidence, but a later witness caused another complication. Mrs Elizabeth Long told the coroner that at 5.30 on the morning of the murder she had been walking through Hanbury Street and at the front of No. 29 she had seen a woman, who she later identified as Chapman, talking to a man. As she passed the couple, she heard the man say, "Will you?" – a way of asking a Whitechapel prostitute if she would give her services – and the woman replied, "Yes". Mrs Long described the man as foreign in appearance. He wore a deerstalker hat and his clothes, although shabby, looked as if they had originally been of good quality.

The inference from Mrs Long's evidence was that after she had passed by, the couple walked through the passage at the side of the house to the back yard, where Chapman was then murdered. This explained why the body had not been in the yard when Richardson went there at 4.45 and would have been completely convincing if the sighting of the couple had been fifteen minutes earlier. If it had, there would have been no dispute at all that Chapman had been killed in the yard because what Cadosche had heard could only have been the murder taking place. Like him, however, Mrs Long was certain of the time – in her case because she had heard the local brewer's clock strike the half hour as she approached the couple.

The coroner, Mr Edwin Wynne Baxter, seemed anxious to reconcile the evidence of the two witnesses when he summed up. Cadosche's evidence could have been dismissed because Mrs Long had apparently proved that Chapman had been alive at 5.30, which was *after* he heard the sounds in the next yard – but Wynne Baxter suggested that he might have mistaken the time. "Had he been out in his reckoning by only 15 minutes", it would explain everything. This was true, but in the time scale of events as Cadosche had described them, a difference of 15 minutes would have been more significant than Wynne Baxter made it sound. He may have felt that Cadosche's evidence, coupled with Mrs Long's, provided such a convenient scenario that he was reluctant to abandon any of it, but it's equally possible that a very simple and relevant question had occurred to him. If the sounds from the other side of the fence had *not* been connected with the murder, what was the true explanation of them?

It might have been that other residents of No. 29 Hanbury Street had been in the back yard at that time, and in that Cadosche heard nothing like a struggle or an argument that prompted him to look over the 5' 6" fence, there might well have been some innocent explanation of what was happening. In that case, however, the police would have known about it from questioning the other occupants of the house. If Chapman had taken her client into the yard, so might another prostitute before her – but in fact, it's very doubtful that Chapman would have done that, and this is one of two very valid reasons for doubting the convenient explanation that Mrs Long's evidence suggested.

Reporting the inquest, *The Times* quoted John Richardson as saying that he had seen "lots of strangers" in the passageway beside the house "at all hours of the night," and had seen "both men and women there and had turned them out".

What this meant was that the passageway beside the house was often used by prostitutes and some experts have suggested that although Richardson was reluctant to say so at the inquest, his real purpose in going to the house on that morning had been to see if any were there, and if so, to send them on their way. *The Times* also reported that it had been established that there was always access to the passageway from the street and that Chapman would have known that she could walk through it to the yard. No doubt she did – and it's quite possible that like the other prostitutes mentioned by Richardson, she had taken her clients into that passageway before, or if not that one, others by similar houses in the neighbourhood. What is questionable, however, is why on that particular morning she would have chosen to go through to the open yard, where she might easily have been seen by occupants of the house. At that time of the year it would have been almost broad daylight by 5.30 in the morning and as she would have known, people in the house would have been up and preparing to leave for work.

If it was unlikely that Chapman would have forsaken the cover of the passageway for the yard, the same must apply to the murderer. Why would he have chosen to kill and mutilate her in a place where at any moment he could have been seen, when he could have done so safely out of sight in the passageway? If he and Chapman had entered it together and she had suggested that it would be a suitable place for their engagement, he would hardly have persuaded her that it would be better to go on out in the yard.

The other reason to doubt the sequence of events suggested by Mrs Long's evidence – and, in fact, the evidence itself – is that Dr Phillips provided good reason for believing that whatever may have been the exact time of her death, Chapman could not have been alive at 5.30 that morning. When the coroner asked him how long it might have taken the murderer to mutilate her body, his answer was –

> "I myself could not have performed all the injuries I saw on that woman, and effect them, even without a struggle, under a quarter of an hour."

Phillips probably mentioned the possibility of a struggle because he believed that Chapman had been half-strangled before she was murdered. When the coroner queried the possibility of her having been gagged, he drew attention to "the swollen face and protruding tongue, both of which were signs of suffocation." Given that it would have taken two or three minutes for the couple to have walked through to the yard after Mrs Long saw them, and for Chapman to have been overpowered and murdered, the mutilation of her body would then have had to have been completed in probably less than half the time that Phillips had estimated. It could only have been a minute or two after he got up at 5.45 that Davis went out and saw the body – his toing and froing with Green and Kent and the journey to the police station would probably have taken about a quarter of an hour but he was still able to arrive at Commercial Street at 6.02 – and with no sign at all of whoever had killed her, she would have been dead for at least a few minutes. The mutilation of her body would therefore have been completed in about seven minutes, probably between 5.33 and 5.40 at the latest, which was half the time that Dr Phillips had suggested.

It's possible, of course, that Phillips overestimated the time that it would have taken to mutilate the body but that would still not mean that it could have been done in the few minutes available if the murder had been committed after 5.30, as Mrs Long's evidence had suggested.

Her testimony is made even more doubtful by Phillips' conviction, which seemed justified by the obvious signs of suffocation that he mentioned, that Chapman had been "seized by the throat" before the fatal wound had been inflicted. If that had happened in the yard at any time after 5.30, John Davis might well have heard the sound of the struggle. He told the coroner that after a disturbed night he had fallen asleep at around 5 o'clock, but woke again after only about half an hour. He was, therefore, awake from the time when, according to Mrs Long's evidence, Chapman and the murderer must have entered the yard, until he finally got up at 5.45. He obviously heard nothing which prompted him to go outside during that period – and unless for some strange reason they failed to mention it to the police, neither did any of the other residents of the house who must have been awake at that time.

What may have been another doubt about Mrs Long's evidence was that questioned by the coroner, Cadosche said that when he left the house at 5.30 that morning, he saw neither her nor the man and woman she had described. It must be said, however, that it would not have taken any of them very long to leave the scene, as Wynne Baxter may have concluded. He would have had a more valid reason to question her evidence if Dr Phillips had stood by his own testimony and said that there would have been no time for the murderer to have mutilated the body to the extent that he did if Chapman had been killed after 5.30.

The Lancet actually reported him as saying that under proper surgical conditions it would probably have taken him "the best part of an hour". Phillips was also strangely amenable over the question of the time of death. The police, also experienced in such things, were inclined to believe his original statement, made at 6.20 a.m., that the victim had been dead for "two hours and probably more." Even without their backing, Phillips was quite capable of arguing a point, as he had shown earlier in the hearing.

Victorian coroners were not men who would allow their authority to be questioned but Phillips had a lengthy disagreement with Wynne Baxter on whether he should give the full results of his post mortem examination. This began when, having made some general remarks, he said that he felt that he should go no further as the full details would be "painful to the feelings of the jury and the public." That was just before the inquest was adjourned for the day but when it was resumed, Wynne Baxter said that he felt that the evidence from the post mortem should be "on the records of the court for various reasons which I need not enumerate."

What he meant – and what he obviously felt that Phillips knew quite well – was that it was necessary for the length, breadth and depths of any wounds found on a murder victim to be recorded. Phillips complained that he had had no notice that the post mortem details would be required – a strange remark from a police surgeon of his experience – but he declined the coroner's offer of a postponement so that he could prepare himself and said he would do his best to give them.

He answered Wynne Baxter's first question, but almost immediately broke off to repeat that he felt that such details were unfit for the public to hear. The coroner reminded him that "we are here in the interests of justice and must have all the evidence before us", but said that he had noticed some women and boys in the court and felt that they might "retire". When they had gone, Phillips made a fresh objection – "I still feel that in giving these details to the public you are thwarting the ends of justice."

It has been suggested that Phillips was attempting to give the police the benefit of "guilty knowledge" – withholding some detail of the murder so that a suspect under skilful interrogation might refer to it, and reveal his guilt. That, however, would surely have been something for the police to put to the coroner and, as the law stood, it could not in any case have been done by withholding any details of the medical evidence. Whatever his opinion of that particular objection by Phillips might have been, Wynne Baxter merely repeated that he was bound to take all the evidence in the case.

Phillips then shifted his ground once again, saying, "I am of the opinion that what I am about to describe took place after death, so that it could not affect the cause of death, which you are inquiring into."

Wynne Baxter overruled him again, so Phillips finally gave his evidence – and having previously complained that he was unprepared, gave a very detailed and apparently fluent account of the victim's injuries. He had obviously been determined to withhold that evidence, yet he must have known that if Wynne Baxter insisted, he would have no choice but to give it. Faced with Mrs Long's dubious evidence, however, he made no attempt to pursue an argument that he could have won and, in effect, admitted to a considerable error of judgement in his estimation of the time of the victim's death.

The doubts about Mrs Long's evidence might suggest that what Cadosche heard at around 5.15 that morning was the murder being committed, but this is also doubtful. Dr Phillips would still have been over an hour out in his estimate of the time of death – which seems unlikely – and there would still have been the strange choice by Chapman and the murderer to go into the yard when the passageway would have provided cover. Also, Phillips had probably been right in his opinion that Chapman had been half-strangled before her throat was cut and Cadosche heard nothing from the other side of the fence which suggested it. After the voice had said, "No", there had been nothing which suggested a struggle or somebody choking – only the sound of something falling against the fence. If that had been the body of the already dead Chapman being placed there and her body brushing the fence, it would explain why she was not in the yard when Richardson went there half an hour after Dr Phillips believed her to have died, and why the fence was smeared with blood.

Chapman's throat was cut in the yard but the small amount of blood suggests that, like Polly Nichols, she was already dead when it happened. The flow of blood might have been lessened because she had been half-strangled but there was no evidence of that when Nichols was murdered and it seems beyond coincidence that in both cases there was this lack of blood at the crime scene. The reason again advanced by the police, that the victim's clothing had soaked up the blood, was not born out in the evidence of Chandler, Phillips or anyone else who saw the body. With the first two murders, there was, therefore, reason to believe that the victims were already dead when they arrived at the places where they were found, and that there had been "staging" in the form of attempts to make it appear that they *had* been killed in those places. If this was true of Chapman, leaving her in the yard rather than the passageway was an error which might deny the local knowledge which some experts have attributed to the murderer.

Another angle on the killing of Chapman was suggested by Wynne Baxter, in his summing up. In the closing stages he seemed to abandon the painstaking approach that had caused the hearing to drag on over several sessions, and one sign of this was his somewhat tendentious attempt to reconcile the evidence of Cadosche with that of Mrs Long. In the opinion of some experts, this was because he was anxious to put forward a theory as to the motive for the murder. It had been reported that the pathology museum of a London hospital had been approached by an American who wanted human organs as specimens for a physiological monograph that he had produced. He intended to distribute twenty copies to interested parties. This prompted Wynne Baxter to think that a market for organs existed and his theory, which provoked angry responses from the medical profession, was that Chapman had been murdered to supply it. In his favour was Dr Phillips's opinion that the murder had been

> "obviously the work of an expert – of one,
> at least, who had such knowledge of anatomical
> or pathological examination as to be enabled to
> secure the pelvic organs with one sweep of
> the knife."

Phillips probably based his opinion on the fact that the uterus seemed to have been quite clinically removed but some authors have pointed out that when he extracted it, the murderer also cut away a considerable part of the victim's bladder, which suggested that the apparently expert removal of the other organ was really accidental. The question of whether or not the Ripper had medical training or anatomical knowledge has never been resolved. Dr Phillips also reported that –

> "the throat was dissevered deeply; ... the
> incisions through the skin were jagged, and
> reached right round the neck..."

One expert, Martin Fido, believed that this had been an unsuccessful attempt to remove the victim's head, and suggested that it ruled out any possibility that the murderer had medical knowledge.

If, as many experts believe, Jack the Ripper was no more than a sexual serial murderer, Chapman's uterus was probably taken as a trophy. Serial murderers often take such trophies and if he had done so in the case of Chapman, the Ripper was following the classic pattern. Having taken the crucial step between fantasy and reality with the murder of Nichols, he had progressed rapidly by mutilating Chapman to a greater degree and taking the trophy from her body. The significance of this would not have been recognised in those early days of detection, but what should have been noted were the various facts which made it doubtful that both Chapman and Nichols had been killed where they were found, and the attempts to make it appear that they had. Knowing the ways of the local prostitutes, the police would certainly have known that Chapman was unlikely to have taken a man she believed to be a client into the yard when she could have used the passageway, as she probably had on many previous occasions.

The evidence of Mrs Long had apparently explained the discrepancy between the evidence of John Richardson and Dr Phillips' original opinion of the time of death, but it's known that the police were still inclined to accept that opinion as correct. Mrs Long might well have been wrong in identifying Chapman as the woman she saw on the morning of the murder, but her description of the woman's companion was similar to that of a man seen with one of the later victims. This suggests a scenario which would be compatible with practically all the various testimonies, with Mrs Long's identification of the woman she saw in Hanbury Street as Chapman the only error.

If, as previously suggested, Cadosche had heard the body of the already dead Chapman being placed in the yard at around 5.15, it would mean that Dr Phillips was probably right in saying that she had been dead for over two hours when he saw her at around 6.30. Also, it would explain why she was not in the yard at 4.45, when John Richardson was there. Mrs Long would have been wrong in saying that the woman she saw at the front of Hanbury Street at 5.30 was Chapman but the woman's companion could have just left the yard by the side passageway, having helped to place the body there. The woman with him could have been another of the local prostitutes, who had approached him as he came out into the street. Seeing Mrs Long approaching, he might have decided to stop and talk to the woman until she had gone by, in the hope that she would think that what she had seen had been just another man asking a prostitute for her services, and that she might even forget the incident.

It would have been in keeping with such a ploy if, as Mrs Long reported, he kept his back to her as she passed by, at the same time asking the prostitute, "Will you?", to leave no doubt as to what they were discussing. They would probably have moved on as soon as the witness had gone past, which would explain why Cadosche saw nothing of them when he left for work at about the same time. It seems unlikely that the man would actually have availed himself of the woman's services as he would have been anxious to be on his way. His best solution would have been to give her some money and make an excuse for not keeping to their agreement.

This is, of course, no more than theory, but the many strange facts and the contadictory evidence suggest that there was far more to the murder of Chapman than even the removal of the uterus from her body implied. It's difficult to believe that the police were not of that opinion – particularly with John Richardson's strong assertion that Chapman's body had not been in the yard at a time when, according to Dr Phillips first reaction and their own belief, she must have been dead. Strangely, there is no evidence of them entertaining such thoughts.

CHAPTER 3

Elizabeth Stride

Known to her friends and fellow prostitutes as "Long Liz", Elizabeth Stride was about five feet five inches in height. That was probably above average height for a woman in the Victorian era but in the East End of those days the epithet 'Long" was likely to be applied to anyone named Stride – a stride is a long step – and therefore had nothing to do with her height. She was born in Sweden, near Gothenburg, where she was known by the name of Gustavsdotter. She married John Thomas Stride in March 1869, and for a while they ran a coffee shop in Poplar High Street.

Often drunk and disorderly, Liz Stride told a number of untrue stories about her past, one of which was that her husband and children had been drowned when a pleasure boat, the *Princess Alice*, collided with another vessel and sank in the Thames in 1878. She claimed that she had a speech impediment because another passenger of the steamer had kicked her, permanently damaging the roof of her mouth, as they struggled in the water. When he examined her after she had been murdered by Jack the Ripper on 30th September 1888, however, Dr Phillips found no evidence of such an injury. John Thomas Stride actually died from a heart attack in the Bromley Sick Asylum in 1884, six years after the "Princess Alice" disaster. He and Elizabeth had parted a few years earlier and he had been living in a workhouse in Poplar.

For some three years prior to her death, Stride had lived with a docker named Michael Kidney, in Dorset Street, near to Crossingham's doss house where Annie Chapman had hoped to stay on the night of her murder. She carried on her trade in the vicinity of Berner Street, which was a little way away from Spitalfields, on the other side of the Whitechapel Road. She was seen with several different men in that area on the night that she was killed. Most of them could be eliminated as suspects and the first of her companions who might have been involved in her murder was one who was with her at midnight, at the shop of a greengrocer named Matthew Packer, at 44 Berner Street.

According to Packer, the man was about five feet seven inches in height, broad-shouldered, "rather quick in speaking – rough voice". He wore a long black overcoat and a "soft felt hat, kind of hawker hat". Packer "put the man down as a young clerk". The police later decided that Packer was unreliable and he was not called to give evidence at the inquest on Stride but there is little doubt that she was the woman he saw. When he described her, he said that she was "playing with a flower like a geranium, white outside and red inside". The police officers who examined her body said that the flower, pinned to her jacket, was a red rose, set in a spray of fern, so although Packer's memory was a little confused on that point he obviously saw the flower. His description of her clothes was very accurate.

The man bought half a pound of black grapes and rejoined Stride outside. Packer said that they stood talking within sight of the shop and he last saw them as he closed for the night at half past twelve. Five minutes later PC William Smith passed them as he made his way along Berner Street on his beat. He described the man as about twenty eight, with a small dark moustache, and wearing a "hard, deerstalker hat" and dark overcoat. Packer made no mention of the moustache but his description of the man's clothing was so like Smith's that it must have been the same man. The constable also said that in one hand the man held a parcel which was about eighteen inches by six, and wrapped in newspaper.

At 12.45, ten minutes after Smith had seen the couple, a Hungarian-born Jew named Israel Schwartz entered Berner Street on his way home. Nearing Dutfield's Yard, the premises of a cart-making firm, he saw Stride and a man standing in the gateway of the yard. As he came up to them he saw the man pull Stride towards the road, then throw her to the ground. In a statement which he later made to the police, Schwartz said that she screamed three times "but not very loudly". Schwartz did not want to be involved in a violent incident so he quickly crossed over to the other side of the street. As he did, Stride's assailant shouted the word "Lipski".

Israel Lipski was a Jew who had been hanged for murder in 1887. There was a lot of anti-Semitic feeling in the East End at that time and a popular way of insulting Jews was to shout his name at them. In correspondence with the Home Office over the incident Inspector Abberline said that Schwartz had "a heavy Jewish appearance" and it was agreed that the man who had attacked Stride had shouted the word at him to send him quickly on his way.

Schwartz had very little English and could have had no knowledge of current idioms, because he misunderstood what the man had said. When he reached the other side of the street he came almost face to face with another man and, assuming that the two of them were together, he thought that Stride's attacker was shouting a warning to his accomplice. He turned and walked away then, seeing that the second man was following him, he ran. He told the police that the man did not follow him for very far.

Schwartz said that Stride's assailant had been about thirty, five feet five inches in height, with a fair complexion, dark hair, a small brown moustache, full face and broad shoulders. He wore a dark jacket and trousers and a black cap with a peak. The second man was aged about thirty-five, five feet eleven inches in height, with a fresh complexion, light brown hair and brown moustache. He was wearing a dark overcoat and an old black hard felt hat with a wide brim. He was almost certainly the man who was with Stride when Packer and Constable Smith saw her. The statements of the three men all included the dark or black overcoat and the wide-brimmed hat although on the latter, their ways of describing it varied.

At 1 a.m. – fifteen minutes after Schwartz saw the attack – Mr Louis Diemschütz, steward at the International Working Men's Educational Club in Berner Street, found the body of Stride, lying just inside the gateway to Dutfield's Yard. Diemschütz was driving a cart into the yard when his pony shied to the left, having seen the body lying there. Unable to see what had frightened the animal, Diemschütz looked down to his right but although he could see something lying there, he could not make out what it was. He felt with his whip, then jumped down from the cart and struck a match. It was a windy night and the match quickly blew out, but Diemschütz could see that it was a woman, apparently unconscious.

He went into the club and informed his wife and some of the members who were still there that a woman was lying outside, then returned to the yard with a candle. He then saw the blood that had flowed from the woman's throat, and set off to find a policeman. Diemschütz had been accompanied into the yard two other members of the club, Morris Eagle and 'Isaacs' Kozebrodsky, who also went off looking for a constable. In the nearby Commercial Road they saw Constable Henry Lamb and reported the murder to him. Lamb quickly made his way to Dutfield's Yard where a crowd of what he later estimated to have been between fifteen and twenty people had assembled.

During his unsuccessful search for a policeman, Diemschütz had met one of the local residents, Edward Spooner, and told him about the murder. Spooner returned to the yard with Diemschütz, and they arrived just before Lamb. When one of the members of the club struck a match, Spooner had lifted up the victim's chin and saw blood still flowing from the wound in her throat. Lamb then arrived, followed almost immediately by another constable who had probably heard the commotion from the yard. Lamb shone his light on the body and when he saw that the throat had been cut, he sent the other constable to fetch Dr Frederick William Blackwell, who lived nearby. Dr Blackwell arrived at 1.10, so all this happened within ten minutes of Diemschütz finding the body.

After some twenty minutes, Blackwell was joined Dr Phillips who, three weeks earlier, had been called to the scene of Annie Chapman's murder. Phillips had been summoned by Leman Street police station when the murder was reported there. By the time that he arrived Inspector Charles Pinhorn had taken charge of the investigation, together with Chief Inspector West, who worked closely on the case with Abberline. When the two inspectors arrived, Constable Lamb was in the process of making a very thorough search of the Club and its surroundings.

Dr Blackwell was of the opinion that Stride had been dead for between "twenty minutes to half an hour" when he saw her at 1.10, which meant that she had died at some time between 12.40 and 12.50. As she was known to have been alive at 12.45, Blackwell's assessment was probably accurate. The only doubt is in Spooner's claim that her throat was still bleeding when he saw her at some time after 1 o'clock, when Diemschütz first discovered the body. This suggested that she had died later than 12.50 but it's possible that by lifting her chin, Spooner had stretched the wound and caused further bleeding, and assuming that Blackwell *was* correct in his assessment of the time of death, it must be fairly certain that she was killed by the man who attacked her at 12.45. If she was not, she was amazingly attacked twice, at exactly the same place, within the space of five minutes.

The wound in Stride's throat differed from those inflicted on Nichols and Chapman, and on the two subsequent victims. It severed the carotid artery but seemed to have been made hastily – deep where it started but progressively shallower, with the knife apparently having been withdrawn before it reached the right jugular vein. This suggests strongly that the murderer, having seen Schwartz appproaching after he had thrown Stride to the ground, killed her quickly and made his escape, no doubt anticipating that Schwartz would report the incident and consequently, the police would soon arrive.

Less than an hour after the murder of Stride, the Ripper killed again. The body of Catharine Eddowes, a forty-six-year-old prostitute, was found in Mitre Square, Aldgate, less than a mile from where Stride was murdered. She was mutilated in a similar way to Chapman but to a greater degree and the post mortem showed that two organs – the uterus and a kidney – had been removed. Accepting that both women had been killed by the same person, another obvious conclusion would be that frustrated at being prevented from mutilating Stride as he had Chapman, he quickly found another victim. If so, his desperation was shown by the risk that he took in killing Eddowes. Knowing that Schwartz had seen him attack Stride, he would have realised that there was a very good chance that her body would have been found before he attacked Eddowes and consquently, the police would already be looking for him. That, it seemed, was no deterrent at all to him.

The murder of Eddowes would have convinced many people that the Ripper's motivation lay in the mutilation of his victims. That view would have been reinforced by the probability that his mania was increased by his frustration at being unable to butcher Stride – but what evidence was there that Stride had been his victim? Some observers would feel that the strongest proof was that the murderer himself had apparently said so. On the day after the two murders the text of a letter sent to the Central News Agency was published. It said –

"Dear Boss,
I keep on hearing the police have caught me but
they wont fix me just yet. I have laughed when
they look so clever and talk about being on the

right track. That joke about Leather Apron gave
me real fits. I am down on whores and I shant
quit ripping them till I do get buckled. Grand
work the last one was. I gave the lady no time
to squeal. How can they catch me now. I love
my work and want to start again. You will soon
hear of me with my funny little games. I saved
some of the proper *red* stuff in a ginger beer bottle
over the last job to write with but it went thick
like glue and I cant use it. Red ink is fit
enough I hope *ha ha*. The next job I do I shall
clip the ladys ears off and send to the police
officers just for jolly wouldnt you. Keep this
letter back till I do more work, then give it out
straight. My knife's nice and sharp and I want
to get to work right away if I get a chance. Good
luck.
       yours truly
         Jack the Ripper
Don't mind me giving the trade name."

At right angles to the rest of the letter was written –

"wasnt good enough to post this before I got all
he red ink off my hands curse it. No luck yet.
They say I'm a doctor now ha ha."

The letter was posted three days before the two murders and on the day
after them, a postcard was sent to the agency saying –

"I was not codding dear old Boss when I gave you
the tip, you ll hear about saucy Jacky s work
tomorrow double event this time number one squealed
a bit couldnt finish straight off. had not time
to get ears for police thanks for keeping last
letter back till I got to work again.
        Jack the Ripper"

The letter had not been published when the postcard was sent, so it was obviously from the same source. For many years experts were prepared to believe that the messages really did come from the murderer. This was largely due to a misconception that the card had been postmarked for Sunday, 30 September, the day of the killings when, it was thought, only the murderer would have known the details mentioned. In 1974, however, Stephen Knight examined it and saw that it was actually postmarked for Monday 1 October. In 1888 there was a Sunday collection and had it been posted on that day, it would almost certainly have been postmarked for the Sunday. Later, Martin Fido pointed out that there was a good prima facie case for believing that a journalist was responsible for the messages. They were posted in the Fleet Street area, already a centre for the newspaper industry, and by sending them to a news agency rather than one particular newspaper which would probably have featured an "exclusive" on them, he ensured maximum publicity.

Soon after his retirement, Sir Robert Anderson, the Assistant Commissioner of the Metropolitan Police at the time of the murders, claimed to have known the name of the "enterprising London journalist" who concocted the messages but a more reliable opinion was that of the former Chief Inspector John George Littlechild, at one time head of the Secret Department, the forerunner of the Special Branch. In 1993, the author Stewart Evans discovered a letter written by Littlechild in 1913, to a journalist of his acquaintance, George Robert Sims. After mentioning another matter relating to the Ripper murders, Littlechild wrote –

> "With regard to the term 'Jack the Ripper'
> it was generally believed at the Yard that
> Tom Bullen [a misspelling of Bulling] of
> the Central News was the orginator, but it
> is probable Moore, who was his chief, was
> the inventor. It was a smart piece of
> journalistic work. No journalist of my
> time got such privileges from Scotland Yard
> as Bullen."

It's most unlikely, therefore, that Stride was accepted as a Ripper victim on the evidence of the messages, so on what basis was it decided? Stride's throat was cut from left to right, like those of Nichols and Chapman, but in a hasty, less confident manner and this, with other marked differences, should have raised some doubts. Dr Llewellyn thought that Nichols was already dead when her throat was cut and if he was right, this may have been because, like Chapman, she had been rendered unconscious in some way. From Schwartz's account of the attack on Stride, it must have seemed very unlikely that her attacker intended to do anything similar with her. His attack was crude and direct, giving the impression that he had nothing more in mind than a quick despatch.

Although there was some doubt about the time and place of death, the official view was that having killed Chapman, the murderer mutilated her in the open yard, oblivious to the risk to himself. In the case of Stride, he had hastily slit his victim's throat, then fled in a way which could not be fully explained by the arrival on the scene of Israel Schwartz – when the full details of the murder of Catharine Eddowes were known, it seemed that she had killed and extensively mutilated in the space of five minutes. If he had been capable of that, he could have done the same to Stride, when Schwartz had gone.

The police were not convinced that the two men seen by Schwartz were together, or even that the man who attacked Stride was her murderer. On the first point it has been suggested that when Stride fell to the ground and screamed, she was calling to the other man to help her. This seems quite likely. It was not very long after they had spent at least thirty five minutes together and she would probably have known that he was still nearby. If so, there must be a very good chance that her assailant also knew that he was there, but apparently had no hesitation in attacking Stride while he looked on. The presence of Schwartz, however, provoked from him the instant and angry response of the shout of "Lipski".

There were, then, grounds for believing that the two men were together and it might be argued that that fact should have made it seem unlikely that Stride had been a Ripper victim. The police, however, accepted from the start that she had been killed by the same man who had murdered Nichols and Chapman, and who killed Eddowes later that night. If they were right, the possibility that two men were involved should have merited, at the very least, serious consideration but it seems to have been dismissed as doubtful, in a very cursory manner. The *Police Gazette* twice issued descriptions of the two men, saying that they had been seen with Stride prior to her murder but giving no indication that they were together at Dutfield's Yard. The description of the man who walked with her from Packer's shop was not, in fact, the one given by Schwartz but by PC Smith, who had seen them ten minutes earlier. This could be construed as an attempt to separate the two men.

The investigation of the murder of Stride was, in other ways, a somewhat strange affair. When the police began to question people living in Berner Street immediately after the murder, Sgt Stephen White spoke to Matthew Packer and received a comprehensive but unhelpful reply. As White reported it, Packer said,

> "I saw no one standing about, neither did I see anyone go up the yard. I never saw anything suspicious or heard the slightest noise, and knew nothing about the murder until I heard of it this morning."

White, however, returned to Packer's shop four days later and a peculiar sequence of events began. White wrote –

> "On 4th inst., I was directed by Inspector Moore to make further inquiry and if necessary see Packer and take him to the mortuary. I then went to 44 Berner Street and saw Mrs Packer, who informed me that two detectives had called and taken her husband to the mortuary. I then went towards the mortuary where I met Packer with a man. I asked him where he had been. He said, 'This detective asked me to see if I could identify the woman.'
> I said, 'Have you done so?'
> He said, 'Yes, I believe she bought some grapes at my shop about 12 o'clock on Saturday.'
> Shortly afterwards they were joined by another man. I asked the men what they were doing with Packer and they said they were detectives. I asked for their authority. One of them produced a card from a pocket book, but would not allow me to touch it. They then said they were private detectives. They

then induced to Packer to go away with them.
About 4 p.m. I saw Packer at his shop. While
talking to him the two men drove up in a hansom cab,
and after going into the shop they induced Packer to
enter the cab, stating that they would take him to
Scotland Yard to see Sir Charles Warren.   From
inquiry I have made there is no doubt that these
are the two men referred to in the attached
newspaper cutting [from the Evening News] who
examined the drain in Dutfield's Yard on 2nd inst.
One of the men had a letter in his hand addressed
to Le Grand & Co., Strand."

The two detectives are believed to have been employed by the *Evening News* and the cutting from that newspaper which White referred to, reported that they had found a grape stem in the drain in Dutfield's Yard. It was probably because of this that White was sent to question Packer again. Sir Charles Warren did interview Packer and personally took the statement in which Packer told of Stride and her companion buying grapes from him, and described the man.

After it was taken, the statement was altered in two places. Packer had said that the couple came to his shop at 12 o'clock that night and, as he said when White spoke to him on the morning of the murder, that he had closed for the night at 12.30. These times were changed, at the insistence of the police, to read 11 o'clock and 11.30. There can be no doubt that the original times given by Packer were correct. PC Smith reported that he saw the couple near the shop at 12.35, corroborating Packer's statement that they had remained in his view until he closed for the night at 12.30. Packer could not, in any case, have been mistaken in the time to that extent and he had no reason to attempt to mislead either White or Warren when he spoke to them.

Some experts have suggested that the police wanted the times changed because they had carelessly allowed the grape stem to be swept down the drain in the yard with other rubbish after the murder, and were embarrassed when it was found by the two detectives. Taking the time back an hour would presumably have made it unlikely that it had had anything to do with Stride.   If the couple had bought half a pound of grapes at 11 o'clock, they would have finished them and discarded the stem long before 12.45, when she was murdered. On the face of it, the stem was not a particularly important clue but it seems that as soon as it was mentioned in the *Evening News* report, White was sent back to Packer. This was probably because of reports that grapes had been found in Stride's hand and it was thought that she must have dropped the stem which the two detectives had found. Packer, as a greengrocer trading near the crime scene, would have been the logical person to question, to see if he had seen Stride – in spite of his forthright statement that he had not seen or heard anything suspicious on the night of the murder.

Stephen Knight attached great importance to the grapes and raised some interesting points concerning them. In his post mortem, Dr Phillips referred to some cachous which the victim had held in her left hand but made no mention of the grapes held in the right. Knight pointed out that *The Times*, which was correct in every other detail when it reported the finding of the body, had mentioned that Stride had had grapes in her right hand. What he also thought to be suspicious was that when Phillips gave evidence at the inquest, he told the coroner that although stains on the deceased's handkerchief "were those of fruit", he was "convinced that the deceased had not swallowed the skin or inside of a grape within many hours of her death". That statement was clearly untrue as she must have eaten the grapes from Packer's shop soon after 12 o'clock, but it was allowed to go unchallenged because Packer was not called to give evidence.

Packer was judged to be unreliable because he had made statements to newspapers, apparently adapting his story to please his interviewers. From his description of the man who came to his shop with Stride, however, the police must have known that it was the same one who was with her when Smith saw her, and who was standing across the street when Schwartz saw her attacked. The grapes in her hand and the stem found in Dutfield's Yard would have removed any doubts that Packer had told the truth about her coming to the shop.

It's possible that Warren, who was being criticised for his handling of the investigation, interviewed Packer to show that he was playing an active part in it, or that the two detectives took it on themselves to take the greengrocer to Scotland Yard because they thought they had stumbled on something significant, but the whole episode was suspicious. The police must have realised that Packer and Smith had seen the same man, whose description they obviously thought worth publishing, but they dismissed Packer. Ably assisted by Dr Phillips, they were then able to hide the fact that Stride *had* eaten grapes before she was murdered – so what was so significant about that mundane fact that it needed to be hidden?

The combined evidence of Packer, Smith and Schwartz could have changed the whole complexion of the investigation because it revealed a sequence of events unlike anything that had happened previously. Packer's man had met Stride, taken her to a shop and bought her some fruit, remained with her for nearly three quarters of an hour, then stood by while she was murdered by another man. The obvious conclusion is that the first man engaged Stride in conversation so that he could lead her to a convenient place where his accomplice could kill her. Two men, therefore, seemed to be involved but apparently the possibilities raised by that idea were never explored. Incredibly, Israel Schwartz, the most important witness to have come forward during the investigation, was not called to give evidence at the inquest.

In correspondence with the Home Office, Sir Robert Anderson made reference to Schwartz and "his evidence at the inquest", raising the possibility that he testified in a private session, but this would have been very unusual. Statements that he made in later years show that Anderson was certainly not above suspicion, but might have expected Schwartz to testify and therefore referred to his evidence in good faith. The handling of that evidence, however, suggests a clear intention to exclude it. It was only in the *Police Gazette* that his description of Stride's attacker was published, with nothing more disclosed than that the man had been seen with her on the night of her murder. With Schwartz and Packer effectively excluded. the only evidence of Packer's man was given by Smith – whose testimony proved nothing more than that the man had been with her at 12.35. He could have been a mile or so away when she was murdered ten minutes later.

Schwartz's statement only came to light when Stephen Knight was given permission to examine the Scotland Yard and Home Office files on the case in 1974. At that time they were closed and not due to be made available to the public until 1991 and 1992. Schwartz also seems to have given an interview to the *Star* newspaper, in which he was not named but referred to as "The Hungarian". As he spoke no English the interview was conducted through an interpreter, which may have accounted for some marked differences between what he told the newspaper and what he said in his statement to the police. In the newspaper report he was reported as saying that he first saw Stride's assailant, who appeared to be slightly drunk, walking ahead of him as he entered Berner Street. He followed him along the street and saw him go up to Stride, as she stood by the gates to Dutfield's Yard.

As no "takings" were found among Stride's other possessions still on her body, some theorists have suggested that she was not killed but merely robbed by the man who attacked her as Schwartz approached. They have also pointed out that Schwartz said that she was thrown down on the pavement *outside* the gates of the yard, whereas her body was found just inside them. In his newspaper interview, however, Schwartz said that she was "dragged back into the passage" clearly inferring that she was inside the yard when she was attacked. The lack of money on her could have been because she had spent her earnings on drink and had had no chance of recouping them in the time she had spent talking to the man by Packer's shop.

In the newspaper interview, Schwartz was reported to have said that the second man came out of a public house, and had a knife in his hand. In his statement, he said that the man was holding a pipe and made no mention of him coming out of the public house, apparently meaning that he was already standing by the road when Schwartz crossed over to his side. This seemed very clear, as Schwartz gave no impression of having seen him until he reached that side of the street and and then apparently came almost face to face with him.

If he had said in the statement that the second man had been holding a knife, the clear impression would have been that he was involved in the murder, although it seems very unlikely that he would have bee in the public house. It may have been that having manipulated Stride to Dutfield's Yard where his accomplice would kill her, he stood in the *doorway* of a public house or of some other building, where he would be unseen but could watch events across the street, then emerged quickly, knife in hand, to deter Schwartz when he saw him arrive on the scene.

With Schwartz having no English there would obviously be a strong possibly of errors in both the statement and the newspaper report. Like Packer, Schwartz might have been persuaded to embroider his story when he spoke to the press – or perhaps the embroidering was done for him, to make the story more exciting. It's just as likely, however, that the knife became a pipe in the statement – which Schwartz would have been unable to correct – because it made it seem less likely that the man holding it had been involved in the murder.

If some sort of cover-up was being operated – which was also suggested by the two alterations in the times in Packer's statement – it was not very well thought out. It would have been very easy to have presented all the available evidence and suggested that Stride had been the victim of two men, working together, whose aim had only been to rob her, but who killed her because she put up too much of a struggle. That would have separated her from the Ripper murders and and it would have been unnecessary to suppress any evidence. As it was, Stride was included as a Ripper victim, on no real evidence, whereas more likely candidates had been dismissed.

Added to the suppression of Schwartz's evidence and the tampering with Packer's, the possibility that the police knew more than they were saying, and had reasons of their own for believing the Ripper had killed her, must obviously be considered. In this context it may be valid to suggest that the releasing of the Jack the Ripper messages had an ulterior motive. From Littlechild's letter it appears that they were regarded as a hoax, but they added to the sense of panic that was sweeping the East End and must have reduced confidence in the police. No attempt to repudiate them was made, however.

Could this have been because they restored the image of the lone, mad murderer which could have been damaged by Israel Schwartz's evidence? Schwartz could be excluded from the inquest and his statement suppressed but he could still tell friends and relations about the two men he had seen at Dutfield's Yard, and who he had believed to be together. When his story was repeated, an entirely different picture of the murders might have emerged and the fact that it did not was probably due in no small part to the Ripper messages. The misconception about the date of posting of the second of them gave them a greater credence, and we may wonder if that misconception was not due to some deliberate misinformation being circulated.

As is so often the case with the Ripper mystery, there are many possible explanations of the various events. Not even the most vehement critics of "cover-up" theories have satisfactorily explained the suppression of Schwartz's evidence, however, and few have even tried. Whatever the answer may be, a strange trend in the investigation began with the murder of Stride, and continued with that of the next victim, Catharine Eddowes.

CHAPTER 4

Catharine Eddowes

The murder of Catharine Eddowes, less than an hour after that of Elizabeth Stride, brought the Ripper's reign of terror to a peak. It was the most horrific of the four murders that he had then committed. The manner in which it was carried out suggested a ruthless audacity which must have made many people wonder if anyone was safe from this evil presence which was stalking the streets of Whitechapel.

Eddowes, a forty-six-year-old prostitute, was born near Wolverhampton in 1842. By what was probably a typical registrar's error in the early days of civil registration, her forename was spelt Catharine on her birth certificate. Catharine was therefore her official name but on all other records it was spelt in the orthodox way. Her father, a tin plate worker named George Eddowes, brought his family to Bermondsey soon after she was born. The exact date of their move is unknown but the 1851 census return for their home in West Street, Bermondsey, shows that Catharine's younger brother Thomas, whose age was given as eight, was born in that area. If his age was accurate – Catharine's was not – the family must have been there in Bermondsey in about 1843.

Eddowes remained in London for the rest of her life. She claimed that she had once been married to a soldier named Thomas Conway and certainly had children by him, but there is no record of the marriage in civil registration. According to her daughter Annie, it was Eddowes' drinking which caused her and Conway to separate. In 1888 she was living with a man named John Kelly and often used his name, sometimes calling herself Mary Jane or Mary Ann Kelly. By what may have been coincidence, Mary Jane Kelly was the name of the next and final Ripper victim.

Eddowes and Kelly parted company at around 2 o'clock on the afternoon of 29 September, just under twelve hours before she was murdered. They had not long returned to London after spending a few weeks hop-picking in Kent and were short of money to pay for lodgings. They split their remaining sixpence (2½p), with Kelly taking fourpence to pay for a bed in a lodging house in Spitalfields and Eddowes having the remaining twopence, which she intended to use for a night's accommodation in the Mile End Casual Ward. She told Kelly that she would go to Bermondsey, where her daughter Annie was then living, to try to borrow some money from her but Annie did not see her at all on that day. She never reached Mile End, either, because she somehow acquired the money to become riotously drunk and was arrested in Aldgate High Street. By 8.45, she was in a cell in Bishopsgate police station.

This was a Saturday night and it was likely that the cells would be overflowing with various other offenders so, according to the custom of the time, Eddowes was discharged when the gaoler, PC George Hutt, considered that she had sobered up sufficiently to be allowed out. That was at 1 o'clock. Discharging her, Hutt asked for her name and she replied that she was Mary Ann Kelly. Before she left she asked Hutt for the time and on learning that it was around 1 o'clock, remarked that she would get "a damn fine hiding when I get home". This probably meant that she intended to join Kelly in Spitalfields because it was then too late for her to be given a bed at Mile End. As he watched her leave the police station, however, Hutt saw that she turned left, towards Aldgate. Spitalfields was in the opposite direction.

At 1.30 that night, PC Edward Watkins of the City Police walked around Mitre Square, in Aldgate, and having seen nothing which merited his attention, went on his way. "Square" was a misleading name for the small, oddly shaped space between buildings. It was bordered on one side by warehouses and there were three entrances to it in those days. To the west was Mitre Street, which led out into Aldgate High Street, quite near to the famous Aldgate Pump, which marks the beginning of the East End. Opposite the Mitre Street entrance was Church Passage, leading out into Duke Street, which also ran down to Aldgate High Street. Diagonally opposite to the Mitre Street entrance was a small alley way, connecting the square with St James Place, which gave access to Duke Street, a little way to the north of Church Passage.

Soon after Watkins had made his patrol, PC James Harvey's beat took him along Church Passage, bringing him up to the edge of the square.

At that point, using his lantern, he could have seen right across to the Mitre Street entrance. He saw nothing which prompted him to go on further into the square. He went back along Church Passage and into Duke Street, where he turned right and went on down into Aldgate High Street.

Constable Watkins was required to patrol Mitre Square at fifteen minute intervals and on that particular night he re-entered it at 1.44 a.m. When he shone his light into the darkest corner, which was behind a building by the Mitre Street entrance, he saw the body of Catharine Eddowes. Although the full horror would not immediately have registered, Watkins obviously saw enough to realise that she had been the victim of the Whitechapel Murderer. He ran to the warehouse of Kearley and Tonge on the edge of the square and asked the watchman, an ex-policeman named George Morris, to help him. Whether or not Watkins knew it, another police officer PC Richard Pearse was at that time in his house at No. 3 Mitre Square. Asleep when the murder took place, Pearse knew nothing about it until the following morning, and neither did George Clapp, a caretaker at No. 5 Mitre Square whose bedroom overlooked the square.

Morris, who later claimed that he could usually hear Watkins's footsteps in the square, had heard nothing at all that night but shocked as he must have been by the constable's news, he reacted quickly. Taking a lantern, he went out into the square and having seen the body, he took a whistle from his pocket and blew it. He then went on through the square into Mitre Street and ran down to Aldgate, where he found PC Harvey and another officer, PC Holland. They returned to the square with him and Morris went back to his warehouse.

Eddowes had been mutilated in a similar way to Annie Chapman, but more extensively. Her stomach had been opened by a cut running up from the pubis to the lower ribs, and her intestines had been taken out and placed over her right shoulder. Two feet of them had become detached and were placed under her left arm. The end of her nose and the lobe and auricle of her right ear had been cut off, and her lower eyelids had been nicked by the tip of some sharp-pointed instrument. On each cheek a triangular flap of skin had been raised. The post mortem examination revealed that her uterus and one kidney were missing.

As modern investigators would have seen it, the murderer had once again taken trophies from his victim, and had revealed another trait of serial killers. He had apparently disfigured or "depersonalised" his victim. "Depersonalising" can also be achieved by covering the victim's face. The murderer had apparently acted in a very disorganised way by rushing off from the scene of Stride's murder, disregarding the risks to himself. Even if Israel Schwartz had not reported what he had seen at Dutfield's Yard, Stride's body might well have been found and the police could already have been looking for him. Added to that, it would have been very risky to commit a murder in Mitre Square, with its three entrances.

Soon after the murder a Jewish gentleman, Joseph Lawende, told the police that he and two companons, Joseph Hyam Levy and Harry Harris, had just left the Imperial Club in Duke Street when, at 1.35 a.m., they walked through Church Passage and saw a man and a woman talking to each other. The woman, who seemed to be accosting the man, was accepted as Eddowes, although Lawende said that he was unable to identify the body because of the disfigurement. He could only say that some of her clothing that he was shown looked similar to that worn by the woman. Levy remarked to Harris, "I don't like going home by myself when I see those characters about," but neither of them thought that they would be unable to identify the couple if they saw them again.

If the woman had been Eddowes, the murderer would have exercised the same rudimentary control over her that he was believed to imposed on Chapman, by approaching her and walking a short distance with her to the place where he killed her. It's extremely doubtful if not impossible, however, that Eddowes was killed in Mitre Square, or that she was the woman seen by Lawende and his friends. The patrols of Watkins and Harvey left only five minutes in which to carry out the murder in the square and in his post mortem report, Dr Frederick Gordon Brown said,

> "I think the perpetrator of this act had
> sufficient time, or he would not have nicked
> the lower eyelids. It would take at least
> five minutes."

Dr Brown, therefore, was saying that all the time available to the murderer was taken up by one small part of the facial mutilation, leaving no time at all for the killing of the victim or the extensive bodily injuries which were inflicted on her.

47

The lack of time was clearly illustrated by Martin Fido in his book *The Crimes, Detection and Death of Jack the Ripper*. He said that Watkins' patrols of the square at 1.30 and 1.44 would have reduced the available time to ten minutes, and this is almost beyond argument. The murderer would have had to wait a couple of minutes for the constable to complete his tour of the square and go on his way – and as Watkins saw nobody there on his return, he would have left by 1.42 at the latest. Fido also believed that Harvey's presence at the Church Passage entrance would have further restricted the time available to the murderer to five minutes.

Harvey said that he reached the edge of the square at "about eighteen or nineteen minutes to two" – that is, five or six minutes before Watkins returned. From where he stood he would almost certainly have noticed anybody moving about in the place where Eddowes was found, even without his lantern. He was only a short distance away from the corner where her body was discovered and it seems more than probable that he would have shone his lantern into the square. The whole purpose of his beat taking him along Church Passage and then back, would have been to allow him to make a further check of the square, after Watkins had gone. The only reservation would be that if the murderer had been there when Harvey reached the edge of the square, he might have heard him approaching and managed to keep still enough to escape the constable's notice. That would have been very difficult, however, because somehow or other he would also have had to hide the body of his victim, who must have been dead by that time.

Harvey's evidence also shows how unlikely it is that Eddowes was the woman seen by Lawende and his friends at 1.35. He made his patrol of Church Passage only six or seven minutes later and, with five minutes occupied by the facial mutilation, the murderer could hardly have taken her into the square, killed and disembowelled her, removed her kidney and got clean away in that time. Lawende's evidence, however, was accepted, perhaps gratefully, as proving that Eddowes must have been killed in the square. There were certainly other facts which suggested it, but which may have been the result of a deliberate attempt to create that impression.

Dr Brown said in his post mortem report that he believed that the wound to the victim's throat was the first inflicted and that it was the cause of death. This, based purely on the medical evidence, was a logical conclusion. The wound was severe enough to have caused death and the doctor said in his evidence at the inquest that blood had flowed from it and clotted on the cobblestones below. He also noted, however, that the blood did not "spurt" as he clearly would have expected, and this could have been because Eddowes had already lost a certain amount from other injuries. In that case, there would not have been the sudden release from the throat which would have occurred if it had been the first wound inflicted. As in the case of Nichols, there was evidence that two attempts were made to cut the throat. Dr Brown said

"The throat was cut across to the extent of about
six or seven inches. A superficial cut commenced
about an inch below...and extended across the throat
to about three inches below the lobe of the right ear."

He also said that he believed that Eddowes was lying on her back when the throat was cut, but he could find no evidence of a struggle having taken place. The question therefore arises of how she came to be on her back if she was not struck or wrestled to the ground or, as in the case of Chapman, half-strangled. The final cut across the throat was not as deep or confident as in the other murders, where the carotid artery was completely severed. As Brown put it

"The carotid artery had a fine hole opening.
The internal jugular vein was opened an inch
and a half – not divided."

What all this suggests is that Eddowes was brought into Mitre Square already dead, and her throat was then cut to make it look as if she had been murdered there. It would have been possible to have felt the throat in the darkness and to have inserted the knife, apparently with difficulty, and then clumsily hacked it across. It was, in fact, the only wound described by Dr Brown which could have been inflicted in the dark. The careful nicking of the eyelids and the raising of the triangular flaps of skin on either side of the face would have been impossible, as would the removal of the uterus and kidney. In his report and at the inquest, Dr Brown said that in his opinion, the removal of the kidney indicated "a great deal of skill and knowledge" as that particular organ is covered by a membrane and "could easily be overlooked". In the darkness of Mitre Square, it would almost certainly have been "overlooked".

There was therefore a strong suggestion of staging in the murder of Eddowes, and it was not confined to the cutting of the throat in the square. Two other doctors, William Sedgwick Saunders and George Sequeira, were present at the post mortem and disagreed with Brown over the question of the murderer's medical knowledge. They could point to some apparently crude hacking and slashing at the victim's lower abdomen, but that in itself did not prove any lack of medical expertise. It could have been that having removed the organs that he required, the murderer became frenzied in his assault on his victim – or conversely, that being a shrewd and calculating person, he deliberately slashed at the body in an apparently inexpert manner in an attempt to camouflage the skilful removal of those organs.

Dr Brown also told the inquest that several buttons were found in the clotted blood that had flowed from the victim's throat. The obvious explanation of that would be that they fell from her person as she struggled with the murderer – Dr Brown, of course, could see no sign of a struggle – and were either torn from her clothing or fell from her pockets, in which a great number of articles were found. These included six pieces of soap, a small tooth comb, a white handled table knife and a metal tea spoon, and a piece of red flannel, containing pins and needles.

It seems very unlikely, however, that the buttons would all have fallen closely enough to have been found in a relatively small patch of blood. If they had been left there to create the impression that Eddowes had fought with the murderer at that spot, they might well have been dropped by the body, but not from a sufficient height for them to scatter, which they almost certainly would have done if they had fallen during a struggle. The person dropping them would have been anxious for them to land near enough to the body to be noticed and, if he had been keeping contact with it with one hand, would probably have released them from the other. He would, therefore, have been bending over the body and would not have been able to release the buttons from a height of more than some two feet.

The extensive list of the victim's clothing and belongings included with the inquest documents makes no mention of any buttons being missing from her skirts, bodice or jacket, so it's likely that they were in her pockets as "spares". No other articles seemed to have fallen from her pockets, which is strange if the buttons fell in a struggle. It may also be significant that the list of clothing specifically mentions, "No Drawers or Stays." Eddowes was less likely to have worn stays than drawers, but either garment might have been removed or cut so that the murderer could begin to mutilate her body. Neither were found by it, however, so they were probably removed at some other place and overlooked when her body was taken to the square.

What might also have been the result of staging was a thimble lying, in Dr Brown's words, "off the finger on the right side". The thimble could have fallen from the finger because Eddowes was murdered in the square and struggled with her attacker, but it might just as easily have slipped off when she was placed there, already dead. What is strange about its presence there is that although Victorian ladies did sometimes wear a thimble almost permanently like a ring or wristwatch, it seems a little unlikely that a woman like Eddowes would have done so. Assuming that she did, however, it's doubtful that she would have been wearing one on that particular night.

The thimble would have been an encumbrance to her when she had been hop-picking and if she had not worn it for the few weeks that she had just spent at that occupation she would probably not have put it on again until she actually needed it. Even if she had been wearing it that night, she might well have lost it during her drunk and disorderly behaviour before she was arrested, or when she was dragged off to the police station. What seems far more likely is that the thimble was in her pocket, with the pins and needles and what were probably spare buttons, which were found by her body. It may therefore have been found in her pocket, with the buttons, and placed by her hand, which could have been located in the dark, to give the impression that it had slipped from her finger as she fell dead in the square.

In his evidence at the inquest, Dr Brown said that a piece of the victim's intestines, about two feet in length, had become completely detached and had been placed under her arm – "apparently by design". It was, of course, highly unlikely that they would have come to be there by accident, but why had the murderer placed them there? It might simply have been a piece of macabre humour on his part but if, as some experts insist, he had had no medical knowledge and had simply hacked indiscriminately at the victim's body – during which process he miraculously chanced upon the invisible kidney – he would surely have lost track of that detached piece of intestine in the dark. If Eddowes had been killed and mutilated at some other place, however, it might well have been placed under her arm to prevent it from falling as she was carried to Mitre Square.

When Constable Watkins had reported the murder, a message was sent to Bishopsgate police station where Inspector Edward Collard immediately sent a constable to fetch Dr Brown, then set off to Mitre Square. He arrived at just after 2 o'clock. He made sure that nobody touched the body until Dr Brown arrived and he ordered an immediate search of the area. At 2.20 a.m., PC Alfred Long entered a tenement building in Goulston Street, some two or three minutes walk from Mitre Square. He saw nothing suspicious but when he made a second check of the building at 2.55 a.m., he immediately noticed a piece of bloodstained cloth, lying in the entrance, near the staircase to the upper floors. On the wall above it was a chalked message – "The Juwes are The men That Will not be Blamed for nothing". It was subsequently found that the piece of cloth had been torn from the apron that Eddowes had been wearing. As the murderer had obviously left it there, the immediate assumption was that he had also chalked the message.

Giving evidence at the inquest, Long at first seemed sure that the piece of apron and the message had not been there when he first went to the building. This was also the view of Detective Constable Daniel Halse, a City Police detective who had accompanied Long to the building. When he was pressed on the point, however, Long wavered and said that he could not be completely certain that the message had not been there on his first visit. The time that the message and the piece of apron were left in the building is of obvious importance to theorists, but it was still a little strange that the coroner, Mr Samuel Frederick Langham, should have queried the original statement of an experienced and observant officer. If he was simply trying to ascertain the accuracy of the evidence, it may be that he felt it more likely that the murderer would have dropped the piece of apron and chalked the message as he hurried away from Mitre Square, immediately after the murder – in which case, they would have been there when Long first went into the building. If they were not, however, a very different scenario had to be considered.

Instead of acting in a predictable manner and making his way from the scene of his crime as quickly as he could, the murderer would have remained in the area, perhaps watching from some vantage point until the police had made their first search of the street, and then left his clues. If he did, the object of leaving the piece of bloodstained apron was obviously to draw attention to the message on the wall – but what was he trying to say? There have been two main suggestions at to what the message meant.

Stephen Knight believed that it had a Masonic meaning, and that the Ripper murders were carried out in the manner of executions as described in the legends of Freemasonry. He thought that "Juwes" meant the "Jubes", three apprentice Masons Jubela, Jubelo and Jubelum who, in the legends, murdered the Master Mason Hiram Abiff. They were punished by execution, in which their entrails were taken out and thrown over their left shoulders – as had happened to the Ripper victims. Other authors believed that "Juwes" was simply a mis-spelling of "Jews" and although the meaning was not completely clear, it was simply an anti-Semitic graffito. While this is possible, it seems unlikely that "Jews" would have been misspelt as it would have been a familiar word, if only from other anti-Semitic graffiti in that area.

Whatever the meaning may have been, Sir Charles Warren, the Commissioner of the Metropolitan Police and a senior Freemason, expressed the fear that the word could have been taken as "Jews" and could provoke anti-Semitic riots. He arrived in Whitechapel, the first time that he been there during the investigation, just in time to prevent police officers from photographing the message. No doubt surprised by this, one of them suggested that it could be done with the offending word or the first line deleted but Warren still refused and insisted that the message should be washed from the wall.

Stephen Knight was certain that as a Freemason, Warren would have known that "Juwes" meant "Jubes" and that he destroyed the clue because he was party to a cover-up. Authors with different theories have tended to take the argument off at a tangent by defending the Commissioner on the grounds that he was probably right in fearing that the message would increase anti-Semitic feeling. It was, in fact, discussed at the inquest, when the Coroner's line of questioning suggested strongly that he saw the word "Juwes" as a misspelling of Jews. This was reported in the next day's newspapers without any riots ensuing, but this is hardly the point. If, as Knight believed, the word "Juwes" had a Masonic meaning, Warren would almost certainly have recognised it and, like everyone else at the time, would have believed that the message had been left there by the murderer.

Constable Long had found it, together with what was definitely a piece of the victim's apron, and at that time was sure that it had not been in the building when he made his first search. Although others who came to the scene disgreed, Constable Halse thought the writing was recent and protested against it being obliterated without a photograph being taken. In an attempt to justify his action, Warren later claimed that it had been an attempt to falsely incriminate certain Jewish radicals, but this still did not explain why he thought there would be any danger in otographing it for the investigating officers to study in private. When it was suggested in the press that "Juwes" was Yiddish for "Jews", he failed to taken advantage of this by issuing a statement that the word did not mean Jews in any known language.

Whether or not the murderer wrote the message, there is no question that he left the piece of apron by it. The only doubt is *when* – but it's probably true to say that if the Coroner had not pressed Long on the point, it would now be accepted that neither it nor the message were in the entrance when the constable first visited the building. Some authors have suggested that Long failed to notice the piece of apron on the first occasion because it was lying near other pieces of rubbish. Long, however, made no mention of anything else being near it and if that really was the explanation, why did he see it on his second visit, when it would still have been obscured?

The reason that Long noticed the piece of apron was obviously because it was somehow conspicuous, enabling him to see the bloodstains on it and instantly realise their significance. Reports of the occurrence say that when Long saw it, he immediately shone his lantern up the stairs, expecting to see another body. He would hardly have noticed it and realised what it was if, as some authors claim, the murderer had taken it simply to wipe his victim's blood from his hands, and having done so, tossed it into the entrance to the building as he passed. The reason that it was so instantly noticeable and recognisable was probably that it was lying in a space and spread out enough for the bloodstains to be seen, even in the uncertain light of a lantern, which it would not have been if it had been carelessly thrown there.

The assumption that the piece of cloth was torn or cut from the apron simply so that the murderer could wipe his hands on it is also questionable. Even ignoring or missing the fact that Dr Brown's report proves that there was simply no time to complete the extensive mutilation of Eddowes in Mitre Square, it must be admitted that the murderer had very little time. Why, therefore, would he have bothered to cut or tear away the piece of apron just to wipe his hands on it? He could easily have wiped them on the apron *in situ*. Even if he did separate the piece, why did he take it with him – and was the Goulston Street building, seven or eight minutes away from Mitre Square, the first convenient place to get rid of it?

One argument against the murderer having chalked the message on the wall has been found in a book written some years later by Chief Inspector Walter Dew who, as a Detective Constable, was involved in the Ripper investigation. Dew wrote –

"Why should he fool around chalking things
on walls when his life was imperilled by
every second he loitered?"

Why then would he have wasted time cutting off a piece of the victim's apron? Dew had obviously accepted that the Ripper had killed Eddowes in Mitre Square, immediately departed from the scene and discarded the piece of her apron as soon as he saw a convenient doorway – but even in those days of unsophisticated thinking, that view of the events should have been questioned. There seems, however, a concerted effort to deny that the piece of apron was taken from the crime scene and left in a way that made it easily recognisable, to draw attention to the message chalked on the wall.

With the murder of Eddowes, the behavioural pattern of a sexual serial murder was well established. With the murder and the comparatively tentative mutilation of Nichols, the gap between fantasy and reality was bridged. With Chapman, the mutilation was more confident and a trophy was taken in the shape of her uterus. Two trophies were taken from Eddowes and the murder had apparently tried to "depersonalise" her by disfiguring her face. Sixteen days after the murder, with the Whitechapel Murderer then firmly established in the public mind as "Jack the Ripper", another gruesome event took place.

Mr Albert Lusk who, some five weeks earlier, had been elected Chairman of the newly formed Whitechapel Vigilance Committee, received a parcel containing a portion of a human kidney. With it was a letter, with the byline "From Hell". It read,

"Mr Lusk,
Sor
I send you half the Kidne I took from
one woman prasarved it for you tother
piece I fried and ate it was very nise
I may send you the bloody knif that
took it out if only you wate a whil
longer
signed   Catch me when
              you can
              Mishter Lusk."

This obviously contained the same attempts to convey illiteracy, and the same inconsistencies, as the "Jack the Ripper" letter and postcard. Stephen Knight pointed out that a person who would spell "Kidney" as "Kidne" would probably have splelt "bloody" as "bludde", and would have misspelt "while" and "knife" as "wile" and "nife", rather than as they were rendered in the letter.

Disputes as to whether the piece of kidney had actually been taken from the body of Eddowes began at the time and have continued into the present century. One argument which has met with acceptance from some experts who previously disagreed, was that of Nicholas Warren FRCS, writing in the *Criminologist* in 1989. He was of the opinion that the kidney *did* come from the body of Eddowes. Warren showed objectivity in doubting two contemporary medical opinions which would have supported his case. These were that the kidney had been taken from the body of a woman, and had been removed within three weeks of it being posted to Lusk. Warren said that it would have been impossible to know either of those things. He believed that the kidney had been taken from the body of Eddowes because – contrary to some contemporary arguments – it showed signs of Bright's Disease, and the disease is always bi-lateral, affecting both kidneys.

The belief that the kidney was affected by Bright's disease was attacked vehemently at the time by Dr William Sedgwick Saunders, one of the two doctors who attended the post mortem on Eddowes and who disagreed with Dr Brown's opinion that the murderer had medical skill or knowledge. As in other instances, such arguments obscured the real point, which was that the piece of kidney might well have been sent by the person who murdered Eddowes or by one who was involved in the crime, and was at some pains to disguise his real identity with exaggerated and therefore obvious attempts to convey illiteracy. This, together with the evidence of Israel Schwartz which suggested that more than one person was involved in the murders, should have made the police at least wonder if they were dealing with something entirely different from what they had first imagined.

CHAPTER 5

Mary Jane Kelly

Mary Jane Kelly was believed to have been twenty-five when she was murdered by Jack the Ripper and was therefore born in about 1863. She came originally from Limerick, but left Ireland at an early age when her father, John Kelly, took his large family to live in Wales. She was married when she was sixteen but her husband, a miner, was killed in a colliery explosion soon afterwards. She became ill, possibly through the shock of her sudden bereavement, and spent some time in an infirmary, then lived for a while with a cousin, in extreme poverty. In later years, she said that she had lived "a bad life", meaning that she had resorted to prostitution in order to survive.

She left Wales for London and was again on the streets when she met Joseph Barnett, a fish porter, with whom she lived until shortly before her murder. According to the evidence of Barnett and other witnesses at the inquest, she had lived with other men who she still knew, and once visited France with "a gentleman". She was said to have preferred the French pronunciation of her forenames – "Marie Jeanette". It was as "Marie Jeanette Kelly" that her death was registered, and that name was engraved on her coffin.

She gave up prostitution when she and Barnett decided to live together but returned to the streets when he became unemployed in 1888 – some three months before she was murdered. People who knew them said that Barnett was unhappy about her earning money for them in that way but the reason that he left her on 30 October, ten days before the murder, was that she had allowed another prostitute to share their room in the lodging house where they lived.

On the evening of 8 November – only a few hours before the murder – Barnett went back to the lodging house in Millers Court, Spitalfields, where Kelly still had the room. In his statement to the police he said that they had been friendly and that he had told Kelly that he was sorry to be unable to give her any money, as he was still unemployed. This meeting was mentioned in the statement of Maria Harvey, a laundress who spent two nights in Kelly's room in the week prior to the murder. Mrs Harvey told the police that she had left some articles of clothing in the room, including an overcoat, two shirts, some children's clothes and a bonnet. The overcoat was found hanging behind the door to serve as a blind, and covered the gap where a glass pane was missing. It was the only article which was returned to her.

At around midnight that night Mary Ann Cox, another prostitute who lived in Millers Court, saw Kelly returning to the lodging house with a man who was carrying a large can of beer. Mrs Cox said that Kelly was "very drunk" and could hardly answer her when she wished her Good Night. Obviously looking for clients, Mrs Cox went out shortly afterwards and heard Kelly singing in her room. She was still singing about an hour later, when Mrs Cox returned.

Kelly seems to have sobered up considerably during the next hour because it was at about two o'clock that an acquaintance, George Hutchinson, met her hurrying down the nearby Commercial Street in the direction of Aldgate. She asked Hutchinson if he could lend her sixpence and when he told her that he had spent all his money on a trip to Romford earlier that day, she bade him a terse "Good Morning" and went off, saying that she had to go and find some money.

Aldgate was where she was said to have found most of her clients, so it seems that like Nichols and Chapman before her, she intended to earn the money she needed by finding one. In her case, the reason was less clear – she was in fact five weeks in arrears with her rent but that was hardly likely to have troubled her in the middle of the night. Whatever the reason may have been, however, her quest for money ended almost immediately.

As she turned away from Hutchinson a man coming up the street touched her on the shoulder and said something to her. As Hutchinson told the police a few days later, he was suspicious of the man because he had seemed too expensively dressed to be the sort of person that Kelly would have known. The description which the police attached to his statement was –

"Aged about 34 or 35, height 5ft 6in,
complexion pale.   Dark eyes and eye lashes.

Slight moustache curled up each end and hair
dark. Very surley (sic) looking. Dress,
long dark coat, collar and cuffs trimmed with
astrakhan and a dark jacket under, light
waistcoat, dark trousers, dark felt hat turned
down in the middle, button boots and gaiters
with white buttons, wore a very thick gold
chain with linen collar, black tie with
horseshoe pin, respectable appearance, walked
very sharp, Jewish appearance."

Hutchinson said that when the man had spoken to Kelly, they both
burst into laughter, and she said, "All right". The man replied "You
will be all right for what I have told you" and he placed his arm round
her shoulders. Quite obviously, Kelly did know him or had met him
before. Hutchinson noticed that in his left hand the man had a small
parcel "with a kind of strap round it." He said that it was wrapped in
American cloth, another name for oil cloth. From his description, it
was very like the long, slim parcel carried by the man with Elizabeth
Stride, who was seen by PC Smith. On that occasion it was wrapped in
newspaper.

Hutchinson said that he stood back near the lamp of a nearby public
house, the Queen's Head, and watched the man. As the couple came
back up the road, in the direction from which Kelly had come, they
passed Hutchinson, who said,

"The man hung his head down with his hat
over his eyes. I stooped down and
looked him in the face. He looked at
me stern."

From this, it seems that the man did not want to be recognised, and
resented Hutchinson's attempt to look at him. This probably increased
Hutchinson's suspicions because he followed the couple as they walked
a short way up the street and turned into Dorset Street, off which
Millers Court ran. They stood at the entrance to the court for about
three minutes then, in reply to something that the man had said, Kelly
said, "All right, my dear – come along, you'll be comfortable."

The man put his arm on Kelly's shoulder again and she kissed him. Hutchinson then heard her say that she had lost her handkerchief and saw the man take out his own, which was red, and give it to her. This was a possible connection with the murder of Eddowes, as the man seen near Mitre Square by Joseph Lawende wore a red handkerchief knotted round his neck. The woman with him could not have been Eddowes, but like the man seen in Hanbury Street by Mrs Long on the occasion of Annie Chapman's murder, he could have been leaving the scene, having helped to place the body.

Hutchinson's statement concluded,

"They both went up the court together. I
then went to the court to see if I could see
them but I could not. I stood there for
about three quarters of an hour to see if they
came out. They did not so I went away."

The time would then have been getting on for three o'clock. Hutchinson was probably the man mentioned in the statement of Mrs Sarah Lewis, who went to Millers Court that night to stay with her friends Mr and Mrs Keyler, because she had had "a few words" with her husband. Mrs Lewis arrived "between two and three o'clock" and said that the man was standing by the lodging house on the opposite side of the street. Her statement continued –

"Shortly before four o'clock I heard a scream,
that of a young woman and seemed to be not far
away. She screamed out 'Murder'. I only
heard it once. I did not look out of the
window."

The scream was also heard by Mrs Elizabeth Prater, who had been awakened by her kitten walking over her at "about 3.30 or 4 a.m." She lived in Dorset Street, very close to the lodging house and,

"Did not take much notice of the cries as
I frequently hear such cries from the back
of the lodging house where the windows
look into Millers Court."

Although the circumstances made it difficult for the doctors who examined the victim to make more than a rough estimate of the time of her death, it seems very likely that what the two witnesses heard was in fact the last Ripper victim being murdered.

Some hours later, at 10.45 a.m., Thomas Bowyer, an employee of John McCarthy the owner of the lodging house, went to Mary Kelly's room to collect her rent. When there was no reply to his knock, he reached through the space where the pane was missing and pulled aside the coat, later identified by Maria Harvey as the one she left in the room, which was hanging inside the door. He saw the body of a woman, smothered in blood, on the bed.

Bowyer immediately ran to tell McCarthy, who was in the chandler's shop that he ran in Dorset Street and which backed onto the lodging house. McCarthy went to the room with Bowyer and he also looked through the broken window. He then sent Bowyer to Commercial Street police station to report the murder. He followed on a few minutes later and arrived at the station as Bowyer was talking to Inspector Walter Beck and Constable Walter Dew. They accompanied McCarthy and Bowyer back to Millers Court and when they also had looked into the room and seen the body, Beck sent for assistance from the station and for the divisional police surgeon Dr Phillips.

The police did not actually enter the room until about 1.30 – some two and three quarter hours after Bowyer first saw the body. This was partly because they had been informed that bloodhounds were being brought from Commercial Street and Dr Phillips advised them that the dogs would have a better chance of picking up a scent if nobody entered the room before them. Later, they received a message that the dogs were not after all being brought there.

Another cause of delay was that the Commissioner of the Metropolitan Police, Sir Charles Warren, had given an instruction that if another Ripper murder occurred, nobody was to enter the scene of the crime until he came to personally take charge of the investigation. He probably issued that instruction because he had been criticised for lack of action and success in the inquiry. Quite what he meant by "the scene" of the crime is difficult to say, as all the previous murders had apparently been committed in the open street. Theorists who believe in a cover-up have naturally wondered if Warren had had some knowledge that the next murder would take place in a room. Whatever the truth may have been, the police waited in vain for him to come to Millers Court, unaware that he had resigned as Commissioner the previous evening. When it was finally decided that they would enter the room Superintendent Thomas Arnold, who had then taken charge, told McCarthy to break in the door with a pickaxe handle. This was actually unnecessary, as the key to the spring lock had been lost for some time and Kelly and Barnett had been in the habit of unlocking it by reaching through the space where the pane was missing and slipping back the bolt.

In his evidence at the inquest, Dr Phillips mentioned that as the door swung open it knocked against a small table that was just inside the room. On that table were lumps of abdominal flesh which Bowyer had noticed when he first looked into the room. Pieces of flesh had also been cut from the victim's legs, which in places had been stripped to the bone, and the arms had been hacked with a knife. With the exception of the heart, which was missing, the major organs were around the body on the bed, together with the breasts which had both been cut off. The face had been completely disfigured and the report of Dr Thomas Bond, who assisted Dr Phillips, said "The tissues of the neck were severed all round down to the bone." As in the case of Annie Chapman, some theorists believe this to have been an attempt to remove the head.

The Ripper had again depersonalised his victim by disfiguring her and he had taken a final trophy in the shape of her heart. As he left the other organs that he had removed, it might be assumed that on that occasion he had particularly wanted the heart. The excessive mutilation that he inflicted on the body might be put down to the fact that the secrecy of the room gave him more time in which to indulge himself, perhaps with added fervour because he had not killed for over five weeks. We may wonder why he had not previously thought of killing a prostitute who had a room of her own but the answer may simply be that he had tried, but was unable to persuade one to take him back to her lodgings.

There was irregularity in the inquest on Kelly, but not as much as writers such as Stephen Knight have claimed. *The Times* reported that on the morning of the murder both local coroners, Edwin Wynne Baxter and Dr Roderick MacDonald, went to Millers Court to claim jurisdiction over the inquest. According to the report, the matter was resolved by the body being removed to a mortuary in Dr MacDonald's district. When the inquest opened at the Shoreditch Town Hall, however, a juror protested at having the inquest, "thrown on our shoulders when the murder did not happen in our district but in Whitechapel."

The Coroner's Officer, a Mr Hammond, immediately informed him that, "It did *not* happen in Whitechapel." Dr MacDonald then rounded on the juror, in what might justifiably be interpreted as a guilty reaction, demanding, "Do you think we do not know what we are doing here? The jury are summoned in the ordinary way, and they have no business to object. If they persist in their objection, I shall know how to deal with them. Does any juror persist in objecting?"

The juror did.

"We are summoned for the Shoreditch district. This affair happened in Spitalfields."

MacDonald then seemed to lose his air of authority and with a note of desperation insisted, "It happened in *my* district."

Another juror added to his embarrassment by stating, "This is not my district. I come from Whitechapel and Mr Baxter is my coroner."

The coroner then apparently resorted to a kind of sulky dignity. "I am not going to discuss the subject with the jurymen at all. If any juryman says he distinctly objects, let him say so."

Some experts have read his last remark as an invitation to any juror who objected to withdraw, but none did. MacDonald continued, "I may tell the jurymen that jurisdiction lies where the body lies, not where it was found."

This could only be taken as a contradiction of his previous claim that the murder had happened in his district, as MacDonald then seemed to be saying that although it *was* committed in Whitechapel, he was entitled to take the inquest, an argument he repeated later in the proceedings. When the jurors had finally been sworn in, they were taken to see the body and the room where the murder took place, which was then the custom with inquest juries. On their return MacDonald announced that he wanted to correct certain reports that he and Mr Wynne Baxter had been in communication over the inquest. In that instance he could have been speaking the truth as although *The Times* report had said that both coroners had been to Millers Court on the morning of the murder, it had not stated that they were there at the same time.

MacDonald then went on to say that a previous murder had taken place in his district but the body had been removed to a mortuary in Mr Wynne Baxter's district and that gentleman had "quite correctly" taken the inquest. He was referring to the inquest on Annie Chapman, who had been found in the backyard in Hanbury Street, which was definitely in Spitalfields. His claim, therefore, sounded highly suspect, but as it happened, MacDonald was correct in what he said.

Shortly before the murders, the boundaries of the coroners' districts had been redrawn and Spitalfields was left in an anomalous position. It then came under the jurisdiction of Whitechapel, for all purposes *except* coroners' inquests. MacDonald, therefore, *was* entitled to take the inquest on Kelly, and would have been entitled to take the one on Chapman. The jurors would no doubt have accepted this if it had been explained to them but instead, MacDonald chose to threaten, to make the apparently false statement that the murder had taken place in his district and then to contradict this by stating that he had a right to take the inquest because the body had been removed to his district.

MacDonald's strange behaviour has been excused by some theorists as simply an example of the "touchiness" of Victorian coroners. Others have suggested that he wanted to complete the hearing quickly because the Shoreditch authorities could have refused to pay the cost of the hearing and the mortuary expenses. In that case, the body would have been returned to Whitechapel – some experts have said that moving it from one district to the other was actually illegal – and another inquest would have had to be held, with Wynne Baxter presiding. A year earlier, the two coroners had fought a fairly bitter contest for the East London and Tower of London district, with Wynne Baxter being elected, so MacDonald might have let his personal feelings overrule his judgement to prevent his rival from taking over the inquest. This would not fully explain his conduct of the rest of hearing, however.

To a great extent, Dr MacDonald went about his duties painstakingly. One witness, a Mrs Caroline Maxwell, had told the police that she had had a detailed conversation with Kelly at about half past eight on the Friday morning. That was some four and a half hours after Elizabeth Prater and Sarah Lewis heard what must almost certainly have been the murder taking place. MacDonald warned Mrs Maxwell before she began to testify that what she had said was at odds with all the other available evidence, and he later queried one particular point with her.

Mrs Maxwell said in her statement that Kelly had told her that she was up early that morning because, "I have the horrors of drink upon me as I have been drinking for some days past." At the inquest, she quoted Kelly as saying, "Oh, I do feel bad – Carry I feel so bad." The use of her name by Kelly suggested a much closer relationship between them than she had previously inferred, and MacDonald rightly commented on this. His notes simply quote Mrs Maxwell as replying, "She knew my name", but newspaper reports show that the point was discussed fully.

Where MacDonald was less stringent was in taking the evidence of Joe Barnett, who told him about his relationship with Kelly. At the end of his evidence, Barnett said –

> "She had on several occasions asked me to
> read about the murders. She seemed afraid
> of someone – she did not express fear of
> any particular individual, except when she
> rowed with me but we always came to terms
> quickly."

Barnett should surely have been asked to enlarge on that statement as it clearly inferred that Kelly *did* fear some particular person in connection with the murders – and probably blurted this out when she and Barnett quarrelled with each other. MacDonald, it seems, asked no further questions and his handling of the important question of the medical evidence was even stranger.

When Dr Phillips took the stand, the coroner told the jury that they would hear only the preliminary evidence on that occasion, and that they would have the opportunity to hear the full details "at the adjourned inquest", clearly inferring that he intended to extend the hearing to at least one further day. Phillips told of how he was called to Millers Court and saw the body through the window, and he described the opening of the room. The only real medical evidence that he gave was when he told the Coroner that –

> "The large quantity of blood on the bedstead,
> the saturated condition of the palliasse,
> pillow, sheet at that corner nearest the
> partition leads me to the conclusion that
> the severance of the carotid artery, which
> was the immediate cause of death, was
> inflicted while the deceased was lying to
> the right side of the bedstead and her head
> and neck in the top right hand corner."

MacDonald heard only four more witnesses, including the Inspectors Beck and Abberline, then informed the jury that he didn't know if they felt they had heard enough to bring in a verdict, but all they had to do was decide the cause of death, "leaving other matters to the police". He added that there was no point in continually going over the same matters. The jury, after a short conference among themselves, took the obvious hint and announced that they wished to bring in a verdict. This, of course, was "Wilful Murder against a person or persons unknown."

Commenting on this in his book, *Autumn of Terror*, the author Tom Cullen pointed out that British common law had for centuries required that at an inquest, all the injuries of the deceased should be viewed and that the "length, breadth and deepness" of all wounds should be recorded. Cullen also pointed out that as a former police surgeon himself, MacDonald knew this perfectly well, "Yet he chose deliberately to suppress this evidence."

As Stephen Knight said, Cullen was trying to prove that the barrister Montague John Druitt had been the Ripper, and Druitt would not have merited a cover-up. It was all the more telling, therefore, that Cullen should have been moved to quote MacDonald's final remark as he closed the inquest –

"There is other evidence which I do not propose to call, for if we at once make public every fact brought forward in connection with this terrible murder the ends of justice might be retarded."

Cullen then queried,

"What did he mean by this extraordinary statement? Was he being guided by Scotland Yard, which had been so anxious to get the inquest out of Coroner Wynne Baxter's hands? What were the police trying to hide?"

MacDonald's remark that "the ends of justice might be retarded" was, of course, reminiscent of one of the reasons put forward by Dr Phillips at the inquest on Annie Chapman, when he argued at length with the

Coroner that his medical evidence should be withheld. Commenting on the strange happenings at the Kelly inquest, the *Daily Telegraph* reported that Dr MacDonald had conferred privately with Phillips before the hearing opened.

The *Telegraph* also stated that while it was possible for the Attorney General to apply to the High Court of Justice to order a new inquest if he was "satisfied that there has been rejection of evidence, irregularity of proceedings, or insufficiency of inquiry", this was unlikely to happen as Dr Phillips "has had a commission from the Home Office for some time and he does not consider himself a 'free agent.'"

Stephen Knight commented,

"Once more the strange Dr Phillips expedites the cover-up by providing a reason for serious irregularities being tolerated. Firstly he succeeded at the Kelly inquest in his determination to withhold evidence and consulted with the coroner only in private (which Baxter had rightly refused to allow). Secondly, he alone was the reason for the inquest not being reopened, as it most certainly should have been. At least, he allowed himself to be used as the excuse for the Kelly hearing not being revived. That he had a Home Office commission would hardly have stopped him testifying at so important a hearing. On the contrary, in normal circumstances the Home Office would have been eager for justice to be done. But with Jack the Ripper they were not. The authorities clearly wanted the murder of Mary Kelly swept under the carpet."

Neither Knight nor Cullen seem to have been aware of the technical factor which entitled MacDonald to hold the inquest but they were both right in saying that it was illegal for the medical evidence to be withheld, and the *Daily Telegraph* seemed to take the same view. Other writers, such as Paul Begg, Martin Fido and Keith Skinner in their *Jack the Ripper A–Z*, have defended MacDonald on the grounds that he felt that the protracted hearings over which Wynne Baxter had presided – the inquest on Annie Chapman was adjourned four times – were undesirable, but whatever his personal feeling might have been, there is no question that MacDonald should have taken the full medical evidence and failed to do so.

Begg, Fido and Skinner acknowledge that the premature closing of the inquest meant that George Hutchinson was not called to give evidence – he made his statement to the police on the evening of 12 November, a few hours after the hearing was concluded – and that he would have been an important witness. Abberline considered his description of the man with Kelly to be important and had it circulated to all police stations in the district, but he abandoned the inquiry soon afterwards. As Stephen Knight observed, he never returned to Whitechapel although several murders occurred during the next few weeks which quite a few people at the time attributed to the Ripper.

Knight commented that Abberline "knew that the Ripper's day was done," which it certainly was. The serial murderer's pattern was broken because, instead of believing that he had become invincible and continuing to murder until he was caught, Jack the Ripper never killed again. The question of why he stopped is one which needs to be answered if any theory as to his identity is to be considered valid.

CHAPTER 6

Profiling

With the five Ripper murders fully covered, it's worth quoting the words of Robert Ressler, in his book, *Whoever Fights Monsters*, to see how those murders fit into the behavioural pattern of serial murderers that Ressler described. Referring to the American murderer Jeffrey Dahmer, he wrote –

> "...Dahmer followed the predictable pattern
> of serial killers. They begin cautiously,
> frightened of their crimes. Then the pace
> picks up, and they progress to become
> effective and efficient killing machines.
> Eventually they become cavalier and careless,
> convinced that they cannot be caught by any
> mortal. They believe they have ultimate power
> and authority over others".

The mutilation of Polly Nichols was, in comparison with that of the later victims, tentative. In just over a week, however, the Ripper had progressed to the stage where he began taking "trophies" from his victims and when he killed Eddowes, he showed the cavalier approach that Ressler mentioned. Eddowes was murdered less than an hour after Elizabeth Stride and when he attacked her, the Ripper would have known that there was a very good chance that Stride's body had been discovered and the police would therefore be looking for him. Added to this, Mitre Square at that time had three entrances and consequently there was a high risk of him being seen as he mutilated his latest victim. Apart from the self-belief that his previous successes had given him, he was probably driven by his frustration at having been unable to mutilate the body of Stride – and if so, he gave full vent to that frustration when he had killed Eddowes. This is, of course, if the scenario generally accepted over the years is correct. If it isn't, we would have to think again before classifying the Ripper as a typically disorganised serial killer.

With three of the murders, including that of Eddowes, there were reasons to doubt that the victim was killed in the place where she was found. This may mean that Jack the Ripper was less successful in his efforts at "staging" than he had hoped, but if the three of them *were* taken to the crime scenes already dead, he was a far more organised murderer than the police at the time apparently thought. The most serious doubt should have been as to whether Eddowes had really been killed in Mitre Square but if the police shared that doubt, there is no indication of it.

The murder of Eddowes was investigated by the City Police, as Mitre Square was within their territory, and there were signs that they were reluctant to disclose details to the "Met". This may have been because of a rivalry which had developed between the then Dr Robert Anderson, Assistant Commissioner of the Metropolitan Police, and Major Henry Smith who was the acting Commissioner of the City of London Police at the time of the murders. The City Police may therefore have suspected that Eddowes was not actually killed in Mitre Square but because of this rivalry, kept their thoughts to themselves.

The "Met" of course, were far from above suspicion, as is shown by Inspector Joseph Helson's radical change of mind over the murder of Polly Nichols. After standing at the crime scene on the morning of the murder and remarking that it was difficult to believe that the victim had been murdered there, he told the Coroner that he was quite sure that she had. What it was that had convinced him is not known, but those who entertain suspicions about a police "cover up" would probably think it significant that by the time that the inquest on Nichols was held, Inspector Abberline arrived in Whitechapel from Scotland Yard, to co-ordinate the investigation.

One of the most debated subjects in connection with the Ripper murders is whether or not the person responsible had medical knowledge, and the answer could obviously give an important pointer as to what sort of person he was. Dr Phillips thought that he detected medical skill in the mutilation of Annie Chapman, and Dr Brown was certain that the kidney was removed from the body of Catherine Eddowes in a manner which showed considerable anatomical knowlege. Two doctors who assisted Brown with the post mortem, William Sedgwick Saunders and George William Sequeira, disagreed. They thought that the mutilation of the victim was crudely carried out and suggested no particular knowledge or skill.

One important point in Brown's favour was that, as he said at the inquest, the kidney is covered by a membrane and "easily overlooked". This convinced him that the murderer had specifically set out to find and remove the kidney, but he did not think that this necessarily meant that he was some sort of medical practitioner. He felt that that knowledge could have been acquired from cutting up small animals. Some theorists have, in fact, suggested that the murderer was a butcher, but one possibility which has not been considered is that in the mutilation of Chapman and Eddowes, the crudeness displayed was deliberate, to hide medical skill. Another is that having obtained the trophies that he had wanted, he might then have given way to frenzy, which could certainly have been the case when he had murdered his final victim, Mary Jane Kelly.

The body of Kelly showed that she had been subjected to the most savage attack, with practically every organ removed from her body, parts of her legs stripped of flesh to the bone and her face totally disfigured as the Ripper made the most of the comparative safety of her room. What was not generally known until 1987, when the post mortem report and other documents which had been removed were returned to Scotland Yard, was that the heart had been taken out. Unlike the other organs which were left on the bed with her, it was missing, presumably taken by the murderer as a trophy. The report actually read, "The pericardium was open below, and the Heart absent", perhaps suggesting that it had been taken out more carefully than the other organs, which had been left on the bed by they body. This, therefore, could have been another instance of the skilful removal of an organ that was particularly wanted.

On balance, then, the evidence does point to the murderer having had medical knowledge or skill, and quite possibly attempted to disguise it. This is another indication of a cleverer and more organised Ripper than the more obvious aspects of his murders suggested. This, of course, is based on deductions from what may or may not be evidence. For a more informed opinion on the likely characteristics of Jack the Ripper, it would be difficult to improve on that of Christopher Missen, an expert on serial sexual murders. Mr Missen contributed to *Who* Was *Jack the Ripper?*, a collection of opinions and observations from experts and other interested parties, published in 1995 by Camille Wolff, one of the country's most experienced dealers in True Crime books. Missen's full list was –

1. Jack would have resided in the immediate vicinity.
2. Jack would have been an habitual drinker, prone to aggressive outbursts after drinking.
3. Married but estranged from spouse. Subject to irrational unprovoked explosions of jealousy.
4. Naturally clever rather than intelligent.
5. Accentuates Philistinism to ingratiate himself with low life characters.
6. Unable to keep any job for long, due to clashes with superiors.
7. Abnormal height. More likely to be tall as evidenced by Liz Stride's shoulder bruises.
8. Well known locally, expecially to police. Burglary, drink, violent or sexual offences etc.
9. May have been institutionalised in early life.
10. Lacked childhood bliss.
11. Childhood overshadowed by dominant mother.
12. Probably Catholic upbringing, some victims were Catholic. Parents may have been displaced persons. Rippers, unlike many other types of carnal predators, are most often intra-ethnic.
13. If Jack was English he may well have been a comparative newcomer to the East End.
14. Most likely to be 28-40 years of age.
15. He would NOT have written any of the missives attributed to him. ALL (so-called) RIPPER LETTERS ARE HOAXES. He was a dweller in the shadows.
16. Jack would not have been described as demented by associates. Maybe Jack only exhibited manic behavioural symptoms when intoxicated. On such occasions he would shun company and disappear.
17. Excessively class and status conscious. Never apologises or admits errors.
18. Likely to have been a regular patron of a class of whore similar to those he butchered.

19. Excessively repressed and tried to ignore or deny his secret vices. Traits may be more or less repressed homosexuality or bisexuality. Maybe suspected of paedophile propensities (even incest).
20. Outwardly sexually normal. Capable of performing conventional sex acts.
21. Will have tried to control chronic and ever intensifying destructive lusts. May be lengthy intervals between outrages.
22. Known fascination with collection of weaponry in general. May have had jobs requiring the use of a knife.
23. Frequent and sudden change of address whilst remaining in same vicinity.
24. Initial violent outburst, March, April, or August 1888 likely to have been preceded by personal crisis.
25. ALMOST CERTAIN TO HAVE BEEN INTERVIEWED AT LEAST ONCE BY RIPPER INVESTIGATORS, perhaps as a known prowler, or partner of whores.
26. OVERTLY RACIST – likely to have been actively ANTI-SEMITIC.
27. History of domestic disturbances.
28. Not suicidal. Sexual serial killers only kill themselves when they know the "jig is up".
29. Likely to have been in custody. Likely to have served in the military within previous five years.
30. NOTABLY CRUEL TO ANIMALS, especially as a juvenile.

Missen's assessment of the Ripper's height was an exercise in normal detection rather than profiling and he may have been basing his opinion on the erroneous belief that Stride herself was almost six feet tall. If so, he was probably wrong because, as stated in Chapter 4, she was actually only about five feet and five inches in height. Her nickname "Long Liz" derived from the name Stride, and not from her height, although she was probably taller than the average woman was at that time.

In assessing some of the major theories with his conclusions in mind, it's as well to remember that he said most of the characteristics he listed were "likely", and not definite. No suspect, therefore, should be dismissed because not all of them applied to him. Missen stated, for example, that the Ripper was probably a Catholic but one of the better theories put forward concerns a Jew – to whom some of the characteristics did apply. It was, in fact, incorrect to say that "some" of the victims were Catholics. Mary Kelly definitely was, but as none of the others were given Catholic funerals, it's probably safe to assume that she was the only one. On the subject of "frequent and sudden changes of address whilst remaining in the same vicinity", Missen might well be correct, but it applied to many of the inhabitants of Whitechapel at that time. Indiviuals changed lodgings and whole families moved house with great frequency. Most people lived in rented accommodation and the habit of "doing a moonlight" – leaving surreptitiously, often at night, when they were in arrears with the rent – was common.

Profiling has been remarkably successful in helping to solve murders in the last two decades but this has been because all the relevant information has been available. Something else which should be born in mind if we try to apply the art to Jack the Ripper is that, excellent as some of the research has been, the evidence is imperfect. The only views of the crime scenes that we have are police photographs of poor quality of the body of Mary Kelly in her room in Millers Court. Not all the information in the statements of witnesses and in Coroners' notes is relevant or well-recorded. It's probably true to say, however, that many of the points listed by Missen are basic and not therefore made any the less valid by possible inaccuracies in the evidence as it has come down to us.

As a final point, the late Stephen Knight believed that for any theory to be acceptable, it must explain why there was a cover-up. The evidence that he produced to support that view has been found to be less convincing than it appeared to be when he published his *Final Solution* in 1976. Notably, the inquest on Mary Jane Kelly was not as "blatantly illegal" as he thought. Even there, however, the Coroner's reaction to objections by the jurors suggested a sense of guilt and his handling of the proceedings caused surprised comments in the press. Other authors have put forward quite valid reasons to explain some of the strange events which took place during the investigation but it's still fair to say that there were a remarkable number of them. Consequently, something else which we should consider when we decide whether or not a theory is valid is whether or not the proposed would have merited a "cover-up".

CHAPTER 7

Nathan Kaminsky

In 1988 the centenary of the Ripper murders caused renewed interest and several authors suggested new solutions. One of the most ingenious and well-researched was outlined in Martin Fido's *The Crimes, Detection and Death of Jack the Ripper*. In pursuing his theory, Fido followed up a lead which was given many years before but had been dismissed or forgotten by most other authors.

In 1910 Sir Robert Anderson, the Assistant Commissioner of the Metropolitan Police and head of the Criminal Investigation Department at the time of the murders, published an autobiographical book, *The Lighter* Side *Of My Official Life*. In it, he claimed that the Ripper's identity had been known. He had been a Polish Jew of low-class origin and "the only person who ever had a good view of him at once identified him". Unfortunately, the witness had refused to testify. As Fido revealed in a later edition of his book, Anderson's memoirs had originally given the reason for the witness's refusal –

> "but when he learned that the suspect was a
> fellow-Jew, he declined to swear to him."

This was when, prior to publication of the book, it had appeared in serial form in *Blackwood's Magazine*. Anderson had removed that statment – allegedly for legal reasons – by the time the book itself went on sale, and it stated only that the witness had refused to testify. Some observers interpreted this as meaning that the suspect had had to be released, which conflicted with a statement that Anderson made three years earlier in another book, which was that the Ripper was then "safely caged in an asylum". That apparent contradiction may have been one reason why

76

Anderson's claim was never accepted and other theories continued to be put forward.

What might have been seen as a degree of corroboration of Anderson's claim was contained in some memoranda by Sir Melville Macnaghten, who joined Scotland Yard as an Assistant Chief Constable in the Criminal Investigation Department in June 1889. In 1894, a newspaper was alleging that a man named Thomas Cutbush had been the Ripper and this prompted Macnaghten to compile some authoritative memoranda on the case.

Various copies of them exist but in 1959 one of them, which had remained with his family, was shown to the author Daniel Farson, by Macnaghten's younger daughter Lady Christabel Aberconway. This was an important discovery for Farson and he used it as the basis of a book in which he suggested that Montague Druitt, a young barrister who was found drowned in the Thames at the end of 1888, had been the Ripper. In 1974 Stephen Knight was given permission to inspect the then closed files and he found that Macnaghten's final version differed in several important respects to the one published by Farson.

Having dealt with the case against Cutbush, Macnaghten went on to list three men who he saw as far more likely suspects and who had actually come to the notice of Scotland Yard at the time of the murders. These were Druitt, a Russian doctor named Michael Ostrog and Aaron Kosminski, who was a Polish Jew. In the version that Knight read, Macnaghten was less definite about Druitt than he had appeared to be in Lady Aberconway's copy, but he still seemed to see him as the most likely of the three. In his book, however, Martin Fido opted for Kosminski, and made the point that it was strange that nobody until then had realised that he had been Anderson's Polish Jew.

The explanation of this might well have been that there were certain inaccuracies in Macnaghten's descriptions of the murders which suggested that his notes had been compiled without liaison between him and Anderson, which was odd. Anderson would have been the ideal person for Macnaghten to have consulted when he became concerned over the newspaper allegations about Cutbush. He was the head of Macnaghten's department and had been in charge of the Ripper investigation from October 1888 until the case files had been closed in 1892. Also, if Anderson had known the Ripper's identity and believed him to have been Kosminski, there should have been no need for Macnaghten to have speculated about Druitt and Ostrog – or indeed for him to have compiled the memoranda.

These anomalies apart, Anderson had said that the Ripper had been a Polish Jew and Macnaghten had shown that Scotland Yard had actually suspected one, in the person of Kosminski. The death of the Ripper soon after the final killing would have explained the perennial mystery of why the murders stopped, so Fido set out to find the death of Kosminski, or a man of a similar name, towards the end of 1888, or in the following years. He was unsuccessful in this but in the records of the Whitechapel Infirmary he found that a twenty-three-year-old Polish Jew named Nathan Kaminsky had been admitted there on 24 March 1888, suffering from syphilis. Kaminsky was then living alone at an address in Whitechapel which was only two or three minutes walk from most of the murder sites. This, together with his race and religion, convinced Fido that he had been the Polish Jew referred to by Anderson, and that he had been Jack the Ripper. As a bootmaker, he might also have been the man known as Leather Apron who, at the time of the murders, was terrorising the local prostitutes by jumping out at them from alleyways and around corners, shouting, "I'm going to rip you up!"

Kaminsky was discharged as cured six weeks after his admission to the infirmary and there is no further trace of him in any records. On 7 December 1888, however, a man was taken to the Whitechapel Infirmary after the police had found him wandering the streets, "no longer able to take care of himself". Described as a "foreign" Jew in the infirmary records, he was found to be violent and was transferred to the Colney Hatch Lunatic Asylum on 21 December. He died there on 20 October 1889. Fido believed that he was actually Kaminsky. Although he did not say so specifically, his theory was obviously that Kaminsky had not really been cured of syphilis when he left the infirmary in 1888 but was in remission. When the disease began to affect his brain he started to take his revenge on the local prostitutes, one of whom had probably infected him. Fido was specific, and convincing, on the reason for the state of bewildered dementia in which the police found Kaminsky (as Cohen) in December 1888. That was a month after his last murder and his instincts would have told him that he needed to kill again to preserve what was left of his mental stability. On that occasion, however, his mind had completely collapsed.

Searching for the death of Kaminsky at the General Register Office, Fido found that two men of his name and of an appropriate age had died during the probable span of his life, but painstaking tracing of their descendants proved conclusively that neither of them had been in Whitechapel in 1888. In Fido's opinion, the absence of any record of the death of the other Nathan Kaminsky was because he had died in 1889 as David Cohen. His original explanation of why Kaminsky had been shown in the infirmary records as David Cohen was that in the accent of those days, "Nathan" could have been misheard as "David" and if the name Kaminsky had been mumbled and the final syllable had not been heard, it might have been mistaken for Cohen. As a number of readers wrote to inform him, however, at that time "David Cohen" had been a John Doe name for any Jew whose name was difficult to spell or pronounce – and quite possibly, therefore, for one who could not be understood.

David Cohen was described in the infirmary records as a tailor, whereas Kaminsky had been a bootmaker. Both could be apprentice trades but they also involved unskilled labour and Fido thought it quite likely that a man might change from one to the other. It would have been just as valid, however, to suggest that in the same way that David Cohen had been a John Doe name for Jews, "tailor" in that instance might have been a John Doe occupation. It was a popular trade among Jews and if some perplexed record keeper had finally decided to "stick him down as David Cohen", he might also have entered the incoherent new inmate as a tailor because he had been recognised as a Jew and "It's what most of them do, anyway."

All this worked out very well but there were flaws in Fido's theory. The fact that Kaminsky was living near the murder sites in March 1888 did not necessarily mean that he was at the same address or even in the same locality five months later, when the murders began. Genealogical research shows that in those times whole families changed addresses quite frequently in areas like Whitechapel. Kaminsky might well have wanted to return to his old address after his spell in the infirmary, but there's no certainty that he was able to. If he had been renting a small house the payments would have lapsed and the place would probably have been re-let. If he was lodging with a family who let out rooms to make some extra money, they might have taken in a new lodger during his absence which, as regards the duration of it, would obviously have been a very indefinite one. Another possibility is that having survived a very dangerous illness, Kaminsky decided to give up his solitary existence in London and go to America or Germany, where some of his relations might already have been living. Unless any steamship company records from that time still existed, there would be no evidence of his departure. If Kaminsky did leave the country it would explain why there was no record of his death in civil registration but Fido's own theory suggests another possibility. If Kaminsky had not been properly cured of syphilis when he left the infirmary in 1888 – which could well have been the case at that time – and became ill again, he would have been unable to work and might have become destitute. In that case, he could have died as an "unknown", as hundreds of people did each year in that part of the nineteenth century. Many of them were tramps and vagrants whose bodies were found under railway arches or bridges and in similar places where they would go for overnight shelter. Others were lucky enough to be taken to workhouses or infirmaries when they became seriously ill, but died without giving their names.

This does not, of course, prove definitely that the man who died as David Cohen was not Nathan Kaminsky, but there are other doubts. Cohen was taken to the Whitechapel infirmary when the police found him wandering the streets in December 1888, some seven months after Kaminsky left the same institution, having spent six weeks there. If he was Kaminsky and had had to be given the John Doe name of David Cohen, it would mean that nobody at the infirmary remembered or recognised him from his previous stay there, or that all the members of the staff who had known him had left. Both possibilites seem slight.

Apart from this, Cohen's death certificate showed that he died of "exhaustion of mania" with the secondary cause phthisis, a kind of pulmonary tuberculosis which was prevalent at that time. There was no mention of syphilis, but if insanity had caused Kaminsky to commit the murders, it would in all probability have been brought on because he was still suffering from that disease.

What neither Fido nor any other expert knew at that time was that some important evidence existed which supported Anderson's claim to have known the Ripper's identity, and which actually named his suspect. When his book was published, Anderson sent a copy to the former Chief Inspector Donald Sutherland Swanson, who had been involved in the Ripper investigation, and in 1980, this came into the possession of his grandson. The book had not been opened for some years but it was then examined and it was noticed that on the page on which Anderson had referred to the identification and the witness's refusal to testify, Swanson had pencilled some notes. Below the text he had written –

"Because the suspect was also a Jew and because
his evidence would convict the suspect, and
witness would be the means of murderer being
hanged, which he did not wish to be left on
his mind. D.S.S."

In the margin on the same page he added –

"And after this identification which suspect
knew, no other murder of this kind took place
in London."

He concluded his remarks on an endpaper –

"After the identification at the Seaside Home
where he had been sent by us with difficulty
in order to subject him to identification and
he knew he was identified.
   On suspect's return to his brother's house in
Whitechapel he was watched by the police (City
CID) by day and by night. In a very short
 time the suspect with his hands tied behind his
back he was sent to the Stepney Workhouse and
then to Colney Hatch and died shortly afterwards.
Kosminski was the suspect. D.S.S."

It was possible to prove that the writing was Swanson's and it was in any case known that he often made notes in books when he knew something of the subject matter. For various reasons his grandson had difficulty in having the notes published but they finally appeared in the "Daily Telegraph" in 1987. In August 1990 they were featured in a London Weekend Television "Crime Special" programme, in which further evidence was produced. Swanson had written a date "March 1890" by the reference to the identification at the "Seaside Home" and it had been found that a police convalescent home had been opened at Brighton at that time. In the records of the officers then in residence, two "specially authorised visitors" were included. It was suggested that these were the suspect and the witness, who had been sent there so that the witness might feel more at ease away from Whitechapel.

The "Swanson Marginalia", as the notes are now called, provided startling evidence. At last there was a first-hand statement by somebody involved in the investigation that explained the feeling, shared by many people over the years, that not everything about the Ripper investigation had been made known. A suspect had been definitely identified but, because it had not been possible to charge him, he could not be named. As he was a Jew in a time of widespread anti-Semitic feeling, it might have been felt that this was just as well, and could have made the various authorites even more tight-lipped.

Martin Fido recognised the significance of Swanson's evidence but he was understandably reluctant to admit that it dismissed his theory about Kaminsky. He suggested that because there were errors in Swanson's narrative, he may have confused the two men and that it was actually Kaminsky who was identified. Swanson was incorrect in saying that Kosminski died shortly after being sent to Colney Hatch. He was sent to the asylum in February 1891 and lived on until 1919, when he died in the Leavesden Asylum. Swanson's other error was in saying that he was sent to Colney Hatch from the Stepney Workhouse. He was admitted to the Mile End Old Town infirmary.

The error about the workhouses was not a significant one. The two districts, which bordered one another, were often confused, as were other East End district. Genealogists often find that births registered in Stepney, Mile End and St George's in the East had actually taken place in other districts.   After over twenty years, Swanson might simply have confused the two districts and David Cohen, who may or may not have been Kaminsky, was in any case transferred to Colney Hatch from the Whitechapel Infirmary.

The mistake about the time of Kosminski's death was admittedly strange, particularly as it seems that Swanson knew Kosminski – or at least, knew of him. He was correct in saying that the man lived with his brother in Whitechapel because Aaron Kosminski was in the care of his brother with his brother Wolf, who was a hairdresser at Syon Square, Whitechapel. It seems that Anderson also knew about him because Kosminski was in the Leavesden Asylum in 1907 when Anderson wrote in his earlier book that the Ripper was then "caged in an asylum". Believing or claiming that Kosminski had been the Ripper, Anderson would probably have made it his business to know what was happening to him over the years.

Swanson's strange but definite statement that after the identification it was the City CID who kept surveillance over Kosminski in what was Metropolitan Police territory, prompted Fido to suspect that there was "poaching" by the City Police. He suggested that they had secretly taken Joseph Lawende to identify Cohen in Colney Hatch. That possibility was supported by the fact that in the earlier version of his book, Anderson said that the suspect had been identified *after* he had been confined in the asylum. However, Anderson did not say that in the final version of the book, so it might have been another statement that he felt it politic to withdraw.

It would in any case have been a strange error if Swanson had set the identification in a south coast convalescent home when in fact, it had been in a Hertfordshire lunatic asylum. It could hardly be explained by Fido's suggestion that after a number of years, Swanson had simply "misremembered" those events. Even less adequate was a quote that Fido obtained from the author and Police historian Donald Rumbelow, who asked "pertinently" why there should have been any difficulty, as Swanson had said, in arranging an identification in a major murder investigation. That bordered on the disingenuous.

The question should have been why there would have been any difficulty, if everything was above board – and there are plenty of indications that it was not. Swanson referred to the suspect being "*sent* by us" for identification rather than "*taken*", so it's likely that he did not actually accompany him and was therefore reporting what those present had said. In his notes there is a definite air of him faithfully repeating what he believed to have been the truth, but there are reasons to doubt that that it was.

As far as we know, there were only two Jewish witnesses who might have been called upon to identify the suspect, and those were Joseph Lawende and Israel Schwartz. Lawende can be ruled out because of his doubts that he would be able to identify the man he saw just before Eddowes was murdered – particularly if Anderson was correct in saying that the witness "unhesitatingly" identified the suspect. This leaves only Schwartz, who came close enough to Stride's attacker to have had what Anderson called "a good view of him". Unfortunately, however, the man who attacked Stride was almost certainly not a Jew.

This is proved by his use of the word "Lipski", at that time a popular anti-Semitic taunt, which he shouted at Schwartz when he saw him and recognised what Anderson, in reply to a query from the Home Office, referred to as his "strongly Semitic appearance". Schwartz, who thought that Stride's assailant was shouting a warning to the second man at the scene of the attack, did not realise its significance. Anderson, however, was well aware of the meaning of the word, as he showed in his correspondence with the Home Office. This should have led him to the obvious conclusion that Stride's attacker was an anti-Semitic gentile, who had no doubt used the "Lipski" taunt on previous occasions. In that instance, he probably intended it to be a warning to Schwartz to be on his way.

Abberline also entered into correspondence with the Home Office on the meaning of the word "Lipski", and should also have deduced that Schwartz's man was a gentile. The same might have been assumed of Swanson, who would have been very familiar with the idioms of the East End at that time, but strangely enough he is said to have believed that the use of the word meant that Stride's attacker *was* a Jew. It's not known why he thought so but it would explain why he was ready to accept the account of the identification which he dutifully reported in his notes. Others, however, were not convinced. Major Henry Smith, Anderson's counter-part with the City Police, dismissed his claim to have known the Ripper's identity as irresponsible and anti-Semitic, and may have disputed other statements that he made.

It's said that it was because Smith warned him that he could face a libel action if he suggested that a Jew had concealed a crime that Anderson removed the original reference to the Jewish witness's refusal to testify from his book. If this is true, it was curious advice. Anderson had named no specific person, which would have made it very difficult for an action to be brought, especially after an interval of some twenty years. Also, if the best defence against an action for libel is to prove the truth of the statement, Anderson should have had no difficulty in defending himself as there must have been at least one surviving witness to the identification. Smith was in any case no friend of Anderson's, and would have been more likely to have taken the view that it would serve him right if he did find himself in legal difficulties through making a dubious statement.

What seems more likely is that Anderson withdrew the statement because in disputing his claim to have identified the Ripper, Smith pointed out that part of his account was barely credible. Anderson had written that the witness had declined to testify when he "learned" that the suspect was also a Jew – in other words, he had not realised that fact until he was told, after he had identified the man. It may simply have been that Anderson had expressed himself badly but there is another possibility. Anderson and Swanson both claimed that the witness was unwilling to testify against another Jew, and this raises one obvious question. Why, therefore, did he not take the easy way out and simply say that he did not recognise the suspect?

Perhaps Anderson anticipated that question and tried to forestall it by saying that it was not until after the witness had made his identification that he realised that the man before him was a Jew – which may have been a good example of what Hannibal Lecter in *The Silence of the Lambs* called "the overelaborations of a bad liar." It's possible, therefore, that what Smith really said was that it would be practically impossible for one Jew to fail to recognise another and realising the truth of this, Anderson deleted the whole reference to the Jewish witness.

Macnaghten wrote with authority about Kosminski's hatred of women and his indulgence in "solitary vice", but he was obviously relying on what other people had told him. Martin Fido's researches showed that apart from an attack on his sister during a family quarrel, Kosminski had had no history of violence. When he was finally certified, witnesses testified that he refused to wash and because he would not accept food from another person's hand, he would sometimes pick up scraps from the gutter and eat them. It should have been obvious from this that not even the Whitechapel women would have accepted such a dirty and deranged character as a client and follow him to places where they could be killed.

It's possible that in those days even experienced police officers believed that Kosminski's eccentricities made him a valid suspect, but it seems more likely that it was felt that the general public could be convinced of it. The artist Walter Sickert claimed knowledge of the Ripper murders and is reported to have said that Montague Druitt was a scapegoat. Whether or not he did say that, various statements made by the authorities at the time can be seen as fairly strong hints that Druitt had been responsible for the murders. It's believed that in March 1889, Mr William Bachert of the Whitechapel Vigilance Committee was told that the Ripper had died by drowning at the end of 1888. Similar statements followed but the rumours and speculation continued. Was Kosminski seen as a better prospect? Macnaghten said that he was a suspect at the time of the murders so it's possible that when the campaign of innuendo against Druitt failed, an attempt to incriminate him was made.

If the witness had identified him as Jack the Ripper he could have been charged. He would almost certainly have been found unfit to plead but his name could have been disclosed and as far as the majority of people were concerned, the mystery would have been solved. What might also have made that idea attractive was that if Kosminski could not be tried, and no evidence in his defence would have been heard. With his lack of English, Israel Schwartz could have been manipulated into identifying him, and if that was the intention, secrecy would have been thought necessary. That would explain why the identification had been held in the convalescent home, no doubt with as few people attending as possible.

If Kosminski's eccentricities actually did make some of the investigating officers think he was a valid suspect, Abberline, the detective in charge, did not agree with them. In later years he said in a newspaper interview –

> "You must understand that we have never
> believed all those stories about Jack the
> Ripper being dead, *or that he was a lunatic
> or anything of that kind.*" (my italics)

In another interview, this time with the *Pall Mall Gazette* in 1903, he said,

> You can state most emphatically that Scotland
> Yard is really no wiser on the subject than it
> was fifteen years ago. It is simple nonsense
> to talk of the police having proof that the man
> is dead. I am, and always have been, in the
> closest touch with Scotland Yard, and it would
> have been next to impossible for me not to have
> known about it. Besides, the authorities would
> been only to glad to make an end out of such a
> mystery, if only for their own credit...I know
> that it has been stated in certain quarters that
> 'Jack the Ripper' was a man who died in a lunatic

asylum a few years ago but there is nothing at
all of a tangible nature to support such a theory."

Perhaps the phrase "for their own credit" is the clue to the whole thing.
It might have rankled with Sir Robert Anderson to have it thought that
Jack the Ripper had beaten the police and, having had some reputation
as a detective, he felt that it reflected on him personally. His story of the
identification, with its unlikely suspect and even unlikelier witness, is
untenable. His honesty has been defended on the grounds that he was
a devout Christian but he actually had some extreme, almost fanatical
views. Martin Fido wrote –

> "As an evangelical fundamentalist, he accepted
> without question that the Devil was the lord
> of this world. But as a hard-headed realist
> he could not deny that organised churches
> formed institutions that were of this world.
> (They owned real estate and investment
> property, for example, and administered it to
> fund ministerial stipends.) These institutions,
> then, were actually and directly under the
> lordship of the Devil, and it followed that
> would-be Christians who adhered to the churches
> would find themselves unwittingly lured into
> worshipping Satan. This had obviously happened
> long ago in the Church of Rome!"

Although this suggests a strict or even fanatical moral code, Anderson
was prepared to bend the rules when he considered it to be justified.
Born and educated in Dublin, his first experiences of police work were in
Ireland and he was actively engaged in combatting Irish terrorism in the
1870s. In this connection, he believed that while Christians should never
lie to their "brothers", men who he regarded as "murderous terrorists"
were not "brothers", and not therefore entitled to hear the truth which,
he thought, "they would misuse".

Few people in the modern era would see anything unethical in
Anderson's approach to such criminals, particularly in matters of
interrogation, but his remarks indicate a readiness to make convenient

deviations from his own code of behaviour. Perhaps it was a facile way of justifying his actions – very near to saying that the ends justified the means, which might have extended to matters other than his detective work. That kind of "convenient" thinking is not all that far from self-delusion, and a man like that could easily have convinced himself of Kosminski's guilt – or that if there was some dangerous truth behind the Ripper murders, it was his duty to hide it and to prevent futher investigation which might reveal a damaging truth. To that end, he might have felt it permissible to implicate a gibbering lunatic who indulged in what Macnaghten called "solitary vice" – and perhaps worst of all, was a Jew. When they were first revealed, the Swanson Marginalia promised to solve the Ripper mystery and to justify a cover-up on the grounds that it was forced upon the authorities for legal reasons. It did neither of those things, nor could the credibility of the explanation they suggested by salvaged by substituting Nathan Kaminsky as the suspect. There is no proof at all that David Cohen really was Kaminsky or that the police attempted to identify him.

Swanson, writing for nobody's benefit but his own, probably believed that everything had happened as he reported but the evidence of the case suggested that he had been misled. Many commentators now seem to reject "conspiracy theories" *per se* – and the term has become a convenient cliché for the unimaginative. However, the very fact that there was an attempt to incriminate Kosminski who, even allowing for the unsophisticated attitudes of his day should never have been regarded as a valid suspect, suggests that it is only by admitting the possibility of a conspiracy theory that the answer to the Ripper mystery will ever be found. As we examine other theories, that becomes increasingly obvious.

CHAPTER 8

Montague Druitt

Montague John Druitt, 1857-1888, was educated at Winchester and New College, Oxford, and trained as a barrister. Probably realising that it would take some time to establish himself in his chosen profession, he took a post as a schoolmaster at a boys' school in Blackheath, run by a Mr Valentine. This provided him with funds while he pursued his legal career and he was called to the bar in 1885. At the end of November 1888, Mr Valentine dismissed him as he was "in serious trouble at the school." He was last seen on 3 December 1888 and his body was recovered from the Thames on 31 December. A letter that he wrote to Mr Valentine referred to suicide and in a note which he left for his elder brother William he said –

> "Since Friday I felt that I was going to be
> like mother (Ann Druitt, his mother, suffered
> from depression and paranoia) and it would be
> best for all concerned if I were to die".

An inquest held on 2 January 1889, concluded with the predictable verdict of "suicide whilst of unsound mind", but some theorists have suggested that he was actually murdered.

Druitt became a suspect when Lady Christabel Aberconway showed her copy of the memoranda compiled by her father, Sir Melville Macnaghten, to the author Daniel Farson. That was in 1959, but until 1965 she insisted that the names of the suspects mentioned by her father should not be revealed. The American author Tom Cullen used the information in the memoranda to write his book *Autumn of Terror*, published in 1965. He set out a case for Druitt having been the Ripper, as did Farson in his book *Jack the Ripper* which was published in 1972.

Macnaghten sounded convincing because he had claimed "private information" that Druitt's family thought he was Jack the Ripper and it has been established that he knew members of the Druitt family. He referred to him, however, as "Mr M. J. Druitt, said to be a doctor", which sounded vague, and was incorrect. The mistake might have occurred because Druitt's father, an uncle and a cousin were all doctors, but it still cast doubt on Macnaghten's apparent claim to have had information from Druitt's family.

The misconception seems to have persisted because in his interview with the *Pall Mall Gazette* in 1903 Abberline, the detective in charge of the Ripper investigation, referred to rumours that Jack the Ripper had been a medical *student*. Possibly it was those rumours, or inaccurate reports, that led Macnaghten to make his error as to Druitt's occupation. On that subject, Abberline said –

> "I know all about that story. But what does it amount to? Simply this. Soon after the last murder in Whitechapel the body of a young doctor was found in the Thames, but there is absolutely nothing beyond the fact that he was found at that time to incriminate him. A report was made to the Home Office about the matter, but that it was "considered final and conclusive" is going altogether beyond the truth...the fact that several months after December 1888, when the student's body was found, detectives were told to hold themselves in readiness for further investigations seems to point to the conclusion that Scotland Yard did not in any way consider the evidence as final."

In an earlier interview he had said that the investigators had never believed the Ripper to have been any sort of lunatic "or dead". In the 1903 interview he enlarged on that. He said that it was "simple nonsense" that the Ripper was known to be dead, adding,

> "I am, and always have been, in the closest
> touch with Scotland Yard, and it would have
> been next to impossible for me not to have
> known about it."

There are many contradictory aspects to the Ripper investigation, and Abberline's statement adds to them. In the months following the last Ripper murder, both Scotland Yard and Home Office officials made statements that the Ripper had died by drowning. Abberline abandoned the investigation just after the inquest on the final victim was completed but although he claimed to have maintained close contact with Scotland Yard, he seems to have been at odds with them on the subject of the Ripper's fate.

Following the publication of the books by Cullen and Farson other, more plausible theories were put forward. In 1987, however, Druitt was again suggested as the Ripper. This was in one of the books written for the centenary of the murders the following year, *The Ripper Legacy* by Keith Skinner and Martin Howells. Their theory was that Druitt had become involved with a group of homosexuals, former Cambridge University men, which included Queen Victoria's grandson, the Prince Albert Victor, now remembered by his later title the Duke of Clarence. Although the police were aware that he was responsible for the murders, they did not arrest him because his relationship with Clarence might have been discovered. He was finally murdered by other members of the homosexual group to ensure that the truth was never revealed.

The authors were able to point to irregularities in the police handling of the case which supported their belief in a "cover up" and revealed that Clarence went to Wimborne in Dorset when Druitt's funeral was held there. However, apart from a lack of conclusive evidence which caused Martin Fido to refer to it as "a mountainous superstructure of speculation", the flaw in the theory was that if it had been known that Druitt was committing the murders, some way of stopping him would surely have been found. At the same time, however, Druitt seems definitely to have been associated with the case and the answer to that may have been in evidence collected by Sir James Monro, once time the Commissioner of the Metropolitan Police.

Until shortly before the murders, Monro was the Assistant Commissioner, under Sir Charles Warren. He resigned because Warren vetoed his proposal that Sir Melville Macnaghten should be appointed as Assistant Chief Constable in the Criminal Investigation. Macnaghten, of course, took up that appointment in 1889, after Warren himself had resigned. Warren's objection to Macnaghten was that when he was in India, he was knocked unconscious during a riot and was therefore, "the only man in India to have been beaten by the Hindoos". It was felt, however, the Warren wanted to be rid of Monro so that he could bring in Sir Robert Anderson, a fellow Freemason, as his assistant. Monro returned as Commissioner when Warren was forced to resign, just before the final Ripper murder.

When he resigned in 1888, a post at Scotland Yard was found for Monro and it was believed that the officers involved in the Ripper investigation preferred to report to him, rather than Warren who was little more than a heavy-handed law and order enforcer.

During his career, Monro amassed a large number of papers relating to various matters, including the Ripper murders. When he died, they came into the possession of his elder son Charles and according to a story circulated, Charles Monro showed them to his brother Douglas, who advised him to "Burn the stuff, Charlie – burn it and forget it." It was believed that although he later regretted it, Charles Monro followed his younger brother's advice.

In 1995, I was provided with corroborating evidence of this. After I'd appeared on the BBC Quiz *Mastermind*, answering questions on "The Whitechapel Murders of 1888", I received a very long letter from Mr Christopher Monro, the son of Douglas Monro, and grandson of Sir James. When Skinner and Howell were writing *The Ripper Legacy*, they contacted Mr Monro concerning a letter that he had written to *The Radio Times*, following a television play about the Ripper murders. He said –

> "Something in the phrasing of my letter had convinced the collaborators (Howells and Skinner) that I *knew*...key matters bequeathed to me by my grandfather which would have settled the whole question of identity, better late than never. Well, they learned otherwise.
> .... All I did succeed in doing for Skinner and Howells was putting them on the track of my first cousin, Dr James Monro in Edinburgh, the old hero's (Sir James) eldest grandson."

Mr Monro said that Howells and Skinner visited his cousin in Edinburgh and he allowed them to examine his grandfathers papers. They contained information about some notable criminal cases but any reference to the Ripper murders was conspicuously absent – due obviously to Douglas Monro following his brother's advice. In his letter to me, Christopher Monro went on to describe the famous meeting between his father and his uncle. No doubt knowledge of that meeting came about because he – Christopher Monro – had reported it. From what was said, it was obvious that neither his father nor his uncle would have leaked it. He wrote –

"I was sent to meet my uncle at the Chesil
railway station (long vanished) to meet my
uncle, who was visiting us at short notice
from somewhere north of Oxford: from the
City (L & SW) station he knew the way to our
house, but not by the other route. I can
recall that although only about sixty he was
wholly white-haired, slow, tottery and nervous.
About two hours later, while weeding a bed under
the window of my father's study, I heard him
(Douglas Monro) suddenly and loudly cry out in
something like a scream, quite uncharacteristic
of him, 'No, no! Burn the stuff, Charlie –
burn all of it.'
　My uncle must have made some reply, and then he
fairly shouted again, 'Think of the scandal to
both Winchester and Trinity.'
　I couldn't understand it at all, but moved away
round a corner of the house for fear of being
seen and suspected of eavesdropping."

Eventually, Mr Monro came to understand the subject of that conversation, as he described –

"Twelve years later, between the outbreak of
World War II and that of Stalin's and
Manneheim's Winter War, my father and I

were bailed up in a dark bungalow at an
Himalayan village called Gurez... fearing
an attack by Shinaki dacoits at any moment
and also fearing to be trapped by snowfalls
on a key pass even if we escaped them, through
having delayed on mission business north of it
a good deal too long. Though he lived in fact
till '58, he was an old man even then and with
nerves shaken by years of quite different
troubles: expecting probable death, he wanted
to get this story off his chest, and it spilled
out uncontrollably. I had known of our
connection with the case ever since asking
him in 1930 what a newspaper meant by referring
to the newly-guillotined mass-murderer Peter
Kurten as 'Germany's Jack the Ripper', but it
had never occurred to me that Uncle Charles's
visit, a few months before his death, could have
the remotest connection with it. I learnt at
Gurez that he had come with a sense of his
approaching end to consult his only surviving
brother...about the disposal of those top-secret
memoranda."

Although he made it clear that no name had been given in his grandfather's
missing papers, it had evident that when Sir James had succeeded Warren as
Commissioner, he had been convinced that Druitt had been Jack the Ripper.
Probably it was no more than that, as Abberline said in 1903, Druitt had
died at the right time to explain the end of the murders plus, perhaps, the
circumstances of his dismissal from the school at Blackheath. Monro, it
seems, was prepared to make his suspicions public but was prevented from
doing so because William Druitt, Montague's elder brother, put pressure
on the Government. He knew that there were homosexuals in prominent
positions in Parliament, the Law, the Army and the Church and said that if
his brother was accused of the Ripper murders, he would reveal this.

Douglas Monro's concern about scandal at Winchester and Trinity
may appear confusing as Druitt did not attend Trinity College, but later
in his letter Christopher Monro, referring to his conversation with his

father in their dangerous situation in India, inferred that there was more involved than the Ripper murders –

"As it was, his disjointed gabble in October
1939 did not enlighten me on the name, but it
told me a lot else, and made it quite clear why
he had been bowled over by the double threat of
scandal to 'Winchester and Trinity'. My father,
born in 1874, had entered Winchester College in
1887 about twelve years after Druitt had left it
for Oxford, and in 1892 had gone on to Trinity
College, Cambridge. Eventually, after years in
missionary work he returned to Winchester as a
member of College staff. What my grandfather
was thinking of in letting him enter that of all
Cambridge colleges I can't imagine for he (James
Monro) had uncovered almost all of the degenerate
'Apostle' cult in which J. K. Stephen was the
high priest: Druitt, though an Oxonian, was
quickly drawn into the circle of Stephen's
disciples when studying for the Bar."

It seems, then, that Douglas Monro was not suggesting that there would be a scandal at Trinity because Montague Druitt had been Jack the Ripper, but because of certain affairs discovered by James Monro, which had begun at the college. These seemed to have involved some sort of perverted religious cult. J. K. Stephen, himself a Ripper suspect, was Clarence's tutor at Cambridge and it could be inferred from this that Stephen had involved him as well as Druitt in these affairs.

All that seems to be in line with what Howells and Skinner had suggested in *The Ripper Legacy*, when they claimed that Druitt had become involved with some homosexual ex-Cambridge men but Douglas Monro seems only to have been concerned that exposure of his father's findings would do damage to Winchester and Trinity. There was no mention of Clarence, however, either in Douglas Monro's remarks, nor in Christopher Monro's letter.

We shall never know if Sir James Monro's writings offered what he regarded as proof that Druitt had been the Ripper. He is said to have remarked in the presence of one of his grandsons that "the Ripper was never caught, but he should have been" but if that particular grandson was Christopher Monro, he did not say so in his letter. It seems, however, that Sir James did suspect Druitt and that sheds some light on the timing of the identification of Kosminski. That was probably not long before he was sent on from the Mile End workhouse infirmary to Colney Hatch in February 1891.

Two full years had elapsed since the last Ripper murder and during that time, Aaron Kosminski had been at liberty. If, as seems likely, Sir Robert Anderson was the instigator having him identified, to what did he attribute the lull in the murders? The answer is probably that Anderson was determined that Kosminski was guilty but was prevented from taking action against him by the fact that Monro was convinced that Druitt had been the murderer. Monro resigned as Commissioner in 1890 to take up missionary work and it seems likely that Anderson then began to move against Kosminski, finally putting him up for identification, early in 1891.

The Scotland Yard and Home Office statements apparently pointing to Druitt, made while Monro was still Commissioner, convinced authors such as Stephen Knight that Druitt was seen as a suitable scapegoat. It may be, however, that believing in Druitt's guilt but prevented from saying so, Monro allowed these statements to be made so that indirectly, the truth might emerge. If there was a scapegoat, it seems more likely to have been the unfortunate Aaron Kosminski.

Place and Date of Inquest.	Parish *Shoreditch*	
	House *Town Hall*	No. *19*
	12 day of *November* 1888	

Deceased's Name *Marie Jeanette Kelly*
Address *1 Miller's Court Spitalfield*

Occupation			Newly Born.
			_____ Days.
		Age	_____ Weeks.
Date of Death *9* day of *November* 1888			_____ Months.
Place of Death *1 Miller's Court, Spitalfield*			_____ Years.

Verdict (as in Certificate) *Severance of Right Carotid Artery*

Wilful Murder against some *Violent* *person or persons unknown*

An Inquisition taken for our Sovereign Lady the Queen, at the House known by the Name of the **Middlesex, TO WIT.** *Town Hall* in the Parish of *Shoreditch* in the County of MIDDLESEX, on the *12* day of *November* A.D. 188*8* [and by adjournment on the _____ day of _____ and the _____ day of _____], before RODERICK MACDONALD, Esquire, one of the Coroners of our said Lady the Queen for the said County of MIDDLESEX, upon the Oath of good and lawful Men of the said County, duly sworn to inquire for our said Lady the Queen, on view of the Body of *Marie Jeanette Kelly* as to h*er* death, and those of the said Jurors whose names are hereunto subscribed upon their Oaths duly administered do say

That on the *9* day of *November* in the year aforesaid, at the *1 Miller's Court* in the Parish of *Spitalfields* aforesaid, the said *Marie Jeanette Kelly was found dead from the mortal effects of*

and so the Jurors aforesaid, upon their Oaths, do further say that *such death was due to*

and the Jurors aforesaid do further say that the said *Marie Jeanette Kelly* was a *fe* male person of the age of *about Twenty Five* years, and a *Prostitute*

In Witness whereof as well the said Coroner as the Jurors have hereunto subscribed their Hands and Seals the Day and Year and place first above written.

RODERICK MACDONALD. ♛ Coroner. ♛ Foreman.

(140 T.D.R.—5-88:) Shaw & Sons, Fetter Lane, E.C.

1. One of the documents from the inquest of Mary Jane Kelly. The inquest was thought to have been illegally moved from Spitalfields to Shoreditch. Document is completed to read 'in the parish of Shoreditch'. The murder was actually in Spitalfields. (City of London, Metropolitan Archives)

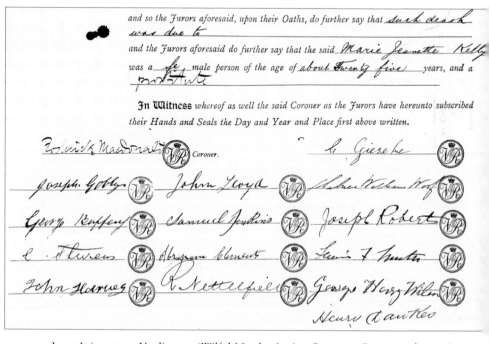

MIDDLESEX, **An Inquisition** taken for our Sovereign Lady the Queen, at the House known by

to wit. the Name of the _Town Hall_ in the Parish of

Shoreditch in the County of MIDDLESEX, on the _Twelfth_

day of _November_ A.D. 188_8_ [and by adjournment on the _____

day of _____, and the _____ day of _____],

before RODERICK MACDONALD, ESQUIRE, one of the Coroners of our said Lady the Queen

for the said County of MIDDLESEX, upon the Oath of good and lawful Men of

the said County, duly sworn to inquire for our said Lady the Queen, on view of the Body

of _Marie Jeanette Kelly_ as to h_er_ death, and those

of the said Jurors whose names are hereunto subscribed upon their Oaths duly

administered do say

That on the _Ninth_ day of _November_

in the year aforesaid at the _1 Millers Court_

in the Parish of _Shoreditch_ aforesaid, the said _Marie Jeanette_
Kelly was found dead from the mortal effects of severance
of the right carotid artery

2. Similar document but this says 'Shotalfields' – combination of both. (City of London, Metropolitan Archives)

and so the Jurors aforesaid, upon their Oaths, do further say that _such death_
was due to
and the Jurors aforesaid do further say that the said _Marie Jeanette Kelly_
was a _fe_ _male_ person of the age of about _Twenty five_ years, and a
prostitute

In Witness whereof as well the said Coroner as the Jurors have hereunto subscribed
their Hands and Seals the Day and Year and Place first above written.

Roderick Macdonald Coroner.   _L. Giesche_

Joseph Gobby   _John Lloyd_   _Walter William Wray_

George Raffery   _Samuel Jenkins_   _Joseph Robert_

E. Stevens   _Abraham Clement_   _Lewis T Hunter_

John Harvey   _R Nettlefield_   _George Harry Wilson_

Henry Dawkes

3. Jurors' signatures. Verdict was 'Wilful Murder Against Person or Persons unknown'
but that has not been entered. The inquest was closed very abruptly without full
medical evidence being given. (City of London, Metropolitan Archives)

4. 1902 census return for Spitalfields, showing John McCarthy, landlord of the lodging house where the final murder took place, still in Dorset Street. (National Archives)

5. 1881 census for Bow, showing the third victim, Elizabeth Stride, living with her husband John Thomas Stride. She claimed that he had died in the *Princess Alice* disaster on the Thames, two years earlier. (National Archives)

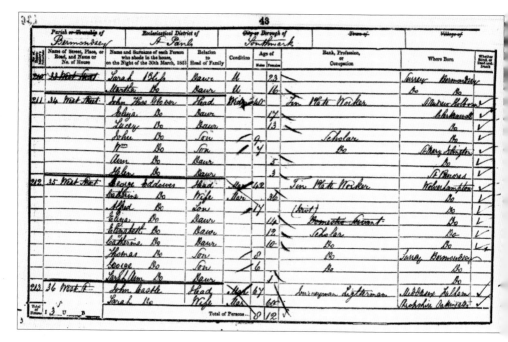

Above: 6. 1851 census return for Bermondsey. Catharine Eddowes, shown as ten, was living with her family. Her age is incorrect as she was born in 1842. (National Archives)

Left: 7. 'From Hell' letter sent to George Lusk of the Whitechapel Vigilance Committee, enclosing part of a human kidney – now thought to have been taken from the body of Catharine Eddowes.

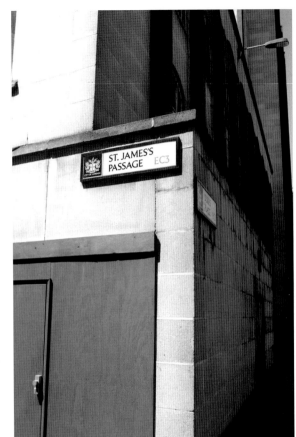

Right: 8. St James's Passage, Aldgate. One of the entrances to Mitre Square, where the body of Catharine Eddowes was found. (Oliver Phillips)

Below: 9. Another view of St James's Passage. (Oliver Phillips)

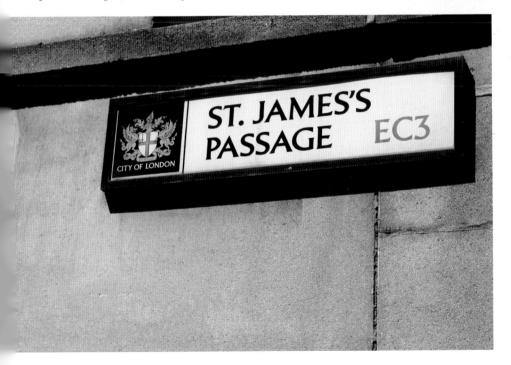

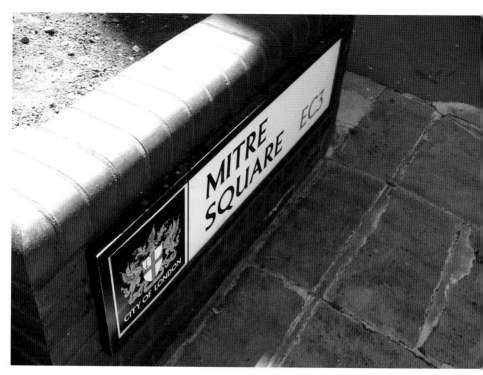

10. Entrance to Mitre Square. (Oliver Phillips)

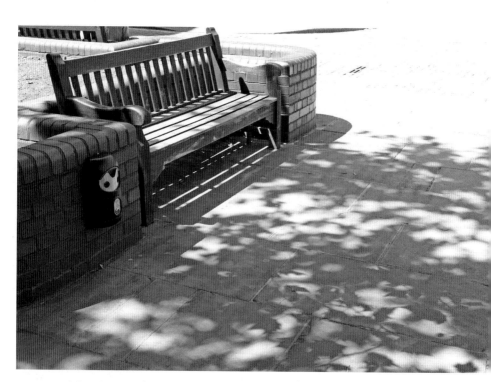

11. Mitre Square. The body of Eddowes was found where the bench now stands. (Oliver Phillips)

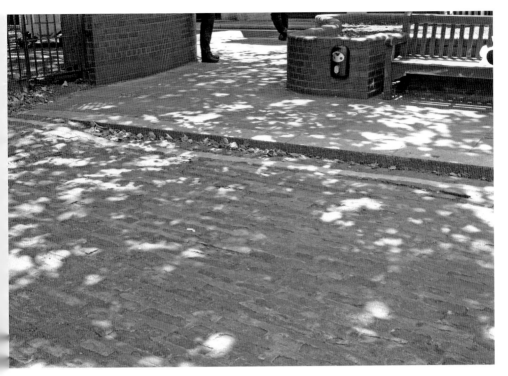

12. Mitre Square. A better view of the crime scene. (Oliver Phillips)

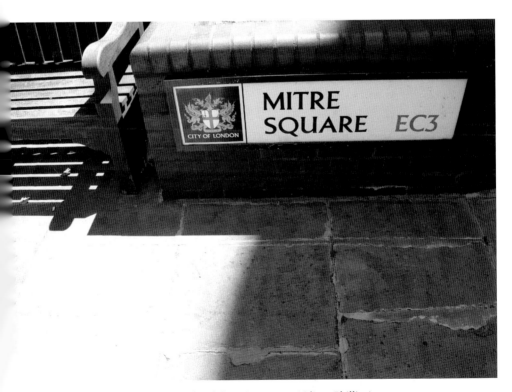

13. Mitre Square. A wider angle of the crime scene. (Oliver Phillips)

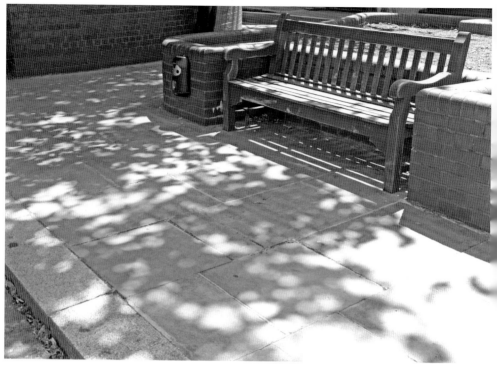

14. Mitre Square with Mitre Street in the background. (Oliver Phillips)

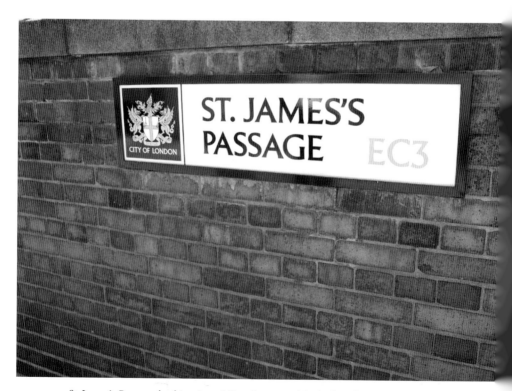

15. St James's Passage looking into Mitre Square, with the bench seen. (Oliver Phillips)

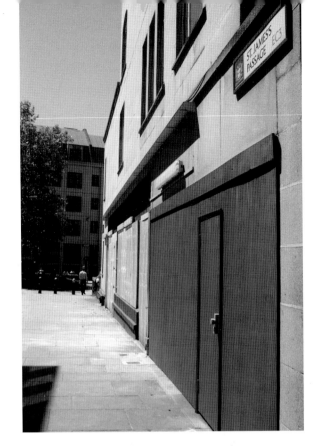

16. Another view of St James's Passage. (Oliver Phillips)

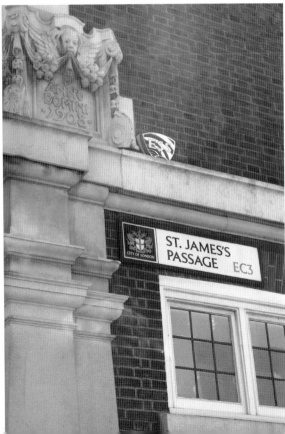

17. St James's Passage again. (Oliver Phillips)

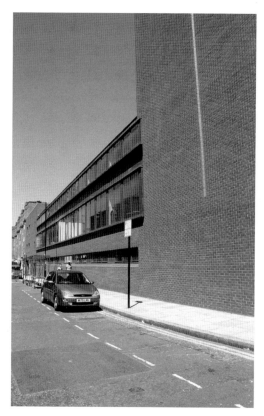

18. Goulston Street. The site of Wentworth Dwellings where the piece of Catharine Eddowes' apron and the chalked message were found. (Oliver Phillips)

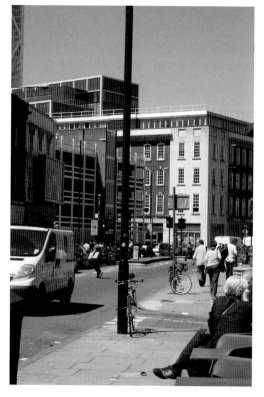

19. Commercial Street shown from the junction of Thrawl Street where Polly Nichols left the doss house shortly before she was murdered. In the distance is the multi-storey car park where Mary Kelly's pub The Britannia stood on the corner with Dorset Street, where she lived in McCarthy's lodging house. It was on that stretch of road that Mary Kelly talked with George Hutchinson, then met the strangely dressed man and walked back to Dorset Street with him. (Oliver Phillips)

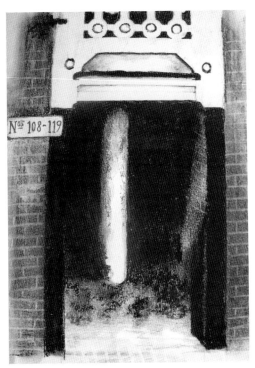
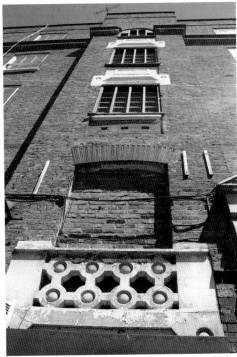

Left: 20. Sketch of the entrance where a piece of the victim's apron and the chalk message were found. (Lawrence Rothwell)

Right: 21. Goulston Street, showing some of the original stonework from the façade of Wentworth Dwellings. (Oliver Phillips)

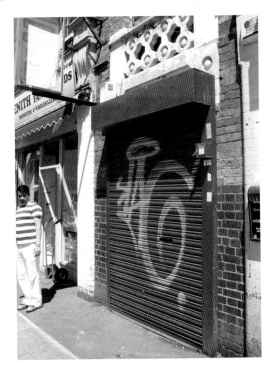

22. Better view of the stonework as on Wentworth Dwellings. (Oliver Phillips)

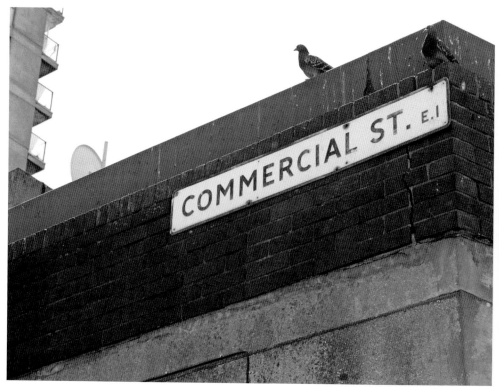

23. Present day street sign of Commercial Street. (Oliver Phillips)

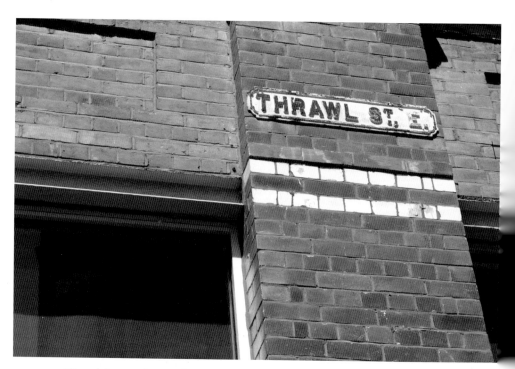

24. Thrawl Street, where Polly Nichols left the doss house. (Oliver Phillips)

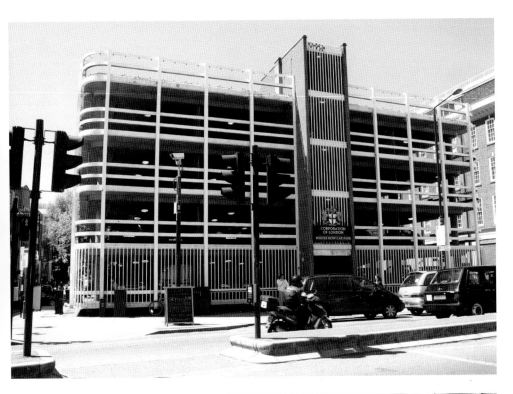

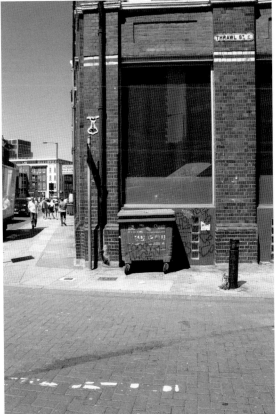

Above: 25. The car park in Commercial Street where The Britannia stood. (Oliver Phillips)

Right: 26. Another view of Thrawl Street. (Oliver Phillips)

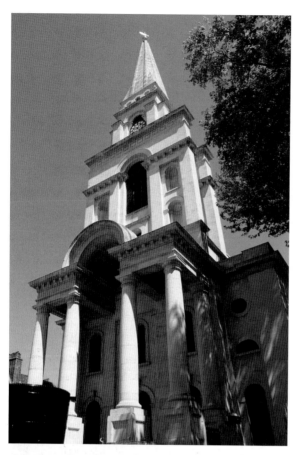

Left: 27. Christ Church, Spitalfields. The local prostitutes met here, looking for clients. (Oliver Phillips)

Below: 28. Spitalfields Market, restored in 1887. The witness John Richardson worked there. He was on his way there when he went into the backyard of 29 Hanbury Street, where his mother lived, and where the body of Annie Chapman was later found. According to the police surgeon's estimate she would have been dead for over half and hour when Richardson went into the yard. The market was almost opposite Christ Church, but a little further up the road. (Oliver Phillips)

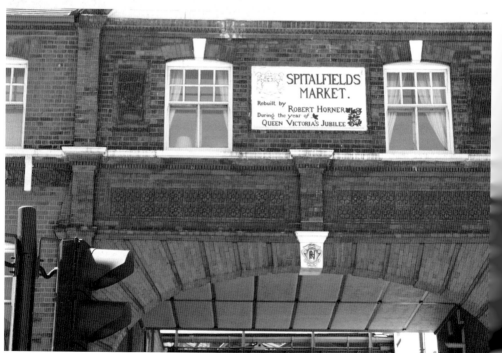

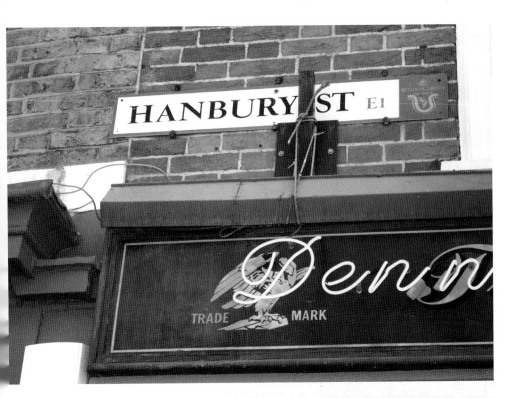

Above: 29. Hanbury Street.
Turning off Commercial Street,
a little way past Christ Church.
(Oliver Phillips)

Right: 30. Truman's brewery on
the corner of Hanbury Street and
Commercial Street. Named after
the brewers Truman, Hanbury and
Buxton who were active in the
area. (Oliver Phillips)

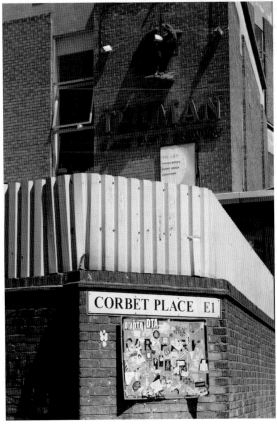

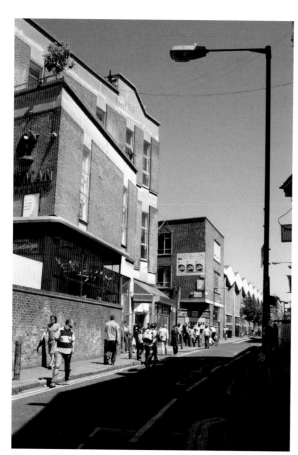

Left: 31. View of Hanbury Street. The building with the diamond shapes in the façade was the brewery that expanded over the site of 29. (Oliver Phillips)

Below: 32. White's Row, the street just beside the car park on the site of the Britannia pub. When Mary Kelly met the strangely dressed man in Commercial Street and walked back to Dorset Street on the night of the final murder, they would have crossed White's Row on their way. (Oliver Phillips)

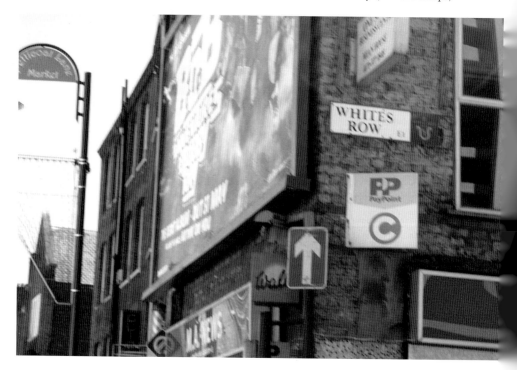

CHAPTER 9

Francis J. Tumblety

The case against Francis J. Tumblety is based mainly on what has become known as "The Littlechild Letter", and some excellent follow up research by Stewart P. Evans, a police officer in Suffolk and a collector of crime ephemera. He was offered the letter, along with some other items, in 1993 by a book dealer who knew of his interest in the Ripper murders. Written in 1913 by the former Chief Inspector John George Littlechild to a journalist George Robert Sims, it was probably the most important "find" since Stephen Knight discovered the statement of Israel Schwartz in 1974.

Littlechild was head of Scotland Yard's Secret Department, which later became the Special Branch, from 1883 to 1893. Although not actively involved in the Ripper investigation, he obviously knew quite a lot about it, as his letter to Sims reveals. It was written in reply to one that he had received from Sims, in which the journalist had apparently mentioned a "Dr D." – which may have been a cryptic reference to Montague Druitt, who was wrongly referred to as a doctor in Macnaghten's notes. Littlechild mentioned other aspects of the Ripper investigation but the reference to Tumblety read,

> "I never heard of a Dr D. in connection with
> the Whitechapel murders but among the suspects
> and to my mind a very likely one, was a Dr T.
> (which sounds very much like D.). He was an
> American quack named Tumblety and was at one
> time a frequent visitor to London and on
> these occasions constantly brought under the
> notice of police, there being a large dossier

97

concerning him at Scotland Yard. Although
a 'Sycopathia (sic) Sexualis' subject he was
not known as a 'Sadist' (which the murderer
unquestionably was) but his feelings toward
women were remarkable and bitter in the
extreme, a fact on record. Tumblety was
arrested at the time of the murders in
connection with unnatural offences and
charged at Marlborough Street, remanded on
bail, jumped his bail, and got away to
Boulogne. He shortly left Boulogne and was
never heard of afterwards. It was believed
he committed suicide but certain it is that
from this time the 'Ripper' murders came to
an end."

If Tumblety was in fact Jack the Ripper, he came near to confirming one
of Christopher Missen's opinions in *Who Was Jack the Ripper?*. Listing
the likely characteristics of the Ripper and some probable happenings
in his life, Missen included, "Almost certain to have been interviewed
at least once by Ripper investigators." Tumblety was arrested by the
police, but as Littlechild told Sims in his letter, it was not in connection
with the Ripper murders. That suspicion came after he had been granted
bail on another offence. The police may, in fact, have narrowly missed
arresting him, as the Ripper, earlier in the investigation. Stewart P. Evans
suggested this in his book, *Jack the Ripper – First American Serial Killer*,
which he wrote when the Littlechild Letter had been full investigated.
Co-authored by a journalist and researcher Paul Gainey, it was first
published in 1995.

Evans and Gainey found a report in the *Daily News* of 22 October
1888 which said that the police were watching "a house at the East End
which is strongly suspected to have been the actual lodging house, or a
house made use of by somebody connected with the East End murders".
The report went on to say that neighbours had made statements that
a lodger had been missing since the Sunday morning of the "Double
Event", when he had returned to his lodgings, in the early hours.
Disturbed by hearing him moving about, the landlady went downstairs
and saw the lodger, who said that he was going away for a while. He had

taken off a shirt that he had had on and asked her to wash it for him, so that it would be ready to wear again when he returned. Examining it, she found that the wristbands and part of the sleeves were wet with blood. When she told her neighbours about it they advised her to go to the police, which she did.

The *Daily News* sent a reporter to the house, where he found a middle-aged German lady, who spoke very little English and was in any case reluctant to tell him anything. The neighbours, however, said that since she had reported the matter, two detectives and two constables had been in the house, waiting for the lodger to return. Several other newspapers carried the story and in a Central News Agency release, the address of the house was given as 22 Batty Street, which was near to all the crime scenes. The general opinion, as given in the various reports, was that with a heavy police presence in the nearby streets following the two murders, the man had decided to leave the area. He left the bloodstained shirt in case he was stopped by the police as he went.

Evans and Gainey agreed with this. They think that Elizabeth Stride was wrongly included among the Ripper victims and suggest that the lodger – who they believe to have been Tumblety – returned to Batty Street after killing Catherine Eddowes in Mitre Square and, unaware of Stride's murder, was surprised to find the streets already full of policemen, hunting for the culprit. They quote a report from the *East Anglian Daily Times* commenting on what appeared to be the deliberately negative responses of the police to any queries from the press, and also a further release from the Central News Agency in which it was stated that the lodger had returned to Batty Street after a week and was questioned at Leman Street police station. It was claimed that he was quite quickly released because he had given a satisfactory explanation of everything that had happened.

The newspapers of that time carried reports of the police questioning and exonerating quite a few men in connection with the murders. Many of those reports would have had some basis in fact because there was such a state of panic in the East End that nervous people were apt to rush to the police whenever they saw anything that seemed at all suspicious. Evans and Gainey, however, believe that the Batty Street incident was regarded as significant, with the Central News Agency release instigated by the police as part of the hush hush policy that they appeared to have adopted. This seems possible, as it may have been hoped that if the incident could be played down, the lodger would think that it was safe for him return to Batty Street. He would then have been arrested by the waiting officers.

The "Double Event", of course, took place on 30 September 1888 and it was not until over five weeks later, on 7 November, that Tumblety was arrested – charged with committing an act of gross indecency with four other men. As this was not a felony but a misdemeanour, he could not be held until he was formally charged in a court and he was granted police bail for seven days. On 14 November, a warrant for his arrest was issued. Evans and Gainey suggest that this was either because he had failed to appear for formal charging on that day as he had been instructed, or that since his arrest the police had begun to suspect that he was guilty of a more serious offence – that is, the Whitechapel murders. Tumblety was formally charged on 16 November, at Marlborough Street police court. It was then the responsibility of the court to decide on the question of bail, which was granted. As Littlechild said, he "jumped his bail" and left the country. Having reached Boulogne on a channel ferry, he returned to America on the liner "La Bretagne", which left Le Havre on 24 November. Littlechild was wrong in suggesting that he committed suicide – he died of natural courses in 1903 – but was obviously correct in saying that the Ripper murders ended at the time of his escape.

The Evans and Gainey theory poses more questions than the basic one of whether or not Tumblety was Jack the Ripper. He could have been the Batty Street lodger but not the Ripper or conversely, the Batty Street lodger could have been the Ripper but not Tumblety – so what is the truth? If the first newspaper reports were accurate, the police seemed to think it quite possible that the lodger was Jack the Ripper and the suggestion that the Central News Agency release was put out at their instigation would be a valid one. The episode of the blood-soaked shirt would obviously have aroused their suspicions but according to the Agency, it was only week later that the suspect gave them an explanation which satisfied them to the extent that they released him "within an hour or two". On the other hand, if he had been the Ripper, returning from Mitre Square, he would have had his trophies, the womb and kidney that he took from his victim's body, on his person. What did he do with them?

The police would have searched his room and probably the whole house, but there is no report of them finding the organs. This could have been because they were trying to keep as quiet as possible about the whole episode but if, as most experts now believe, Nicholas Warren was correct in saying that the part of a kidney sent to George Lusk was taken from the body of Eddowes, the murderer obviously retained his trophies. If he had been the Batty Street lodger, therefore, he abandoned his blood-soaked shirt but risked going out through streets heavily patrolled by the police, with the two organs still on his person. This is unlikely, and it also seems unlikely that if there had been anything untoward about it, he would have given his shirt to his landlady to wash when it would probably have been quite easy to conceal it in the house. Suspicious though the incident undoubtedly seemed, the Central News Agency release was probably a true account of what had happened and the man had satisfied the police with his story.

As there is nothing but supposition to link him with Batty Street, the unlikelihood of that man having been Jack the Ripper does not harm the case against Tumblety. Evans and Gainey are probably wrong in suggesting that it was because he was suspected of the Whitechapel murders, that the warrant for Tumblety's arrest was issued on 14 November. If that had been the case, he would surely have been refused bail and their research suggests that it was not until after he left the country that he was suspected. In many respects, however, Francis Tumblety was a suitable character to have been Jack the Ripper and the final murder could have been triggered off by his arrest and subsequent release.

If Tumblety was Jack the Ripper, he murdered Mary Kelly while he was on police bail, and it would be understandable that that murder showed signs of frenzy and perhaps anger. To have killed again with the police already interested in him would have been an act of great audacity and the frenzy might have resulted from his realisation that it would be his last chance, at least for a while. Anger might also have come into it because it's known that whenever Tumblety was accused of anything, he denied the charges with great vehemence, and often with fury. Most of the accusations brought against him over the years were probably justified – as Littlechild told Sims, Scotland Yard had a large dossier on him – but once Tumblety had made his denials he probably believed himself to be innocent and felt that his anger was justified. Christopher Missen thought that Jack the Ripper – "Never apologises or admits errors" – probably meaning that he could never accept that he was in the wrong about anything.

There was another aspect of Kelly's murder which could have fitted in with Evans and Gainey's theory but the two authors showed integrity in resisting any temptation they might have felt to suggest that Tumblety, known for his flamboyant appearance, was the opulently dressed man who met Mary Kelly on the night of her murder. They were unconvinced about Hutchinson's reliability as a witness and no doubt because of their scepticism, avoid another point that they might have made in favour of Tumblety having been the Ripper. Kelly seemed to know the man who approached her and then went into Millers Court with her, and Tumblety's Irish ancestry might have made it possible for him to strike up a friendship with her and so gain her confidence.

It's also true to say, however, that with his dislike of women, it must be doubtful if Tumblety would have managed the show of affection that Hutchinson reported, even to help him to murder Kelly. As they stood by the entrance to Millers Court the man put his arm around Kelly's shoulders and she kissed him. It seems likely that there had been at least this degree of intimacy between them before and with his known feelings about women, it's difficult to believe that Tumblety would have managed it. The counter argument to this would be that if he made a supreme effort to lull any suspicions that Kelly might have had by pretending affection for her, his resentment would have given him even more reason to revenge himself on her body when he had finally killed her, but the point is really unimportant. Whether or not he was Hutchinson's man, it's still possible to make out a strong case for Francis Tumblety to have been Jack the Ripper.

As Littlechild obviously thought significant, the murders ended when Tumblety left the country, so his flight could answer the perennial question of *why* they stopped. Also, as a herb doctor he was unlikely to have had any surgical skill but he might well have acquired some knowledge of anatomy – perhaps enough to remove organs that he wanted and knew where to find, but not sufficient to avoid crude mutilation as he extracted them. He once showed some acquaintances in America a large collection of women's wombs which he kept preserved in specimen jars – and as we know, the Ripper took the wombs of Annie Chapman and Catharine Eddowes.

Edwin Wynne Baxter, coroner at the inquest on Chapman, spoke of reports that an American had approached the sub-curator of the Pathological Museum in London and "asked him to procure a

number of specimens of the organ that was missing in the deceased"
– and not surprisingly, Evans and Gainey suggest that that American
was Tumblety. Moving on to events after the murders, it's definitely
known that Scotland Yard detectives went to America after Tumblety's
departure and that killings similar to those in Whitechapel took place
in Central and North America in a way which suggested that if he had
indeed been the Ripper, he continued his murderous practices as he took
a carefully indirect route home. His hatred of women would have been
an additional motive for the murders and is one that theorists have often
attributed to the Ripper.

These points give quite powerful support for Evans and Gainey's
theory but, as ever, there is the other side of the coin. The Ripper made
no attempt to remove the uterus from the body of Polly Nichols, whose
murder and mutilation showed the typically tentative approach of the
serial killer as he first bridges the gap between fantasy and reality. There
was no sign of him seeking any particular organ, whereas Tumblety
would probably have attacked his victim with confidence and known
exactly what he wanted from her. If he had been seeking wombs, he
would hardly have taken the kidney from Eddowes and the heart from
Kelly and, unless he was in a state of mental exhaustion after the long
and frenzied mutilation of his final victim, he would not have left her
womb on the bed, among the other organs that he had extracted from
her body.

The case for Francis Tumblety having been Jack the Ripper is therefore
finely balanced, particularly in respect of the charge brought against him
on 7 November. He did not appear before the magistrates again until 16
November and might therefore have been in custody when Mary Kelly
was murdered, on 9 November. Evans and Gainey, however, contend
that on that particular charge, Tumblety could not have been held in
custody without a magistrate's warrant or charges being brought, and
he would been granted police bail which, because it would have been
automatic, would not have been recorded.

The case probably because of a weakness that it shares with those
accusing all the other suspects so far mentioned. Neither Tumblety nor
any other solo murderer could have killed and extensively mutilated
Catherine Eddowes in the darkness of Mitre Square, within the five
minutes available to him if, as Dr Brown's post mortem report suggests,
all that time would have been occupied in the one act of nicking the

lower eyelids. The acid test of any theory is probably whether or not it can explain how and where the murder of Eddowes took place and it's unlikely that any solution which suggests one completely unassisted murderer will ever do so.

The Littlechild Letter was an important find for reasons other than it's introduction of Tumblety as a plausible suspect. It practically settles the question of whether or not the original Jack the Ripper messages were fakes by supporting Sir Robert Anderson's statement that an "enterprising London journalist" was responsible. It gives another reason for doubting Anderson's statements and motive, however, as in a final, handwritten sentence Littlechild says,

> "...I knew Major Griffiths for many years.
> He probably got his information from Anderson
> who '*only thought he knew*'."

Some experts, notably Begg, Fido and Skinner in *The Jack the Ripper A–Z*, have interpreted that final, emphasised phrase as a quote from Anderson, referring to the identity of Jack the Ripper, and have felt that Littlechild was mistaken in inferring that. Had he intended to convey that Anderson had been careful to say that he "only thought he knew", Littlechild would certainly have been in error, but it seems very unlikely that that was his meaning. His letter was written three years after Anderson's book, *The Lighter Side Of My Official Life* was published and he could hardly have been unaware that in it, Anderson had made the categoric statement that Jack the Ripper had been a Polish Jew. What seems more likely is that Littlechild was saying that Anderson was guilty of reporting conjecture as fact, and in that he referred to Tumblety as a "very likely" suspect, he could not have taken his claim seriously.

What also seems obvious from Littlechild's letter is that he, like Macnaghten, seems to have had no idea that the identification of Kosminski had taken place. Admittedly, he did not actually take part in the investigation but in the way in which he wrote of the Jack the Ripper messages, saying that it was generally accepted at Scotland Yard that two particular journalists were responsible, he made it quite obvious that he was au fait with what was going on. Anderson could not have told him, any more than he told Macnaghten, that Kosminski had been identified as Jack the Ripper. Anderson would not have confided in every officer but Littlechild, like Macnaghten, was a man of considerable seniority at Scotland Yard. It seems, however, that he could only speculate about the Ripper's identity when according to Anderson, it had been firmly established.

What also seems definite, is that Anderson would have known about Tumblety. Littlechild's letter leaves no doubt that the doctor was regarded as a suspect and in their book, Evans and Gainey establish quite firmly that detectives followed him to America. That would hardly have been simply because he had jumped bail, and as the man in charge of the investigation Anderson would probably have been responsible for sending them. Evans and Gainey suggest that the police instigated a conspiracy of silence because they believed that Tumblety had been the Ripper and they had allowed him to escape. If they are right, there is yet another possible reason for Aaron Kosminski being seen as a suitable and convenient scapegoat.

If Anderson, whose fanatical religious views have been outlined, had decided that Kosminski was a more likely suspect than Tumblety, it was because he preferred to believe it. It would not have been his personal responsibility if Jack the Ripper in the person of Tumblety had slipped from the hands of the police, but it would probably have embarrassed him and, for all his Christian principles, it would have been a blow to his ego. If so, he might well have convinced himself, as the years went by, that Kosminski had been the Ripper – irrespective of the fact that the case against Tumblety was much the stronger.

The Littlechild Letter may not prove that Francis J. Tumblety was Jack the Ripper but it contains the most authentic evidence regarding the authorship of the original Ripper messages. It also demonstrates, again, the lack of liaison between Anderson and other Scotland Yard officials which was at best odd, and at worst highly suspicious.

CHAPTER 10

The Masonic Theory

Most authors dealing with Stephen Knight's *Final Solution*, which was first published in 1976, begin by mentioning an article which appeared in the *Criminologist* in 1970. This is because it's very difficult to separate the two things – and those of us who are still tolerant towards Knight's theories would say that it was a classic case of one thing following another.

The *Criminologist* article was "Jack the Ripper – A Solution?" by Thomas Edward Alexander Stowell FRCS. It caused an instant sensation because Stowell seemed to be accusing the Duke of Clarence, Queen Victoria's grandson and, until his death in 1892, heir to the Throne. Stowell said that he preferred not to name his suspect but gave enough details of him – including a nickname that he had had at college – to leave no doubt that he was referring to Clarence.

Basically, his explanation was that the suspect had contracted syphilis during a cruise of the West Indies, and committed the murders when it began to affect his brain. He was "apprehended" within minutes of the fourth murder and taken to a private asylum in the Home Counties, escaped after a few weeks and killed Mary Kelly but was re-captured almost immediately. Thanks to the expert care of Sir William Gull, the Queen's Physician, he enjoyed a period of remission and made a brief return to public life, but finally succumbed to the disease.

What Stowell seemed to be suggesting was fantastic, but it was probably given some credence because of the longstanding suspicion that there had been more to the Ripper murders than had ever been officially admitted. Stowell had suggested a reason. Also, he seemed to have had inside information. He had been a close colleague of Theodore Dyke Acland, the husband of Sir William Gull's daughter Caroline, who had told him of an entry in her father's diary in November 1889 –

"Told – (the suspect's father) that his son
was dying of syphilis of the brain."

Stowell's article was reprinted or discussed in some 3,000 newspapers
in many different countries and a few days after it first appeared he was
interviewed on BBC Television. He was then eighty, and in the excitement
of it all, he was no doubt feeling stressed. Another few days passed and,
as one author put it, his nerve broke. A letter from him appeared in *The
Times*, stating –

"I have at no time associated His Royal
Highness, the late Duke of Clarence, with
the Whitechapel murderer, or suggested
that the murderer was of royal blood."

Later on the day that his letter appeared, it was announced that he had
died. According to his wishes, all the papers concerning the Ripper
murders that he collected during many years of interest were later
destroyed.

It should have been quite obvious that somewhere in all this, Stowell
had not been completely honest. He must have known that his description
of his suspect would be recognised as Clarence, so why had he denied it?
What was not known at the time was that ten years earlier, he had told
the author Colin Wilson quite categorically that Clarence *had* been the
Ripper. Stowell, having read some of Wilson's writings on the murders,
had invited him to lunch at the Athaeneum Club in London. During their
conversation he inferred that they had been thinking along similar lines.
Wilson had mentioned that a witness had said that a man she had seen
near one of the murder scenes had spoken "like a gentleman." Wilson
saw no significance in this, and pointed out that he had only quoted
what the witness had said. Stowell's reply was, "Your instincts led you in
the right direction – Jack the Ripper was the Duke of Clarence."

Not long afterwards Wilson had contracted to write some articles on
the Ripper case and telephoned Stowell to ask if he could quote him on
his Clarence theory. Stowell declined, saying that "Her Majesty" might
not approve, but Wilson was left with the feeling he hoped it might be
mentioned. Stowell, he said, had been "sitting on the thing for thirty
years" and would have welcomed the chance of testing public opinion.

In a way, it was understandable that Stowell should be reticent. In those pre-Camillagate days, accusations against even dead members of the Royal Family would have been unpopular – and yet why would anybody in effect give away a theory, particularly one which he had apparently believed in for so long? A possible answer was given a few years later, when Stephen Knight published his *Final Solution*.

Knight's book was really a by-product of a television series which the BBC planned in 1973, as a result of the new interest in the Ripper murders which Stowell's article had helped to arouse. Involved in it were Paul Bonner, a BBC producer, and Elwyn Jones, who had created the classic *Z-Cars* series. Their task was not likely to be made any easier by the official Scotland Yard line that all known facts concerning the case had been published. Bonner was reluctant to believe this, so he and Jones decided to explore a new avenue. As Stephen Knight put it –

"They had lunch with a senior Yard man, whom Jones already knew. Though his name cannot be disclosed, he is regarded as an impeccable source. They quickly outlined their plans. A tense hour followed during which they underwent a long grilling about the intentions behind the proposed documentary. The contact was anxious to be assured that their treatment of the murders was to be conscientious in the extreme, and that they genuinely hoped to provide the definitive account of the Ripper murders. Once satisfied that this was the case – and it was no easy task convincing him – he produced a scrap of paper from his pocket. It bore several handwritten notes. He would not specify the source of the information he was about to give, but attributed it to 'one of our people'. He also requested that what he told them would be in confidence.

He asked if they had had any contact with 'a man named Sickert who has some connection with the artist'. He said the man knew of a marriage

between the Duke of Clarence...and an Alice Mary
Cook. The clandestine ceremony had taken place
in 'St Saviour's' and two witnesses present were
later to become victims of the Ripper. Alice
Mary died in 1920. No other information was
given."

The BBC team tried to verify the facts given, but were unable to do so.
Efforts to find the registration of the alleged marriage were pre-doomed
as royal marriages were not shown in civil registation and it was, in any
case, unlikely that such a marriage would be registered. Ian Sharp, a
research assistant with the BBC team, told Knight what happened next.

"So it was decided that we should try our Scotland
Yard man for more information, and preferably the
whereabouts of Sickert if he still (or even)
existed.
    I remember very clearly Paul Bonner ringing the
informant and in urbane and diplomatic tones
informing him that we had found nothing, without
actually saying so. He then asked if Sickert
was still around. And then to Paul's
astonishment he provided him with Sickert's
phone number within a couple of seconds.
Since this was a fortnight after their meeting
and there had been no contact during that time,
it appeared very odd that he should now lay
hands on the phone number instantly. He may
well have had it on the slip of paper, but why
hadn't he given it to them at the time?"

Sharp phoned Sickert that evening. The conversation was a difficult
one as Sickert suffered badly from deafness and Sharp's side of it had
to be relayed to him by another man. A meeting was arranged for the
following morning, however, and this took place at an artist's studio
in Islington. This was the home of an elderly gentleman named Harry
Jonas, the man who had helped Sickert with the telephone conversation
the previous evening.

Joseph Sickert, born Gorman, claimed to be the illegitimate son of Walter Sickert the artist and that his mother, Alice Margaret Crook, was the illegitimate daughter of the Duke of Clarence. He believed that he inherited his deafness through Clarence, from Queen Alexandra, who suffered from the same affliction. When Sharp had told him of the meeting at Scotland Yard, he conferred with Jonas and they agreed that what had been said was, in essence, correct but some details were wrong. Only one witness to the secret marriage had been murdered by the Ripper and this was Mary Jane Kelly, who was the final victim. Clarence's secret bride had not been Alice Mary Cook, but Annie Elizabeth Crook.

Sickert supplied a possible answer to Sharp's question as to why the Scotland Yard contact had not given his telephone number to Bonner and Jones at their meeting. He suggested that some of the details had deliberately been given inaccurately so that the BBC would in future go to him rather than the Yard for their information. Stephen Knight believed that this was a carefully contrived 'leak'.

Joseph Sickert said that the story of the secret marriage and the Ripper murders had been told to him by Walter Sickert, when he was about thirteen. At that time Walter was nearing the end of his life and felt that Joseph should know the real story of his birth and ancestry. He said that the whole thing had begun when the then Princess Alexandra had asked Walter Sickert, who was already known in Court circles, to befriend her son Albert Victor, later Duke of Clarence and Avondale, and known in the Royal Family as Eddy. She believed that he had artistic leanings and that if he could develop some ability that direction it might offset any loss of confidence through his many short-comings in other ways.

Eddy began to visit Sickert's studio in Cleveland Street, in the Tottenham Court Road area, which was then the centre of an artists' community. He would leave Buckingham Palace in an official coach but at a prearranged place he would transfer to a closed carriage, driven by a man named John Charles Netley. Later, Netley was to be involved in the Ripper murders. It was at Cleveland Street that Eddy met Annie Elizabeth Crook who was then working in a tobacconist's shop there.

Eddy was a very susceptible young man and being instantly attracted to Annie, he began an affair with her. She became pregnant and her daughter Alice Margaret was born in April 1885. Soon after the birth Walter Sickert arranged for a Roman Catholic marriage to be conducted for them. Mary Kelly had also worked in the tobacconist's shop but when Alice Margaret was born, Sickert paid her to give up the job and act as nurse to the child.

Kelly had left her native Ireland when her father took his family to Wales, where she had been married at the age of sixteen but widowed shortly afterwards She came to London seeking a better life but became a prostitute in Whitechapel. She was offered the job in Cleveland Street by a friend of Sickert's who did charitable work in the East End. In the months following the birth of Alice Margaret Crook she visited Sickert's studio in Dieppe with Annie and the baby. It was there that she became fond of the French pronunciation of her forenames and afterwards liked to be known as Marie Jeanette. It was under that name that her death was registered when she was murdered by the Ripper.

Eddy had been introduced to the Cleveland Street set as Sickert's younger brother but a number of them knew his real identity and his affair with Annie Crook became an open secret. When news of it reached Buckingham Palace, Queen Victoria ordered the Prime Minister Lord Salisbury to take action over it. While police officers dressed as ruffians staged a fake brawl at one end of the street to cause a diversion, Annie was dragged from the basement where she lived and taken off to Guy's Hospital in a closed carriage. She was certified insane by Sir William Gull, the Queen's Physician, and held there until she was physically and mentally broken. She spent most of the rest of her life in infirmaries and institutions and died insane in 1920.

With the removal of Annie, Mary Kelly realised the danger in which her knowledge of the affair had placed her and immediately left Cleveland Street. Taking Alice Margaret with her, she returned to Whitechapel, where she was first given shelter in a convent. Later, when the child had been returned to Walter Sickert, she resorted to prostitution to make a living. After a while she met a Billingsgate porter named Joseph Barnett and they decided to live together but she took to the streets again when he became unemployed. When she and some of her friends were threatened by one of the Whitechapel street gangs that preyed on the local prostitutes, she took the desperate step of attempting blackmail to pay them off, and threatened to reveal her knowledge of the secret marriage.

The victim of the blackmail attempt was never named but it was obvious that she was behind it and the letter, sent from Whitechapel, revealed her whereabouts. Sir William Gull was entrusted with the task of silencing her and her friends and it was no doubt assumed that he would have them removed in the same way as Annie Crook. Gull, however, had been deranged by a minor stroke that he had suffered and began to kill the women. He had always been known as a man who combined great kindness to his patients with a sadistic cruelty. There are two documented instances of him removing organs from deceased patients, contrary to the wishes of the families, in one case blatantly and in a manner calculated to cause distress. He probably did this because he regarded the relations' reluctance to permit removal of the organs as ignorance – which he was known to regard as the greatest of all evils – and felt that it should be punished.

Gull's victims were lured into a coach, driven by Eddy's former coachman Netley, given grapes impregnated with arsenic, then murdered in the manner of an execution described in the legends of the Freemasons' cult. This entailed taking out the victim's intestines and placing them over the left shoulder. Gull and Netley were accompanied by Sir Robert Anderson, then the Assistant Commissioner of the Metropolitan Police. Anderson, also a senior Freemason, helped Netley to carry the bodies to the places in which they were found and to arrange them in the correct Masonic manner.

Catherine Eddowes had not been part of the blackmail plot but was murdered by mistake because she sometimes used the name Mary Kelly. Arrested for drunkenness on the night of her murder, she was released from Bishopsgate Street police station just three quarters of an hour before her mutilated body was found. When she was discharged, she told the duty gaoler that her name was "Mary Ann Kelly".

This was the story that Joseph Sickert told on the television programme but as Stephen Knight said, it was one which 'defied precis' and in the few minutes allotted to him, Sickert was unable to give more than an outline. Some experts derided it as the most far-fetched solution to the Ripper mystery that had ever been suggested. Knight, then a reporter with an East End newspaper, visited Sickert shortly after the broadcast, merely because the story had had local interest. He was still sceptical when he had heard the full version but when he investigated it, he became convinced that it was indeed the true answer to the mystery. He persuaded Sickert, who was at first reluctant, to collaborate with him in the writing of a book on the subject, and this was how his *Final Solution* came to be written. When it was published it made an instant impact and appeared in serial form in the London *Evening News*.

During his research for the book, Knight obtained permission from the then Home Secretary Roy Jenkins to inspect the files on the case which had been closed throughout the century and were not due to be open to public inspection for another seventeen years. Knight found some remarkable evidence which supported Sickert's story, in particular the statement of Israel Schwartz. Sickert had said that Elizabeth Stride had been drunk and could not be persuaded to get into the coach. Netley parked the vehicle in a quiet street and he and Anderson followed her on foot. With Anderson watching from across the street, Netley approached her, then threw her to the ground and with a single vicious stroke, cut her throat. Schwartz's statement, which Sickert could not have known about, gave an uncannily similar account of her death, although having left the scene he did not actually see her killed.

Joseph Sickert's story explained a lot. If it were true, it solved mysteries such as the strange handling of the investigation, the lack of blood at the crime scenes, the amazing speed at which the victims seemed to have been murdered and mutilated, and why their bodies had been treated in that way. It also suggested a reason for Stowell's strange behaviour. The theory that Clarence himself had been the Ripper was easily disproved. It was only necessary to check the suspect's movements, which could be done quite simply through Court Circulars, and it could be seen that on the day following the "Double Event" which included the fourth murder, he was a member of a shooting party at Balmoral. He could not, therefore, have been arrested within minutes of that murder and taken to an asylum in the Home Counties, as Stowell professed to believe.

It seemed from this that Stowell could never have believed that Clarence was the Ripper and, as Stephen Knight put it, was actually "pointing a camouflaged finger" at Gull. In his article, he dismissed as nonsensical the claims that the Ripper had been a surgeon, then went on to say that in that context, it was only natural for the "rumour mongers" to pick on Sir William Gull – but as Knight said, it was not at all natural and as far as anybody knew, Gull had never been a suspect. Stowell also said that there had been reports that Gull had been seen in Whitechapel on the nights of Ripper murders, and suggested that he had been there to certify the murderer.

What he was saying, therefore, was that it had been suspected that a royal prince had taken to going to the East End to murder prostitutes but it had been thought necessary to "catch him in the act" before anything could be done about it. In Clarence's case certification would anyway have been unnecessary. One of its purposes is to make it legal to confine the person but as it would obviously have been done secretly – as Stowell himself suggested in his theory about the suspect being taken to a private asylum in the Home Counties – no offical documents would have had to be produced to justify it. Apart from that, unless there had been some prior knowledge of the Prince's intentions, why would Gull have been seen in Whitechapel only on the nights of the actual murders? There would surely have been many nights when he was there, waiting for the suspect to show up and be caught.

Having made one damaging statement about Gull, Stowell went on in the same apparently innocent way to make another. There had been a belief, retold over the years in several different versions, that the famous Victorian medium Robert James Lees had tracked Jack the Ripper to his home. When he managed to find a police inspector who would believe him, they visited the home of the man, who was a very distinguished West End physician. The inspector first questioned the doctor's wife, who was obviously annoyed at being confronted by two men who had called without first making an appointment. She gave a series of terse and non-committal replies, but finally admitted that she had been worried for some time about her husband's mental state and had noticed that he had been absent from the house on the nights of the murders in Whitechapel.

The doctor then joined them and he told the inspector that for some time he had been aware that something was wrong with his mental faculties. He would sometimes feel that he had just emerged from a trance-like state and find that he was unable to remember what he had been doing for the previous few hours. On one of those occasions he had found his shirt heavily stained with blood and supposed that his nose had been bleeding, and on another he had found scratches on his face. Lees said that after their meeting, the doctor was secretly certified and it was announced that he had died. A fake burial was carried out and the funeral attracted a great crowd of mourners, which included some of the most eminent men in the world of medicine. That sounded like a description of Gull's funeral, held in 1890 at Thorpe-Le-Soken in Essex, where his family had originated. All the leading figures in the British medical profession attended, and so many mourners travelled from London that special trains were needed to carry them all.

Having recounted the Lees story, Stowell went on to tell an even more remarkable one. He said that Gull's daughter, Caroline Acland, had told him of how two men, one a police inspector and the other calling himself a medium, had called unexpectedly one night at her parents' home in Mayfair. They had spoken first to her mother, who had been somewhat short with them, and her father had then come down from his room and told the inspector of having had lapses of memory and finding blood on his shirt after one of them. This seemed to identify Gull quite clearly as Lees' "famous doctor".

It's doubtful if Lady Gull actually said that her husband had been absent on the nights of the Ripper murders, or that Lees in his own version of the story had claimed that the doctor's wife had said so. Stowell was quoting from a book by a well-known psychic investigator of his day and that part of the story was probably an embellishment that had been added as it was re-told over a period of years. Caroline Acland could not have heard her mother make such a statement or she would surely have seen a lot more significance in the incident, and would not have talked about it. As Stowell reported it, she seemed to have related it as a curious incident which remained in her memory because she had never quite understood the reason for the visit by the two men.

Stowell's interpretation of why Gull found the blood on his shirt was that he had examined the murderer after one of the killings, and the blood had been the victim's – and so what could have been a sequence of thinly disguised accusations against the royal physician was completed. Gull had been a suspect – but nobody had known of that except Stowell. Gull had been seen in Whitechapel on the nights of Ripper murders – but only to certify the murderer, which would have been highly unlikely and unnecessary if he was Stowell's suspect. Gull had been the famous physician in the Lees story – but he was not, as the medium had said, Jack the Ripper – simply the real murderer's doctor. All the accusations against him could be therefore be explained – as long as Stowell's theory stood up. As he should have known in advance, it did not.

If, as Stephen Knight suggested, Stowell's intention had been to incriminate Gull while pretending not to realise that he had done so, the approach to Colin Wilson in 1960 had probably been an earlier and more tentative attempt. Stowell would not have let somebody else take over a theory that he believed in, but he might have been prepared to let Wilson take the stick for an unpopular suggestion involving the Royal

Family if it brought Clarence into the picture and prompted other people to look further. Wilson said that Stowell had had the theory in his mind for thirty years when they talked in 1960, and that was roughly the time that had elapsed since the death of Theodore Dyke Acland, Gull's son-in-law and Stowell's close colleague and friend. Contrary to a long established covention under which a doctor is precluded from certifying the death of a relation, Dyke Acland had been one of the doctors who signed Gull's death certificate in 1890.

Stephen Knight naturally suggested this as more evidence that Gull was the doctor whose death, according to Lees, had been faked. When his book was published in 1976 it was not known that Stowell had made his approach to Colin Wilson and, more significantly, that his theories dated back to roughly the time of Theodore Dyke Acland's death. If Knight had been aware of that he might have wondered if Stowell's interest in the Ripper murders had begun because Acland, realising that his life was nearing its end, confided some secret to him. If it was the answer to the Ripper mystery, he would have put Stowell in a dilemma.

Whatever the real intention of his article may have been, there can be no doubt that in one way or the other, Stowell was being devious. This is shown by his conversation with Colin Wilson and his later denial that Clarence was his suspect. Some of that deviousness might have been forced on him, however, if he had been in the difficult situation of wanting to respect Acland's confidence but knowing that if he did, the true solution to the mystery would be lost forever when eventually he himself died. It's likely, of course, that if he did confide in Stowell, Acland had similar feelings. Having then begun his study of the Ripper murders and satisfied himself that what Acland had said had been true, Stowell would then have begun to look for some way of passing on the secret without feeling that he had betrayed his old friend's trust. Stephen Knight believed that as a senior Freemason, Stowell would not have openly revealed the secret as he would have felt that he was breaking his oath of loyalty to the Brotherhood.

When his meeting with Colin Wilson failed to achieve its purpose, Stowell would have looked for some other way and when another ten years had passed and he knew that time was running out for him, he decided on the *Criminologist* article. At the time, that also failed. In apparently accusing Clarence, Stowell had caused a sensation and any debate which resulted from it was centred on whether or not the young

Prince could have been the Ripper. Stowell's letter of denial to *The Times* could have been a vain effort to divert attention from Clarence himself when his plan had obviously misfired but later, in 1973, the Scotland Yard officials who sent the BBC researchers to Joseph Sickert might have been influenced by the article. However clearly Clarence's innocence was proved to interested parties, he was permanently linked with the Ripper mystery and it seems possible that the feeling of those men at the Yard was that as he had now been brought into it, the real truth might as well be revealed. At the same time, it would finally destroy the belief that Jack the Ripper had made fools of the police, because it would be seen that they had never had any real chance of catching him.

Whether or not it was prompted by Stowell's article, the Scotland Yard tip off is a very important factor in assessing Stephen Knight's *Final Solution*, particularly in view of events which followed the publication of the book. Whereas Walter Sickert had apparently said that it was Sir Robert Anderson who had helped Netley to place the bodies in the places chosen for them by Gull, Knight became convinced that Sickert himself and not Anderson had been the "Third Man". Anderson was, in fact, on holiday abroad when two of the murders were committed.

Knight based his opinion mainly on descriptions of men who were seen, sometimes with victims, near the crime scenes. On that basis, he made out a reasonable case. Something else which could have supported his contention but which he apparently failed to notice, was an unusual gap in the otherwise detailed account which Walter Sickert was said to have given. It was said that the name of the recipient of Mary Kelly's blackmail letter was never disclosed. When the *Final Solution* was first published, my feeling was that if the story were true, the most likely person was Sickert himself. In 1990, this was suggested in a book *Sickert and the Ripper Crimes* by Jean Overton Fuller whose mother, Violet Overton Fuller, knew the artist Florence Pash, who was a close friend of Walter Sickert.

In her book, Ms Fuller states that Florence Pash knew Mary Kelly and told Violet Overton Fuller many details about her life which were in accordance with Joseph Sickert's story. She is also reported to have said that Kelly tried to blackmail Walter Sickert – who, if Kelly did resort to that solution when she herself was being threatened, would have been the obvious person. Kelly, a young and illiterate Irish girl in London, would have known nobody else who was worth blackmailing, and Sickert would have had a lot to fear from her threat. He would already have been unpopular for helping to arrange Prince Eddy's visits to Cleveland Street which had caused so much embarrassment to the Royal Family. Any further repercussions from it could have been damaging to him in the career that meant so much to him because they might have cost him his carefully cultivated friendships with a number of people in high place – including Eddy's father, the then Prince of Wales.

When Stephen Knight's book was published Joseph Sickert contributed an Afterword, in which he acknowledged that Knight's suspicions that Walter Sickert had been the "Third Man" were probably correct. He was of the opinion that the artist was forced into assisting with the murders but in fact, Sickert might have offered to do so. If he was in fact the person blackmailed by Mary Kelly, he may have panicked and reported her threat to somebody in authority, feeling that with this latest echo of the unfortunate affair, he had better show willingness to undo some of the harm that he had helped to cause. It may be that he quickly regretted his action and did his best to help Kelly escape – Stephen Knight suggested that he had deliberately allowed Eddowes to be killed in place of her – but initially, he might have offered to track her down and he would have been an ideal person to do so. He often went to the East End to paint "low life" scenes and had an intricate knowledge of its tiny streets and alleys. He also knew many of the women there as he used them for models, finding in their looks and postures an authenticity that professional models could never provide.

Unfortunately, there was inconsistency as to what was supposed to have been the purpose of the Ripper killings, as explained in the story that Joseph Sickert claimed to have heard from Walter. When he appeared in the final programme of the 1973 television series, Joseph Sickert said that Gull's plan was to kill some women and mutilate them in accordance with the Masonic ritual. This would be unrecognised by most people and the murders would have been seen as the work of a dangerous lunatic. When Kelly was murdered, which was the purpose of the operation, it would be assumed that she was just the latest victim and nobody would look for any other reason for her death. When he told the story to Knight, however, Sickert said that Nichols, Chapman and Stride had been involved with Kelly in the blackmail plot, and the intention was to find and kill all of them. Knight obviously accepted Sickert's second version, as that was how he reported the story in his book.

If Sickert's story was true, Mary Kelly would have needed help to write her blackmail letter because she was illiterate. At her inquest, Barnett said that she was interested in the Ripper murders and asked him to read the newspaper reports to her, so obviously she could not do so herself. This in itself may appear to make another aspect of the story doubtful. Kelly was supposed to have worked in the tobacconist's shop in Cleveland Street with Annie Crook, but although illiteracy would have been a handicap to her it would not have made it impossible for her to have followed that occupaton.   On the birth certificate of her daughter Alice Margaret, Annie is described as a "tobacconist's assistant from Cleveland Street", which confirms that she worked there, and the fact that she was unable to sign as informant but made her mark shows that she also was unable to read or write. As she was obviously able to carry out her duties in spite of this handicap, there was no reason why Kelly couldn't have managed.

Kelly's illiteracy does not, of course, prove that Nichols, Chapman and Stride were involved with her, but the timing of the murders suggests that they could have been specific rather than random victims. Knight believed that Kelly, the real culprit in the blackmail plot, was to be the last victim and that that was why Eddowes, who was murdered in her place, received the full ritual. Apart from the disembowelling, she had Masonic symbols cut on her face and her body was left in Mitre Square, the most Masonic site in London, with its name incorporating the mason's two basic tools, the mitre and the square.

If Knight was correct in his conjecture, Gull and his accomplices would have begun by looking for any one of the other three women – Nichols, Chapman and Stride. Having found and dealt with Nichols, they would have looked for Chapman and Stride and after an interval of eight days, managed to find Chapman. With Stride the only target left before Kelly, it took them three weeks to catch up with her, and that would not have been at all surprising. At the time of her death Stride had been cohabiting with a waterside labourer named Michael Kidney, who told the coroner that when she was drinking, she would disappear for days on end and he would have no idea of where she was. Another witness, PC William Smith who saw her with a man in Berner Street ten minutes before she was murdered, said that it was unusual to see prostitutes in that particular area. It would not therefore have been one of the places where the traditional Ripper – the man who was out to murder *any* prostitute and, according to most modern experts, had local knowledge – would have hoped to find his next victim.

If the timings of the murders support Joseph Sickert's claim that Nichols, Chapman and Stride were specific rather than random victims, the number of murders must throw some doubt on any theory that Jack the Ripper was out to kill prostitutes whenever he encountered one at some conveniently secluded place. There were thousands of them in Whitechapel alone and he could have trebled his total of five victims with no difficulty at all. What must make Sickert's claim suspicious is that he changed his story, with the obvious implication that he had sensed a sympathetic listener in Stephen Knight and ventured an even more fanciful version. There could have been another reason – he might, for example, have been asked to shorten the story for the television programme – but what is certain is that if that story is true, Walter Sickert's knowledge of the East End and the women there would have made him just as useful to assist Gull, whether it meant tracking down four particular women or simply luring any potential victims that he might encounter into the coach.

There is another gap in the story that Walter Sickert is said to have told, and it could also point to his participation in the murders. It was claimed that Elizabeth Stride was killed quickly because the three men had heard that "Mary Kelly" had been arrested for drunkenness and knowing that she was likely to be released from the police station at any time after one o'clock, they saw the opportunity to waylay her when she left. The narrative seems to have been uncharacteristically vague on the point of *how* they knew and it may be that if Sickert did tell that story, this was deliberate. Eddowes was arrested at 8.30 that night and Walter Sickert could have known about it. If the murders took place in the way that Stephen Knight envisaged, Sickert would probably have been in Whitechapel, where he often rented rooms, ahead of Gull and Netley. He might have witnessed the arrest of Eddowes or been told about it by another of the local prostitutes who had seen her being taken to the police station.

Knight believed that Sickert was responsible for leaving the piece of Eddowes' apron in the doorway at Goulston Street and chalking the strange message above it. He was convinced that the word "Juwes" meant the three apprentice masons who, in the Freemason's legend, murdered the Master Mason, Hiram Abiff. He thought that Sickert left those clues as a pointer to the involvement of Freemasonry, but he could have had an additional reason. If Sickert did allow Eddowes to be murdered in place of Kelly, he would have been left with a considerable feeling of guilt. Leaving the clues could have been an act of remorse and of resentment at what he had been forced to do. It would have been very rash of him, because it would have been obvious that he had been responsible but at that time, he might well have been past caring. In any case, if it had been accepted that Eddowes was Kelly, the affair would have been at an end and he might have hoped that the men behind the conspiracy would feel that any reprisal would then have been pointless. The words of the message have an air of finality about them – the murders, hopefully, had been completed and the question of blame could be discussed, but would never be really resolved.

In dealing with the Goulston Street clues, some authors have seemed anxious to take advantage of PC Long's wavering when he gave evidence at the inquest on Eddowes. Long had said that the message had not been on the wall when he first went into the building at 2.20 a.m. but pressed by the coroner, Mr Samuel Frederick Langham, he said that he could not be completely sure. The point was important because until then, it had been supposed that the murderer killed for the pleasure of it, whenever there was an opportunity, then disappeared as quickly as he could. If he had placed his clues *after* Long made his first search of the building, however, it might suggest something different. It could have meant that the man was still at large for perhaps as much as an hour from the murder and if so, there was probably a lot more to the crime than anybody had previously suspected. Langham probably realised that and wanted to be completely sure that Long had been right in what he first told the inquest, but with the constable's backtracking, he succeeded only in creating uncertainty.

Some theorists have taken advantage of that uncertainty to suggest that PC Long was totally mistaken in his original evidence. It would have been logical for the Ripper to have simply thrown the piece of apron into the doorway as he hurried by, a few minutes after he had left Mitre Square, and *both* clues were there when Long first entered the building. No doubt it would have been logical for the type of suspect that most of these theorists have suggested to have acted in that way but Long's evidence can hardly be dismissed on the very shaky premise that because he *might* have failed to notice the message on his first visit, it's permissible to assume not only that he *did*, but that he also failed to notice the piece of apron. As I pointed out in Chapter 4, however, when Long returned to the building at 2.55, he immediately recognised that bloodstained strip of cloth for what it was – probably because it had been spread out so that the blood was easy to see. If, as has been suggested, it was obscured by rubbish on his first visit, he would surely have missed it for the same reason when he came back.

If the piece of apron had been placed in a way that made it instantly recognisable, the purpose could have been to draw attention to the message on the wall. The doubts as to whether the Ripper chalked that message have centred on the slightly unlikely possibility that 'Juwes' was a misspelling of 'Jews', which was a familiar enough word at that time. On that basis, it had often been dismissed as an anti-Semitic graffito – as Warren professed to believe. Martin Fido suggests that it could have been written by a disgruntled Gentile who had been cheated by a Jew and refused reparation. Using Cockney double-negative, he was saying, "The Jews won't own up to nothing they've done" – and if this is true, and Long did fail to spot the bloodstained cloth at 2.20 a.m., the whole thing is quite simple. The Ripper cut or tore away a piece of his victim's apron to wipe the blood and other matter from his hands and he tossed it into the doorway as he passed. The objections to that belief have also been mentioned in Chapter Four, however, and are worth repeating.

If the Ripper took the piece of apron solely to clean his hands, he would probably have dropped it by the body as soon as he had done so. He could, in any case, have wiped his hands on the apron – assuming that he could have seen it clearly enough in the darkness – without detaching a piece. That would have been easier to do and would have saved time. Taking the piece of apron away with him would have been dangerous, as the police would already have out in the streets, following the murder of Elizabeth Stride. As he walked from Mitre Square to Goulston Street there must have been other places to lose that incriminating piece of evidence, if that was all he intended. It's also worth emphasising that PC Long would have been trained to be observant, so if he spotted the message and the bloodstained cloth on his second visit to the building, he would probably have seen them when he made his first search some thirty five minutes earlier – had they been there.

There is, then, a reasonable case for believing that the piece of apron was taken for some reason other than for the murderer to clean his hands, and that the person responsible knowingly took a considerable risk in retaining it until he reached Goulston Street. If that person was Walter Sickert, he might have returned to the room he was renting at the time, waited until he had heard the police go by on their first visit, then left his clues in the doorway. Stephen Knight thought that the writing on the wall had some similarities with Sickert's but he was, of course, referring to a copy of the message, made when it was first discovered. On the face of it other authors were correct in saying that the copy, no matter what effort was made to reproduce the writing on the wall, could hardly be used as a comparison. In his book, however, Knight showed the copy with a specimen of Sickert's writing, both of which contained the word "not" – and they are identical.

None of this can be taken as evidence against Sickert, and nor can the fact that he was known be deeply interested in the Ripper murders. A close friend, Marjorie Lilly told Stephen Knight that late in his life, after he had suffered a stroke –

"Sickert would have 'Ripper periods' in which
he would dress up like the murderer and walk
about like that for weeks on end. He would
turn down the lights in his studio and
literally *be* Jack the Ripper in word and
mood."

All these things, however, may have been in Joseph Sickert's mind because in his Afterword to Knight's book he said that secretly, he had probably suspected the truth long before Knight told him of his conclusions. He may also have noticed the significance of the old artist having declined to go into details about the murder and mutilation of Mary Kelly, saying that having known her as a friend and helper, those details were still painful to him. Why would he have known them, however, unless he had witnessed those horrific events? This is something else which may have weighed with Joseph Sickert when he reluctantly agreed with Knight, but two years later, in 1978, he wrote to the editor of *The Sunday Times* saying that he had made up the whole story. All that he stood by was that Walter Sickert had been his father and that his mother, Alice Margaret Crook, had been the illegitimate daughter of the Duke of Clarence. He had never expected the story to go further than a local newspaper – presumably the *East London Advertiser* for whom Knight was working when they met – and now he wanted to clear his father's name.

CHAPTER 11

After the Final Solution

When Joseph Sickert "confessed" to having made up the story of how the Duke of Clarence's secret marriage had caused the Ripper murders, Stephen Knight said that he was not surprised. When he had insisted on publishing his conviction that Walter Sickert was actively involved in the murders, Joseph Sickert had said that he would "find some other way, even if it meant going back on the whole story."

The confession, however, was greeted knowingly and in some cases, it was sensed, gratefully. Two points that were apparently considered irrelevant were why the Scotland Yard official had sent the BBC to Sickert for what he had called the "definitive version" of Jack the Ripper, and how Sickert had described the attack on Elizabeth Stride in a way that coincided so closely with what Israel Schwartz had said in his then unknown statement.

The nearest that anyone came to attempting to explain Sickert's story of the Stride murder was in *Jack the Ripper – The Bloody Truth*, by the late Melvyn Harris, published in 1988. Harris claimed that there was nothing remarkable about it as it was known that there were two men in Berner Street at the time of the murder. That was why the *Police Gazette* had published descriptions of two men. Sickert must have concocted his story from contemporary newspaper reports.

It was true that the *Police Gazette* published descriptions of two men but only one was by Israel Schwartz. That was of the man who attacked Stride. The other was by PC Smith who passed Stride and her companion, the other man at Dutfield's Yard, in Berner Street ten minutes earlier. There was nothing to indicate that the two men had been together at Dutfields Yard – possibly it was a deliberate attempt to separate them. Apart from one obscure newspaper report in which Schartz was referred to as "the Hungarian", there was no newspaper coverage that Joseph Sickert could have used to concoct his account of the attack on Stride, and errors in his story suggest that if he did carry out any research, it was not to any great depths.

One of those errors concerned the coachman, John Netley. Sickert told Stephen Knight that Netley developed an obsession about Alice Margaret Crook, allegedly Clarence's daughter, and more than once tried to kill her. The final attempt was in Drury Lane when Alice Margaret, still a child, was being accompanied by a relation, who later described the incident to Walter Sickert. Netley drove his coach at the girl but the wheel stuck a kerbstone and was damaged. An angry crowd gathered and Netley was forced to escape them on foot. He ran to Westminster, where he jumped into the Thames and drowned.

John Netley actually died in an accident in 1903, when he was thrown from the cab of a horse van that he was driving. It happened, perhaps significantly, by the Clarence Gate to Regents Park. Stephen Knight's researchers found a newspaper report of how a man who gave his name as Nickley was rescued from the Thames at Westminster, by the pier master, in 1892. He was taken to hospital but quickly discharged himself. Nickley is not a name listed in the British Dictionary of Surnames, so it might have been a spur of the moment attempt by Netley to disguise his real name or simply a misheard version of his real name, quite understandable if he had just been pulled out of the river. The real point, of course, is that Joseph Sickert would not have found any contemporary report that would have convinced him that Netley died just after the Drury Lane incident. Walter Sickert, however, might have heard some rumour that "the man who nearly ran down that little girl in Drury Lane" had fallen in the Thames and drowned. Such incidents have always been subject to "Chinese Whispers".

When Joseph Sickert made his confession, he said that as far as he was concerned, "Jack can go back to the Ripperologists", but it was not his last word on the subject. In 1991 he performed a complete u turn when he cooperated on another book, *The Ripper and the Royals* by Melvyn Fairclough. Sickert then claimed that his original story was, after all, true. He had repudiated it "to clear my father's name". He said that Stephen Knight had been "misunderstanding" the information he was giving him, they had quarrelled and consequently he had only given him half the story. The new version, contained in Fairclough's book, was that

Gull had been acting under the instructions of Lord Randolph Churchill, father of Sir Winston, who had masterminded the whole operation. Even more dubious was his stated reason for going back on his 1978 confession.

On New Year's Eve 1985 – coincidentally, Stephen Knight had died a few months earlier – he had watched a televison showing of the film *Murder By Decree*, which told the story of the Ripper murders, based on Knight's *Final Solution*. He was shocked by the way that Clarence and his grandmother, Annie Elizabeth Crook, were shown in the film. "Didn't they suffer enough in their lives without them doing that to them when they were dead?"

In the case of Annie Crook, he might have received some sympathy. He was a Roman Catholic and the film had Annie committing suicide in a lunatic asylum. To him, that would have been a mortal sin. His anguish over Clarence, shown in the film as callously abandoning Annie, was somewhat inconsistent with previous remarks. In the Afterword that he contributed to Knight's book he had said that while some people took pride in their Royal connections, he found his "disgusting". He regarded Clarence as an interloper in his family and his blood a "taint". Even stranger was that *Murder By Decree* was made in 1978 and Sickert claimed to have been an adviser in the production – so apparently, he had had no idea of how his alleged grandparents were to be portrayed and in the seven years since the film's release had made no attempt to see it.

It's stated that in the film Annie Crook was played by Genevieve Bujold – "with a marked French accent". With his impaired hearing, Mr Sickert might have thought that because Annie was shown as the inmate of an asylum, with her speech halting and slurred. Also, like a lot of transatlantic actors – Ms Bujold is a French Canadian – she seemed to struggle a little with a London accent. Her natural accent is transatlantic, which she has often used playing American roles but she managed an impeccable English accent playing Anne Boleyn opposite Richard Burton in *Anne of the Thousand Days*. What seems likely is that Sickert did not actually see the film but used it as an excuse to re-enter the Ripper field to repudiate Stephen Knight's accusations against Walter Sickert. If so, he probably assumed from her name that Ms Bujold is French and there has a French accent.

The Ripper and the Royals revealed Sickert's talent for adapting real events into his stories when he referred to a Scotland Yard announcement in 1988. In 1987, some Ripper documents, including the original "Jack the Ripper" letter, had been returned anonymously to the Yard. As the case documents had then been phased in at the then Public Record Office at Kew, they were all recalled, to ascertain how many of them were actually still there. When the check had been made, Scotland Yard made their announcement.

Their explanation was that one of their officers had borrowed the documents when the file was still at the Yard, to show when he gave True Crime lectures in his off duty hours. He had died in 1987 and his relations had found that those documents were still in his house. Realising the significance of them, they had decided that the best thing to do was put them in an envelope and post them, without any covering letter, back to Scotland Yard.

Sickert, however, claimed that those documents had been in his possession, as Abberline had given them to his mother, many years earlier, in case she ever needed to prove her identify as Clarence's daughter. When Fairclough's book had reached the First Draft stage, he had sent a copy to the Crown Prosecution Service in case it was thought that some of his claims of acquaintanceships with with members of the Royal Family were "seditious". Soon afterwards, some Special Branch officers had descended on him, ransacked his house and taken the Ripper documents.

Not long after *The Ripper and the Royals* had been published, I was looking at the printed list of documents referring to quite a few well-known cases in the MEPO (Metropolitan Police) files at Kew. I noticed that in the list of Ripper documents, there were several hand-written additions, each marked "Returned Anonymously in 1987". These were obviously the documents referred to in the Scotland Yard announcement. I then noticed that among the Crippen case documents, there were similar hand-written additions, also marked "Returned Anonymously in 1987". The only inference from this was that the Scotland Yard version had been correct, but their official had also borrowed Crippen case documents for his lectures. Because these were not a topical as the Ripper ones in 1988, the year of the centenary, they had not been mentioned when the return of the documents had been announced. Unintentionally, Scotland Yard had set a trap and Sickert had walked into it.

I met Joseph Sickert late in his life and shared the general opinion among interested parties, that he was a very different man from the one who had appeared on the original television programme in 1973. Until his death in 2003, he determinedly clung to his claim to be descended from the Royal Family and in the last few years of his life, managed to have himself listed in the local telephone directory as "HRH Joseph Sickert". I think he was affected by years of telling a story that, in some quarters, was openly derided and mistakenly thought that by adding to his story he would make it more believable. It was not long after *The Ripper and the Royals* had been published that Melvyn Fairclough admitted that the information Sickert had given him had been "confused".

I also think that Sickert believed everything that he told Stephen Knight. He had, after all, made no attempt to tell his story before the BBC contacted him and had it been an elaborately concocted and researched hoax, he surely would have done. It probably rankled with him that because of differences with Stephen Knight he had repudiated it, and it was possible to see elements of a revenge motive in Fairclough's book. By the time that book was published, several flaws in the original story had been detected and these were often blamed on Knight's "misunderstandings".

It was orginally claimed that the police raid on Cleveland Street that ended with Annie Crook being taken off to Guy's Hospital had been in April 1888, with Mary Kelly's flight and subsequent blackmail attempt following. However, he statements of Barnett, Kelly's common law husband, and McCarthy, the owner of the lodging house where the final murder took place, reveal that Kelly had been living with Barnett in the lodging house from the beginning of that year. With other writers, I suggested that the raid and abduction of Annie Crook might have taken place two or three years earlier, and Fairclough's book showed that Mr Sickert had been pleased to agree. What was said, however, was that it was Stephen Knight who "set" the date of the raid as April 1888.

Anyone who had read Knight's book would doubt that accusation. Knight said that Annie Crook was held in Guy's Hospital for some five months before being transferred to another hospital, during the lull between the fourth and fifth murders. That would take the date of her incarceration there back to April 1888. As Knight actually quoted the exact number of days that she was at Guy's, it was obviously what he had been told, as no "misunderstanding" or imagination on his part would have made him think that.

The revenge motive seemed to be evident in another context, and this may have been something that had he thought about it more, Sickert would not have had included in Fairclough's book. Stephen Knight died of a brain tumour at the age of thirty-seven and there were suggestions that he had actually been murdered by the Freemasons. Apart from the Masonic connection that he had suggested in his *Final Solution*, he had written a best-selling expose of Freemasonry, "The Brotherhood." Joseph Sickert did not directly abscribe to that theory, but apparently couldn't resist dropping a hint in that direction.

In *The Ripper and the Royals*, it was claimed that on the day that Knight died, a piece of paper was pushed through his letter box. On examination, it proved to be an agreement on royalities from Knight's book, that Knight himself had made out on his portable typewriter. Some of those royalaties should have gone to charities for the deaf, which Joseph Sickert supported, but they were never paid. Possibly this had something to do with the disagreement between Knight and Sickert, and may answer another objection that was made to the veracity of Sickert's 1978 "confession".

Why, if Sickert's motive in repudiating the story had been to "clear my father's name", had he waited two years to do so? Quite obviously, he could have prevented publication of the book if he had gone back on the story when Knight accused Walter Sickert. As it was, he was only drawing further attention to a story which by 1978 had become regarded as just one more attempt to solve the Ripper mystery. The answer may be that Sickert waited two years in the hope that the royalties would be paid but finally accepted that they would not, and made his confession, hoping that it would considerably reduce the amount that Knight was receiving from the book.

Joseph Sickert was obviously an unreliable source – some people who knew him well have said that he took a certain pleasure in persuading the gullible to believe his fantasies – but the theory that Clarence's secret marriage was the catalyst for the Ripper murders does not actually rely on his testimony. There were reports of that affair as early as 1915, and in 1990, Jean Overton Fuller's "Sickert and the Ripper Crimes" supported much of what Joseph Sickert had originally told Knight. As stated earlier, it filled in one gap in Sickert's orignal narrative, which was that nobody knew who the victim of Mary Kelly's blackmail attempt. The logical answer, supplied by Miss Overton Fuller, was that it was Walter Sickert.

Jean Overton Fuller was already an established author when her book was published and she had an impeccable background. Her mother, Violet

Overton Fuller, knew Walter Sickert's close friend and fellow artist, Florence Pash, who told her that Sickert had been able to describe the bodies of the Ripper victims in a way that convinced them that he had seen them at the crime scenes. That led Violet Overton Fuller to suspect that Sickert had carried out the murders himself, which was the basis of her daughter's book. It can never be definitely proved if Florence Pash did make the statments attributed to her but as Begg, Fido and Skinner in *The Jack the Ripper A–Z* acknowledged, the book was potentially powerful corroboration of Stephen Knight's theory as set out in his *Final Solution*. Florence Pash was also said to have confirmed that Joseph Gorman was the natural son of Walter Sickert and that Sickert had infiltrated clues to the Ripper murders in some of his paintings. *Sickert and the Ripper Crimes* did not have the impact that it would have done even five years earlier. Partly due to the books published to mark the centenary in 1988, the subject had suffered from overkill and interest in it had dwindled.

The only reason that Begg, Fido and Skinner could find to doubt that evidence presented in the Overton Fuller book was that it repeated a story included in Stephen Knight's *Final Solution*. This was that after the murders the Marquis of Salisbury, then Prime Minister, had suddenly appeared at Sickert's studio in Dieppe and paid him £500 for an unfinished painting. Obviously this was a bribe. It was doubted because in a collection of Walter Sickert's writings published under the title *A Free House* by Osbert Sitwell, Sickert told the story, but said that the £500 was paid to an artist named Vallon or Vollon. Salisbury had commissioned the painting but was dissatisfied with the finished effort and made the payment as an expression of his disgust. It was further claimed that the painting and the bill or sale were still at Hatfield House, the country seat of Salisbury's family, the Cecils.

Knight's reply to this was that Sickert had invented at least one "cover story" about the Ripper murders, to allow him to talk about the subject with authority – as a well-known talker and raconteur he was used to being the centre of attraction and it irritated him to hear other people discussing the murders when he knew the answer but was unable to speak of it. The story that he definitely made up was of lodging with an elderly couple in Islington, who told him that they believed that the previous occupant of the room, an young veterinary surgeon, had been Jack the Ripper. Possibly he had told the story of Salisbury's bribe for the same reason, but had had to make another artist the recipient.

The problem about the Vallon or Vollon story is that it has been too easily accepted. The subject of the painting has been referred to as a boating scene in Dieppe, a landscape and a family group – so there is at least some uncertainty about it. Nobody seems to have wondered why Salisbury, who could have commissioned any of the well-known artists of his day to produce a painting for him, gave the task to an apparently unknown artist. Also, the some of £500 would have had an equivalent value of over £30,000 in today's money so as a gesture of "disgust" it was an extremely expensive one.

What also suggests that Sickert might have told a "cover story" is that there was a well-known and extremely gifted artist of his day named Antoine Vallon. Accomplished though he was, he never became one of the household names of the world of art but it's very likely that Sickert would have known of him. Perhaps it appealed to his sense of humour to name him as Salisbury's "unknown artist", knowing that nobody without an intricate knowledge of art would recognise it or query the story.

While Jean Overton Fuller produced remarkable but unfortunately third hand evidence that appeared to confirm most of Joseph Sickert's claims, it's hard to accept her contention that Walter Sickert committed the murders. The evidence, particularly that from the murder of Catharine Eddowes, in any case rules out a solo murderer. Much more likely is the possibility that he was an unwilling accomplice, and as will be shown in the next chapter, there is a very strong case for believing that.

CHAPTER 12

Walter Sickert

There is no doubt at all that Walter Sickert was deeply interested in the Ripper murders, as his close friend Marjorie Lilly revealed in her book *Sickert The Painter and His Circle*. As well as relating how, late in his life, he had "Ripper periods", in which he would sit in his darkened studio, dressed according to the popular image, Ms Lilly also wrote of how he would use his famous red handkerchief as a focussing point when he was painting his "Camden Town Murder" series –

> "While he was reliving the scene he would assume the part of a ruffian, knotting the handkerchief loosely around his neck, pulling a cap over his eyes and lighting his lantern. Immobile, sunk deep in his chair, lost in the long shadows of that vast room, he would meditate for hours on his problem. When the handkerchief had served its immediate purpose it was tied to any doorknob or peg that came in handy to stimulate his imagination further, to keep the pot boiling. It played a necessary part in the performance of the drawings, spurring him on at crucial moments, becoming so interwoven with the actual working out of his idea that he kept it constantly before his eyes."

As Stephen Knight pointed out, this must remind us of the description, published in *The Times*, of a man seen with a woman near Mitre Square just before the body of Catharine Eddowes was discovered –

"He is of shabby appearance, about 30 years of
age and 5ft 9in in height, of fair complexion,
having a small fair moustache, and wearing a
red neckerchief and a cap with a peak."

There is no real evidence that the woman who was with that man was
Eddowes – and the impossibility of Eddowes having been murdered in
Mitre Square suggests that when the couple were seen, she was already
dead – but the man could have been leaving the Square, having helped
to take her body there. Seeing Joseph Lawende and his two friends
approaching and noticing a prostitute nearby, he might have engaged
her in conversation until they had passed, and a similar thing could have
happened in Hanbury Street on the morning when Annie Chapman was
murdered, when Mrs Elizabeth Long saw a man and a woman standing
outside No.29 at 5.30.

Mrs Long was almost certainly wrong in identifying the woman as
Chapman. A few minutes earlier, Albert Cadosche had heard what was
probably the body of Chapman being dumped in the backyard. Also,
Dr Phillips' estimate that it would have taken at least 15 minutes to
inflict the injuries he saw on Chapman's body means that there was
insufficient time to have killed and mutilated her between 5.30 and 5.50
when John Davis discovered her body. In both instances, however, the
man could have been Walter Sickert, with the red handkerchief that he
wore at Mitre Square – like the one that Hutchinson's man gave to Mary
Kelly – the obvious pointer. *The Times* description of the man at Mitre
Square includes a small, fair moustache and in later years, a friend of
Sickert remembered his moustache as being "like a little frizzle of gold".

In a recent biography of Walter Sickert, it was stated that he was out
of the country when two of the murders took place but from what we
know of Sickert, it would be very difficult to prove his whereabouts at
any given time – just as it would with anyone at that time. Marjorie Lilly
spoke of his sudden and inexplicable departures to Dieppe, where he had
a studio for many years, and of his equally inexplicable returns, when he
would sudden reappear among his friends in London. What evidence
was there that he had actually been in Dieppe during his absences, and
not in one of the many East End rooms that he rented?

Whatever arguments against it may be advanced, it's likely that
Walter Sickert will always be associated with Jack the Ripper and the

assertion by Joseph Sickert, supported by Jean Overton Fuller, that the Sickert paintings contained clues to the murders was the basis of what Colin Wilson considered to be the most impressive chapter in Stephen Knight's *Final Solution*. Sickert had the habit of giving his paintings strange titles and alternative ones which bore no apparent relation to the subjects of those paintings. Some that Knight mentioned in his book were reported to him by Joseph Sickert, who claimed to have been told about them by Walter, but one was the result of his own deduction. He wrote –

"It is a disturbing painting about which he made
no comment to his son. It depicts a gaunt
Victorian room with a high ceiling. On the wall
in the centre of a fireside alcove is some sort of
ornament whose definition is indistinct but which
can be nothing but a death's head. This age-old
harbinger of impending doom is gazing down on a
woman dressed poorly in a blouse and long skirt.
She is averting her face from its baleful gaze, her
hand has been brought to her cheek in despair. In
suggesting that the woman is Marie Kelly with Death
staring her in the face, I could be justly accused
of allowing my imagination to run riot, except for
one thing – the mysterious title of the picture.
Like so many of Sickert's paintings, it has never
been explained. He gave it two names. "X's
Affiliation Order" and "Amphytrion". Remembering
That an affiliation order fixes paternity of an
illegitimate child, can we escape the conclusion
that Sickert was recalling the events of Cleveland
Street? And who is X? Bearing in mind Sickert's
story about the highest in the land disguising
himself as a lesser being and in that form seducing
an ordinary girl and making her pregnant,
(Clarence was said to have been introduced to the
Cleveland Street set as Sickert's younger brother)
consider the alternative title to this picture
"Amphytrion". The legend of Amphytrion tells how

Jupiter, King of the gods, *the highest in Olympus
disguised himself as a lesser being to seduce an
ordinary woman who became pregnant by him.*"

Knight cited other paintings. "Blackmail" or "Mrs Barrett" was a picture of a square-chinned woman which Knight said was like drawings of Mary Kelly that appeared in newspapers, following the final Ripper murder. A second "Mrs Barrett" showed the subject with her eyes in a shadow, like a skull. According to Joseph Sickert and Jean Overton Fuller, Mary Kelly set off the murders with her attempt at blackmail and Knight suggested that the title "Mrs Barrett" was the result of faulty memory. Kelly's common law husband until just before her murder was Joe Barnett. A second painting titled "Blackmail" was of a woman with the tip of her nose missing – as Kelly's was, among other facial disfigurements, after she had been murdered by the Ripper. Jean Overton Fuller specifically mentioned features of Sickert's painting "Ennui" as an example of his clues. In it, a man and a woman are shown in a room, both expressionless, and behind them on the wall is a picture of Queen Victoria – with a bird, a gull, fluttering near her head.

Sickert's "Camden Town Murder" series had a second title, "What Shall We Do For The Rent?" Mary Kelly was five weeks in arrears with her rent when she was murdered and the paintings were inspired by a murder which had similarities with her own . A prostitute was found lying on her bed with her throat cut, a few hours after she had been murdered – as Kelly was. The paintings show a naked woman laying on a bed, as Kelly's was – although it was not naked as contemporary newspaper reports said – when it was found. A man is near her, as Knight described it "In some he is sitting on the end of the bed wringing his hands, in others he stands over the body of the woman." Sickert knew Robert Wood, who was tried for the murder and acquitted, and was a model for some of the pictures. It may have been his acquaintanceship with Wood that prompted him to create those painting in spite of his often stated belief that an artist cannot paint a subject if he has no experience of it – Knight believed that he was moved by his involvement in the Ripper murders.

Knight made out his case convincingly but he made one serious error in presenting it. In 1988, one of the books published to mark the centenary of the murders was *The Ripper Legacy* by Keith Skinner and Martin

Howells. In it was a letter by Dr Wendy Baron, an expert on Sickert and his paintings, which she wrote in reply to one by Knight, seeking her opinion on the "inexplicable" titles of the paintings. Dr Baron said that although those titles were strange, they were not inexplicable. Sickert was "cocking a snook" at the habit of Victorian artists, such as James Whistler, of giving "titles that told a story" to paintings. She gave as an example "When Did You Last See Your Father?", in which the son of a fugitive Cavalier is being questioned by a panel of Roundheads, following the Civil War.

Knight made no mention of Dr Baron's letter. Even if he felt that a debate on it would occupy too much space in his book or he simply believed Joseph Sickert's assertion that his alleged father had told him the meanings of the strange titles, he would have done better to have said so and thereby avoid the charge of suppressing evidence. It would also have been the wiser course because, even acknowledging Dr Baron's expertise, her opinion could have been challenged. Her reason for citing "When Did You Last See Your Father?" may have been that Sickert himself once mentioned it, perhaps because he thought that to a certain extent, it depended on its title. The picture was famous in Sickert's day and during the twentieth century was often referred to in school history lessons on the Civil War, but without its title or an explanation, it could have seemed meaningless.

It could well have been Sickert's idea of a joke to give his paintings meaningless titles which in later years, self-styled experts might debate and attach meanings to, but it must be possible that something – perhaps some train of thought – suggested them to him. Those titles do not seem to be plucked out of the air and in the case of paintings like "Ennui", it was the details rather than the title which gave the clue. Skinner and Howells said that the painting "Mrs Barrett" was actually a portrait of Sickert's housekeeper – but why the alternative title "Blackmail"? Perhaps Sickert deliberately confused the name, and what in any case must have been the housekeeper's reaction to the second "Mrs Barrett", in which her face was shown shrunken into a skull?

Skinner and Howells also disputed Joseph Sickert's claim that there were echoes of the Ripper murders in a 1935 painting "George V and Queen Mary", in which the King and his wife were shown in a car. The Queen is shown partly obscured by the window-frame of the car and Joseph Sickert claimed that the picture was painted that way because until his death in 1892, Mary had been engaged to Clarence and in Walter's view, still "half belonged to him". Skinner and Howells revealed that the picture was based on a newspaper photograph, but that in no way disproved Joseph Sickert's contention. He obviously saw the photograph and might have decided to make it into a painting because he felt it was symbolic.

It might be argued that Sickert would not necessarily have intended the picture to infer some link with the Ripper murders because the death of Clarence was not, as far as anyone knows, connected with them. It has been suggested, however, that Clarence, probably bi-sexual and definitely involved in a scandal centred on a male brothel – interestingly in Cleveland Street – was removed, either by murder or incarceration, because he was becoming too much of an embarrassment to the Royal Family. Following the publishing of his book, one of Knight's correspondents pointed out that while Clarence had officially been a victim of the influenza epidemic of 1892, final reports said that his fingernails had turned black. That should not have been a symptom of influenza or of complications such as pneumonia setting hin but it could have been the result of poisoning by arsenic.

If Sickert had suspected that there had been something untoward about Clarence's death, he would probably have felt some responsibility. He had abetted the Prince's affair with Annie Crook and according to Joseph Sickert's orginal story as told to Stephen Knight, he quickly realised that the sudden ending to it by the Establishment had been inevitable. It would have been just one of the embarrassing episodes which prompted the decision to remove him from the scene but Sickert would have felt a pang of conscience about it, prompting him to paint the portrait of the King and Queen in the way that he did. It would also be easy to see conscience in the clues that he allegedly included in his paintings and Stephen Knight believed that he also left clues at the crime scenes and at Goulston Street when the strange message was found over the piece of Catharine Eddowes' apron. Knight also suggested that Sickert allowed Eddowes to be murdered in an attempt to save Mary Kelly. As he said, Sickert would never have mistaken Eddowes for Kelly.

Apart from the fact that she was not found with her arm across her body like the other victims, Eddowes was given the most Masonic treatment of all of them. She was left in Mitre Square, a place with strong Masonic associations and its name a combination of the Mason's tools, the Mitre and the Square. Her lower eyelids were nicked with the point of a knife – as shown in the Hogarth etching, "The Reward of Cruelty" which is said to depict a Masonic execution – and the Masonic symbol of a double triangle was carved on her face. It would have been understandable if that treatment had been reserved for Kelly, who would have been seen as the arch-culprit in the blackmail plot.

When Joseph Sickert described the murder of Elizabeth Stride he said that the conspirators had made the decision to quickly kill her in the street because they had "somehow" heard that Mary Kelly – actually Catharine Eddowes – was in Bishopsgate Street police station, having been arrested for drunkenness. It was one of the only two vague points in the otherwise detailed narrative – the other was that the victim of Mary Kelly's blackmail attempt was never named. Jean Overton Fuller, and common sense, tell us that if the story was true, it was Sickert himself. It's likely that on the night of the "Double Event", when Stride and Eddowes were both murdered, he would have met Gull and Netley in Whitechapel and being there before them, he might well have seen Eddowes being arrested. Knowing the local women as he did, he probably knew that Eddowes sometimes used the name Mary Kelly and when Stride would not be lured to the coach, he suggested that they should leave her and take the opportunity to pick up and murder "Mary Kelly" when she left the police station, later that night.

Stewart P. Evans and other authors have queried whether Stride really was a victim of the Ripper. The knife used to cut her throat was thought to be different from the one used on the other four women and the behaviour of the man who Israel Schwartz saw attacking her was not typical of the type of serial murderer some experts believe the Ripper to have been. A murderer of that kind would not have shown the aggression that he did – i.e. the shout of "Lipski" when he recognised Schwartz as a Jew – when he was observed by a witness. These things can be explained within Joseph Sickert's story of how Netley followed Stride, probably volunteering to kill her himself rather than postpone her murder until another night, and cut her throat after he had thrown her down by the gates of Dutfield's Yard. Netley would probably have used his own knife to kill her – and if his behaviour was untypical of a serial murderer it was because he was not one. As allegedly described by Walter Sickert, he was desperate for advancement and would have done anything he could to please his "betters".

On the face of it, Israel Schwartz's account of the attack on Stride does not comply with the original story, attributed to Sickert, of how she was drunk and refused to get into the coach. Schwartz said that he followed her attacker, who seemed to be drunk, along Berner Street then saw him with Stride by Dutfield's Yard – which doesn't suggest that she was ever anywhere near a coach. The descriptions by Matthew Packer, PC William Smith and Schwartz all point to the second man at Dutfield's Yard having been with Stride at around 12 o'clock, when Packer sold him some black grapes, and at 1.35 when Smith passed him with Stride in Berner Street. Significantly, Smith said that it was unusual to see prostitutes in that area – a random murderer who was out to kill a prostitute if the opportunity presented itself would surely have gone to a place where they were more likely to be found.

It's far from impossible that Sickert met Stride at some time before 12 o'clock, when she was already drunk, did his best to persuade her to go to the coach with him – even buying her fruit from Packer's shop – then finally reported back to Gull, to tell him he had failed in his task. When he made his suggestion that they could find "Mary Kelly" that night and murder her, Gull would probably have agreed, but if Netley offered to deal with Stride himself before they went on their way to Bishopsgate Street, he might have taken him up on it. That would have completed the whole operation that night. Within this scenario, the second man at Dutfield's Yard would have been Sickert and it's not inconceivable that he would have gone back there, separately, to make sure that Netley killed the right woman.

In describing the murder of Stride, Sickert might again have been deliberately vague. If he had told the whole story, he would have revealed a more detailed knowledge than he was implying when he told the story that Joseph Sickert relayed to Stephen Knight. What makes this more likely, as well as strengthening the case against Sickert, is Matthew Packer's account of how Stride's companion came into his shop and bought the grapes from him, while Stride stood outside playing with the flower pinned to her coat. Packer said that the man spoke with a rough, local accent but "I put him down as a young clerk". That probably meant that Packer felt the accent was assumed because it didn't go with the man's appearance. Before he became an artist, Sickert was a professional actor and would have known how to use different accents.

When Joseph Sickert told Stephen Knight the story that he claimed to have heard from Walter, he said that Walter declined to give any details of the murder and mutilation of Mary Kelly. Having known her as a friend and helper, the memory of it was still painful to him. This would have been understandable – but if he had not been personally involved, nobody would have expected him to have given a detailed account. He was alleged to have told the whole story of the Ripper episode from Clarence's affair with Annie Crook through to the actual murders but he gave no explanation of how he knew of Mary Kelly's blackmail attempt. If, as it was claimed, the name of the recipient of her letter was never disclosed, it's difficult to see how he could have known about it.

Sickert, then, could have been careful to avoid saying anything that might have suggested his personal involvement in the murders, but as far as the murder of Mary Kelly is concerned, there might have been another reason for him declining to give details. On the morning of her murder, Inspector Abberline took statements from a number of her neighbours. One of them was from a Mrs Caroline Maxwell, whose husband was a deputy in a lodging house in Dorset Street, very near to John McCarthy's. She said –

> "I have known the deceased woman during the past
> four months, she was known as Mary Jane, and that
> since Joe Barnett left her she had obtained her
> living as an unfortunate. I was on speaking
> terms with her although I had not seen her for
> three weeks until Friday morning, 9th instant,
> about half past 8 o'clock. She was then standing
> at the corner of Millers Court in Dorset Street.
> I said to her, 'What brings you up so early?' She
> said, 'I have the horrors of drink upon me as I
> have been drinking for some days past.' I said,
> 'Why don't you go to Mrs Ringer's (meaning the
> public house at the corner of Dorset Street called
> The Britannia) and have half a pint of beer?'
> She said, 'I have been there and had it, but I
> brought it all up again.' At the same time she
> pointed to some vomit in the roadway.
> I then passed on and went to Bishopsgate on an
> errand and returned to Dorset Street about 9 a.m.
> I then noticed deceased standing outside Ringers'

public house. She was talking to a man, age I
think about 30, height about 5ft 5in, stout,
dressed as a Market Porter. I was some distance
away and am doubtful whether I could identify him.
The deceased wore a dark dress, black velvet body
and coloured wrapper round her neck."

Mrs Maxwell's assertion that she had seen Kelly alive at 8.30 in the morning caused a certain amount of confusion as to the exact time of the murder. Two other witnesses, Mrs Elizabeth Prater and Mrs Sarah Lewis, were both in nearby buildings and told the police that they had heard a woman's voice screaming "murder" from the direction of McCarthy's lodging house in the early hours of the morning. Neither of them could give the exact time but roughly agreed that it was towards four o'clock. As it was not unusual to hear such cries in the night in Whitechapel, neither woman took much notice.

On 10 November, *The Times* reported that "great difference of opinion" had arisen, as to the time of the murder. The police surgeon Dr Phillips made a proviso to his initial estimate of the time of death, just as he did in the case of Annie Chapman, when he was faced with John Richardson's evidence. Originally of the opinion that Kelly had been murdered at about the time when the screams had been heard in the small hours, Phillips said that with the body having been "cut all to pieces" and left in a stone cold room for several hours, the woman might have appeared to have been dead for longer than she actually had. The implication, therefore, was that Kelly could have been killed when she returned to her room, after her conversation with Mrs Maxwell. *The Times* in fact noted that Mrs Maxwell had said that when she talked to her in the street, Kelly had been wearing a dark red knitted crossover shawl which "she had not seen her wear for some time" and later that morning it had been found by the police had later found it in Kelly's room.

As some experts have acknowledged, Mrs Maxwell's account of her conversation with Kelly was too detailed to be dismissed as imagination or faulty memory. Others have suggested that she could have been mistaken as to the day on which the conversation took place, or that the woman she spoke to was not Kelly. Both explanations seem unlikely. The report in *The Times* said that Mrs Maxwell had been able to "fix" the time of the meeting because she had gone on to a shop where she had not been for a while and bought some milk. When the police checked at the shop, her visit that morning was confirmed. At the inquest on Kelly she recalled taking some plates from her husband that had been borrowed by the lodging house where he worked and were being returned that morning. What is more conclusive is that Mrs Maxwell made her statement to Abberline on the morning of the murder, which would have been at the most three hours later. She could hardly have become confused about the day on which she had spoken to Kelly during that time.

As to whether it actually was Kelly who she met that morning, Mrs Maxwell made no claim to have had a close acquaintanceship with her, but seemed to know a lot about her. She was wrong in saying that Kelly had only returned to the streets when Joe Barnett left her, but she obviously knew Barnett and that he and Kelly had separated. Stephen Knight said that in claiming to have talked to Kelly at 8.30 that morning, Mrs Maxwell might have been drunk, lying or simply mistaken – but what was certain was that she was wrong. In 1888, people in Whitechapel were sometimes drunk in the early morning but Mrs Maxwell seemed to have been enough in control of her faculties to carry out her shopping trip, she had no reason to lie, and the facts seem to rule out any error in time or identification. As regards lying or drunkenness, the then Detective Constable Walter Dew regarded Mrs Maxwell as a "sane and sensible woman with an excellent reputation". Like most of the investigating officers, however, he thought that she was wrong in what she had said.

It has been suggested that Kelly might have been murdered in her room *after* she had spoken to Mrs Maxwell but several facts make this very doubtful. According to Mrs Maxwell, Kelly was talking to a man in Dorset Street at 9 o'clock. If she had returned to the lodging house and been killed and mutilated after that time, the Ripper would have completed his work in something like an hour and a half, that is, before Thomas Bowyer went to the room at 10.45. It had been estimated, however, that the mutilation of the body would have taken over two hours. For the Ripper to have killed in daylight would have broken the pattern of murders in the early hours of the morning, and would have been extremely risky. The lodging house was full of people, anyone of whom could have gone to the room while he was there. The extensive mutilation of the body suggests that on that occasion, he indulged himself to the full because of the time available in the cover of the room. It's in any case unlikely that the screams in the night heard by Elizabeth Prater and Sarah Lewis at around 4 o'clock were anything but the murder being committed. That time *did* fit in with the previous pattern.

The only other explanation for the mystery of Caroline Maxwell's reported meeting with her – in view of the evidence, some might say the only explanation – is that Mary Kelly was not the woman whose mutilated and totally disfigured body was found in McCarthy's lodging house. This is not a suggestion that has been found favour with most experts because it resurrects that possibility of a conspiracy theory. If Kelly was not murdered by the Ripper she must have been quite happy to let it be thought that she was, and the most likely reason for that would be that she knew that she was the intended victim and that if it had been discovered that she was still alive, a further attempt on her life would probably be made.

In her statement, Mrs Maxwell mentioned the knitted crossover shawl that Kelly was wearing when they spoke in the street, and which the police found in her room, after the murder. If Kelly had later told somebody about the meeting and they had agreed that it would be to her advantage to let it go on being assumed that she had been murdered, her confidante might have decided to take the shawl back to the room – either to create the impression that she had been murdered after she had spoken to Mrs Maxwell, or to cast doubt on the woman's evidence. It can never be proved but if somebody helped Kelly to maintain the belief that she was dead and then disappear, the most likely person was Walter Sickert.

CHAPTER 13

Prime Suspect?

The case for believing that Walter Sickert was involved in the Ripper murders is not watertight but has quite a lot to support it. The existence of John Netley, said to have driven the coach in which the murders were committed, has been proved and as a carman, he could have driven a coach. He died of a fractured skull in 1903, having being thrown from his van. He was found by the Clarence Gate, Regents Park, which prompted Stephen Knight to wonder if this was a piece of ironic Masonic humour. He suggested that Netley had been trying to exact some reward for his services in helping to deal with Kelly and her friends and was silenced, just as they had been.

Sir William Gull was said to have devised and committed the murders but before assessing his suitability as a serial murderer, other possibilities need to be considered. Violet Overton Fuller believed that Walter Sickert carried out the murders so it could be that he brought Gull into the story that he told Joseph, to cover his own involvement. It's also possible, however, that he admitted the truth and Joseph decided to substitute Gull when he told the story on the television programme and later when he collaborated with Stephen Knight. The evidence of the timing of the police patrols in Mitre Square and of the post mortem report makes it impossible for Catharine Eddowes to have been murdered in the square and with the strong doubts about Nichols and Chapman having actually died at the crime scenes, it seems that more than one man must have been involved. Help would have been needed to take those three victims to the places where they were found.

The suppressed evidence of Israel Schwartz proves that two men were present when Elizabeth Stride was attacked by Dutfield's Yard and Schwartz's descriptions of them could fit Sickert and Netley. Stride's assailant was a short man, as Netley was said to have been, he wore a peaked cap, which Netley might have done when he was driving his coach, and he had powerful shoulders which could have been developed by controlling teams of horses. It's possible to imagine that Sickert, fearful of the consequences when he received Mary Kelly's blackmail letter, did initially decide to murder her and her accomplices and recruited Netley to help him. Netley was said to have assisted Clarence in his clandestine visits to Cleveland Street and if he was the ruthless pursuer of "betterment" that he was said to have been, he would probably have been pleased to assist.

The scenario, therefore, does not need Gull – particularly if Violet Overton Fuller's suspicions were correct. It seemed, in fact, that the first murder was carried out in the manner of a serial killer beginning in a tentative, disorganised way, rather than Gull starting the ruthless programme that he was alleged to have plotted and executed. On the other hand, Gull is said to have given no indication that he intended to kill the women before that first murder, so it may be that, like any other serial killer, he turned fantasy into fact with his first killing. Even before he suffered his stroke in 1887 there were facets of his character that could have developed into a serial murderer's mentality – and there are some very good reasons to believe that Stephen Knight was correct in his theory that Thomas Stowell was surreptitiously trying to incriminate Gull in his *Criminologist* article of 1970.

William Withey Gull, 1816-90, was the youngest of eight children born to John Gull, an Essex barge-owner, and his wife Elizabeth. John Gull died from cholera in 1827, leaving Elizabeth to bring up their six surviving children. Two had died in infancy. Elizabeth Gull gave her children a strict religious and moral upbringing, with one of her watchwords, "Whatsoever is worth doing, is worth doing well."

William Gull always saw her as the stongest guiding influence in his early life but whereas her approach was no more than properly industrious, his own was egotistical and competitive. In his formative years he was particularly fond of the rhyme, quoted by Stephen Knight –

"If I was a tailor, I'd make it my pride
The best of all tailors to be.
If I was a tinker, no tinker beside
Should mend an old kettle like me."

When he decided to study medicine he was a determined and brilliant student and after a distinguished and successful career as a doctor he became Physician In Ordinary to Queen Victoria. He was remarkable, not merely for his achievements, but for his ability to overcome his orthodox religious indoctrination and evolve a philosophy of his own. He often said that "Morals and religion have no true and firm basis" and with this approach it's hardly surprising that he was a complete law unto him himself. One of his contemporaries is on record as saying of him –

> "Having once formed an opinion and determined
> upon a line of action, he carried it out
> unhesitatingly, uninfluenced by any thought of
> consequences. He was unswerving in his ideas
> of right and wrong, uninfluenced by other
> people's views and opinions.
>   His insights into truths which lesser minds
> were blind to see and powerless to grasp, and
> a life-long experience that his vast capacities
> generally placed him in the truest relation to
> things, developed in him an absolute confidence
> in the infallibility of his own judgement on
> certain points."

He is also said to have believed that ignorance was the worst of all evils, and in his views lay an obvious potential for danger. A man who believed that he was always right and had no regard for the consequences of his actions would be inclined to dismiss opposition as the ignorance of "lesser minds". He was capable of great kindness to his patients, but he could also be sadistically cruel, and in one instance of this he probably felt that he was punishing what he saw as ignorance.

On the death of a patient with a heart disease he was anxious to perform a post mortem but met with opposition from the deceased's family. It was finally agreed that he could carry out the examination but on the condition that no part of the body was "taken away". It was also stipulated that the dead man's sister should attend to see that that condition was met. When everything was ready, Gull walked up to the body, cut the heart out and placing it in his pocket, walked out. As he went, leaving the opened corpse on the dissecting table, he told the horrified sister, "I trust to your honour not to betray me."

That strange remark hinted at megalomania. Gull had acted against the wishes of the family and laid himself open to a charge of grave misconduct but appeared to think that the woman would be acting dishonourably if she reported his offence. It was as if he felt that although he had acted unethically by Society's standards, his own rules – and perhaps his motives, which were no doubt good – were more important. Therefore, if she subjected him to the judgement of mundane "lesser minds" which could not see the real priorities of the case, it would be she who was in the wrong.

Gull and many of his contemporaries in the medical world would often have met with opposition from the families of deceased patients when they wanted to perform post mortems. At times this would certainly have been frustrating but whereas most doctors would have understood the reticence of the bereaved relations and made allowances for their grief, Gull apparently could not. He obviously regarded their reluctance as stupidity and on that occasion at least, it triggered off an angry response in him. It was not the only time that he acted unethically in regard to deceased patients.

Another example is described in *A Biographical History of Guy's Hospital* by Samuel Wilks and G. T. Bettany. This story relates to a young man, referred to as "Charles W." – a patient's full name could not be revealed – who was admitted to Guy's Hospital with symptoms of a suprarenal disease. Gull was then an assistant physician and was very interested in the disease, following the discovery of it by Thomas Addison. When the young patient grew weaker and it became obvious that he would not live for very long, his father removed him from the hospital so that he could spend his last days at their home. This was some way from London but Gull kept himself informed about the case through the family doctor.

When he heard that the young man had died, Gull went to the family home with the intention of making a post mortem examination. He was accompanied by a colleague, a Dr Bealey, who related the incident to Samuel Wilks. When he entered the house, Gull stated the purpose of his visit and received a flat refusal from the deceased's father. Wilks wrote –

"Gull talked in his most persuasive manner
but without effect. He then sat down,

as if determined not to leave the house.
After an interval he spoke to the man
(presumably some kind of servant but Wilks
does not say so) saying that he should feel
sorry if the latter broke his word, seeing
it was clear that he was sworn to a refusal.
Under these circumstances, Gull said, he
would ask his permission no more, but go
upstairs and do the little operation he
wanted. The man said nothing to him, but
told an old woman who was present to follow
the doctors upstairs to see that they took
nothing away. After the usual incision,
the capsules (membranes surrounding organs)
were taken out and found to be
characteristically diseased; whereupon
Gull took out a bottle from his pocket and
put them into it. The old woman looked at
him with amazement and said, 'You are surely
not going to take that away; what will Mr W.
say?'

Gull looked at her and replied, 'He will say
nothing; I came down here on purpose to fetch
this away. I shall not tell Mr W., and surely
you will never be so foolish as to do so.'"

There are obvious similarities between that story and the one concerning
the heart patient, with the condition that no part of the body should be
"taken away" occurring in both. When such tales are passed on by word of
mouth over a period of years there is always the possibility of distortion.
Dr Bealey's account of Gull removing the capsules from the young man's
body would have been accurate and it might be wondered if the story of
the heart patient is not merely an exaggerated version of it. The difference
between the two stories are just as obvious, however, and it would have
taken an unusual amount of distortion and misunderstanding to convert
one into the other. Wilks and Bettany do not mention the heart patient
but the occurrence was reported in "In Memoriam, Sir William Gull",
one of the tributes to him published after his death.

It must be admitted that in reporting how Gull removed the capsules from the dead patient, Wilks and Bettany reported that Gull returned to London with his "well-earned prize", suggesting that at that time other doctors might secretly have approved of his action. As the family never knew of it, there was no actual harm in what he did, and probably some good if it aided research. It's also true, however, that he was in no way concerned about the feelings of the old woman, who would have been distressed, not only by what he had done but also by the thought that she had let down the deceased's father. She might also have been worried about the consequences for her and her fellow servant if the removal of the capsules was discovered. The father would, of course, have been upset as well as angry if he had found out what had happened but, ignoring such considerations, it was possible to present the episode as a triumphant for the single-minded and determined Gull. The incident with the heart patient could not be seen in the same way and this may be why Wilks and Bettany made no mention of it in their book.

The two incidents confirm Gull's lack of concern for the consequences of his actions. Serious complaints could have been made against him in both instances and when he removed the capsules from the young patient's body he was at the beginning of his career, with no "name" or official position to protect him. If such thoughts had even occurred to him, they could not have deterred him in any way, so fanaticism and ruthlessness had been part of his character for many years when the Ripper murders took place. There may have been a hint of things to come in a letter which, long before his stroke, he wrote to one of his friends, a Dr Hooper.

> "To me, life in all its phases seems but a
> revelation of more than it seems, and
> demonstrably so when I see the moral law
> dominate the physiological law. Hence
> suicide; hence the law of duty *and the
> high sacrifice of life to it.*" (My italics)

Gull was referring to the sacrifice of life by the person following "the law of duty" but it's easy to imagine him condoning the sacrificing of another person's life. Many unpleasant and unethical deeds have been committed in the name of duty and if he really was responsible for the deaths of Kelly and her friends, Gull would probably have told himself that killing them had been a form of duty.

Gull, as we know, was first mentioned in connection with the Ripper murders in 1970, in Thomas Stowell's famous *Criminologist* article. In his *Final Solution*, first published in 1976, Steven Knight made out a strong case for his suggestion that Stowell had been "pointing a camouflaged finger" at Gull, and he would probably have been even more convinced of it if he had known of Stowell's meeting with Colin Wilson, ten years before the article appeared. He would almost certainly have seen the significance in Wilson's statement that Stowell had been "sitting on" his theory for some thirty years – i.e. roughly the time that had elapsed after the death of Theodore Dyke Acland. That suggested that Stowell's interest in the Ripper mystery might have been sparked off by some late in life confession by Acland. He did, of course, remark on the fact that Acland, contrary to convention, signed Gull's death certificate. In the course of his article Stowell, in his usual apparently ingenuous way, suggested a reason for that.

There was a well-known story, quoted in many books on the Supernatural, alleging that the famous Victorian medium Robert James Lees had tracked down Jack the Ripper. It was claimed that Lees had located the murderer's home, which turned out to be the West End residence of very famous doctor. After a lot of unsuccessful approaches to the police, Lees finally persuaded an Inspector to give him some credence and they both went to the house. The Inspector spoke first to the doctor's wife who was evasive and off-hand, answering most of his questions with replies such as "You must ask my husband about that." Finally, however, she admitted that she had begun to be concerned about her husband's state of mind. She had been particularly alarmed to notice that he had been absent from the house whenever there had been a Ripper murder. The doctor then joined them and confessed to having become subject to the sensation of emerging from some kind of trance, unable to remember what he had been doing for the last few hours. On one of those occasions he had found there was fresh blood on his shirt and on another there had been some scratches on his face.

Stowell claimed that Caroline Acland, Gull's daughter, had identified the doctor as her father. She said that two men, a police Inspector and another who said he was a medium, had once called unexpectedly at her parents' home. They had spoken first to her mother and then her father had joined them, and made the admission about the lapses of memory and the blood on his shirt. Mrs Acland, it seemed, had not connected the incident with the Ripper murders but remembered it merely as something strange that had once happened, and which she did not fully understand. She apparently put no date to the occurrence but Stowell obviously thought that it was during the time of the Ripper murders. He suggested that the blood Gull had found on his shirt had been the result of him examining the murderer shortly after he had killed one of the women in Whitechapel.

According to Lees, the doctor was secretly certified insane. His death was announced to explain his disappearance and if he was Gull, there was an obvious reason for Acland signing his death certificate. Lees said that a fake burial took place and due to his fame, the funeral was something of a celebrity event – which was certainly true of Gull's. Special trains had to be put on to take the mourners from London to Thorpe Le Soken in Essex, where he was interred in the graveyard. Knight believed that when his death actually took place at some later date, Gull was secretly buried in the plot that he had bought for him and his wife. When he was researching his book, he visited Thorpe Le Soken and was shown the grave by the verger, a Mr Downes. He had inherited the position from his father, who remembered Gull's funeral. Describing their conversation, Knight wrote –

> "Downes had no idea why I was interested in
> Gull, so I was astonished when he said, 'This
> is a large grave, about twelve feet by nine,
> too large for two people. Some say more than
> two are buried there. It's big enough for
> *three*, that grave.' He fell silent for a
> moment or two, then said pensively, 'Burial
> places for two just aren't normally that big.'
> Then, half jokingly, he mused, 'Of course, it's
> *possible* that somebody else is buried there,
> without anyone knowing who.'"

In his contribution to *Who* Was *Jack the Ripper?*, the expert Christopher Missen wrote –

"Serial sexual killers feel they have nothing
to lose. That rules out dissolute Royals or
their medical appointees."

This was clearly intended to rule out Gull, but with all the respect that
Mr Missen's expertise demands, it's a rather wide generalisation which
doesn't allow for a changed state of mind. In the preface to his book
The Crimes, Detection and Death of Jack the Ripper, first published in
1987, Martin Fido wrote, "there is no further excuse for anyone giving
a moment's credence to flights of fancy concerning Sir William Gull...",
a view echoed by Stewart Evans and Paul Gainey in *Jack the Ripper
– First American Serial Killer*, eight years later. It's possible, however,
that these opinions are based mainly on the obvious flaws in Stephen
Knight's theories and take no account of the character traits which even
before he had suffered the stroke that possibly unbalanced him, made
Gull a suitable candidate.

With his ruthlessness and total disregard for the consequences of
his actions, he was already near to the mentality which Robert Ressler
described as typical of a serial murderer – believing himself to be
invincible. The stroke may have had the effect of allowing that almost
fanatical side of his nature to dominate, although physically it appeared
to make no difference to him. On that topic, it's worth quoting Wilks
and Bettany's *Biographical History of Guy's Hospital*. Probably the most
authentic description of Gull's condition after the attack, this refutes the
claims of some authors that it left him almost totally incompacitated,
and must remind us of his alleged admission to the police officer who
visited him with Lees.

"He recovered in great measure and returned
to London, where he remained for some months
comparatively well. Friends who then saw
him did not discern much difference in his
looks and manners, but he said he felt
another man, and gave up his practice."

It could obviously be argued that when Gull said he "felt a another
man", which might not have been his own phrase, he meant in the purely
physical sense. He was in his seventies but his well-known powers of

stamina and his natural strength had no doubt helped him to resist the "slowing down" process which would have begun to affect any man of his age. It would have advanced during the necessary period of inactivity following the stroke and he would have found it difficult to resume a full range of duties when he returned to work. It would probably have been in character if, rather than play a lesser role, he preferred to give up completely. On the other hand, the implication of Wilks and Bettany's account is that Gull felt a difference in himself that others had failed to notice and it was hardly surprising that Stephen Knight believed that it was the visit of Robert Lees and the police officer which made him acknowledge that difference.

Knight was of the opinion that Gull's withdrawal from practice was because he had been made to realise that he was no longer of sound mind and was preparing for the time when that fact would become obvious. He revealed that Gull's last will was dated 27 November 1888, only 18 days after the final murder and, even more significantly, almost a year from when he had suffered the stroke. Had Gull believed that the stroke was likely to have any permanent effect on him, he would probably have made the will immediately. As it was, the date of it convinced Knight that the encounter with Lees had prompted Gull to put his affairs in order while he was still capable of rational thought.

Although he did not specifically say so, Knight clearly thought that Gull committed the murders as a "another man", and it could also be suggested that when he removed organs from the victims it was some echo of his past battles with the families of deceased patients. With the ordinary serial murderer it would simply have been the taking of trophies, but for Gull it could have been an extension of the sadism that he had shown in at least two cases.

After the skilful removal of those organs, the apparently frenzied mutilation of the bodies might have been a giving way to anger at the ignorance of those who earlier had opposed him, which he still carried in his mind. The whole thing could therefore have been punitive – towards Kelly and her friends who had threatened the very centre of the established way of life, and also towards those people long ago whose squeamish ignorance had stood in the way of his pursuit of knowledge. There is, however, another possibility. Joseph Sickert said originally that the murders were carried out in the way that they were to create the impression that a maniac was about in Whitechapel. Once that was established, the murder of Kelly would have been seen as just another of his crimes. That might also have been in Gull's mind if the murders really were his conception.

Additional support for the "famous doctor" theory was provided by an article which appeared in an American newspaper in 1895. The incident was described fully in the *Jack the Ripper A–Z*:

> "In 1895 the Chicago "Sunday Times-Herald"
> published an article attributing the capture
> of Jack the Ripper to Robert James Lees.
> The newspaper explained that the truth had
> 'recently been told by Dr Howard, a well-
> known London physician, to William Greer
> Harrison, of the Bohemian Club in San
> Francisco'."

The article said that Dr Howard, perhaps "under the influence of too much wine" had said that he had been one of twelve doctors who had been called as a court of medical inquiry and commission in lunacy on a fellow physician. The article said –

> "Jack the Ripper was no less a person than a
> physician in high standing and in fact was a
> man enjoying the patronage of the best
> society in the West End of London.
> When it was absolutely proved beyond
> peradventure that the physician in question
> was the murderer, and his insanity fully
> established by a commission *de lunatico
> Inquirendo* , all parties were sworn to
> secrecy. Up to the time of Dr Howard's
> disclosure this oath has been rigidly
> adhered to.
>   He was a physican in good standing, with
> an extensive practice. He had been ever
> since he was a student at Guy's Hospital,
> an ardent and enthusiastic vivisectionist."

As Stephen Knight said, everything in the final paragraph applied to Gull. The article also said,

> "In order to account for the disappearance
> of the doctor from society a sham death
> and burial were gone through."

Knight said that the Dr Howard mentioned must have been Dr Benjamin Howard, an American physican who was based in London, but spent a lot of time in the USA. His London address was the St George's Club in Hanover Square, which ran the hospital at 367 Fulham Road, where Annie Elizabeth Crook died. The story had a follow up, as Knight was informed before his book was published. He received the information from Richard Whittington-Egan, a well-known writer on Jack the Ripper, who contributed the Foreword to Knight's book. As the final version of the manuscript was then with the publisher, Knight could not include it in the body of the text but mentioned it as a footnote to the relevant chapter. It appeared that a London newspaper *The People* had printed an article based on the Chicago *Sunday Times-Herald* feature, and had referred to the doctor mentioned as "Anglo-American". Whittington-Egan had found a copy of a letter written by Dr Howard to the editor of *The People*, furiously denying that he was the doctor in question, and threatening legal action.

The letter was reproduced in Martin Fido's *The Crimes, Detection and Death of Jack the Ripper*. Mr Fido found it, with its eccentric punctuation and almost frenetic denials, "absolutely convincing". My own reaction was that it was the work of a man in a considerable state of panic who, had he waited a little while until he had taken a calmer look at the whole matter, might have felt that it would have been wiser to have ignored the article, rather than definitely identify himself with it. Knight disagreed with Whittington-Egan's opinion that the denial undermined his case. As he said, if Howard had in fact become drunk and betrayed his oath of secrecy, he would have been bound to deny it. A classic case, in fact, of "He would say that, wouldn't he?"

The debate continued. Donald Rumbelow accused Knight of "calmly pooh-poohing evidence", which was a strange reaction from a serving police officer, used to dealing with unsubstantiated denials. More importantly, this type of argument overlooks the fact that the Chicago

Sunday Times-Herald must have felt justified in publishing the story. Dr Benjamin Howard might not have been the doctor mentioned in the story – although, significantly, he seemed to think he was – but the parallels with the Lees story are obvious, and the details of the "famous doctor" all definitely applied to Gull. There is no record of Lees saying that the physician in his story was a keen vivisectionist but Gull certainly was, as he made clear more than once. What Rumbelow and the other experts seemed to imply was that if Dr *Benjamin* Howard was exonerated by his frantic but unsupported denial, the whole story could be conveniently forgotten – which was not the approach that any painstaking investigator would have adopted. Whoever he might have been, a doctor with such a burdensome secret might well have felt the need to confide in a friend, and that friend might also have found the secret difficult to keep.

Gull's will was an important factor in Stephen Knight's case, but it also showed a weakness in it. Knight wrote confidently of when Gull decided to become a Freemason and what an important step in his career it had been, but the will included no bequests to the Brotherhood or its various charities. This would have been unusual for a senior Freemason, and particularly one as wealthy as Gull whose fortune in today's terms would have been in excess of twenty million pounds. Also, when Stowell died he was careful to leave instructions for the disposal of his Masonic regalia but there was no mention of any such thing in Gull's will. The Freemasons have said, in fact, that there is no record of Gull having been a member of their organisation.

The lack of a record is not irrefutable proof that Gull was never a Freemason and it has been pointed out that with a number of prominent people, including the then Prince of Wales, being quite open about their membership, Gull would have been something of an odd man out if he had not become one. It has also been suggested that had he not been a Freemason, he would never have achieved the position that he did in the field of medicine. As a man with an individualistic nature, however, it would have caused Gull no great worry to differ from many of his contemporaries by declining membership, particularly as he had gained everything that he had in life by his own efforts and ability. Many Freemasons prospered through the influence of their "Brothers" and it would no doubt have angered Gull if it had been thought that he owed any of his success to nepotism. Stephen Knight thought that one of the most significant steps in his career was engineered by the Freemasons, but there is actually evidence to the contrary. This was in 1871, when he saved the life of the Prince of Wales who was dangerously ill with typhoid fever. He was rewarded with his barontcy.

Knight suggested that it was through Masonic influence that Gull, then virtually unknown, took over the case from Sir William Jenner, the Royal Physician, but his account of the event was very much at odds with that of Wilks and Bettany in their history of Guy's Hospital. Their version was that when the Prince was taken ill at Sandringham he was first treated by a local doctor who quickly telegraphed a specialist, Dr Oscar Clayton, and it was Clayton who brought in Gull. Jenner was called shortly afterwards, presumably as a courtesy because the Prince was officially his patient. Wilks and Bettany's account had the ring of authenticity but even if Knight was correct in saying that Gull took over from Jenner, it was only conjecture on his part that it was through Masonic influence. There is, then, no concrete evidence that Gull was a Freemason but even if it could be proved beyond all doubt that he was not, it would not mean that he could not have committed the murders.

Gull would not have had to have been a Freemason himself to know the rituals of the Brotherhood and such factors as the arrangement of the victims' bodies, the marks on Catharine Eddowes' face and the finding of her body in Mitre Square, could have derived from Masonic lore. Gull was possessed of what has been called a "strong sense of the bizarre", and it might have amused him to commit the murders in the manner of Masonic executions. Although he had a theatrical side to his character – on being told that he bore a certain resemblance to Napoleon he took to combing his hair in a way that accentuated the likeness – he was essentially a practical man and it would have been understandable if the Freemasons' posturing rituals aroused a certain contempt in him. It might therefore have appealed to him to present them with actual executions in the form that they enacted in those rituals, to see the reaction of senior Freemasons like Warren and Anderson when they were required to deal with them.

When all this has been said, however, the case against Gull rests on the fact that he was a man of strange character with a cruel and ruthless side to his nature, his medical knowledge, what may or may not have been a very strong hint from Thomas Stowell and the very doubtful testimony of Joseph Sickert. Like other people involved in the history of Ripperology,

Stowell destroyed his own credibility. The approach to Colin Wilson in which he stated quite firmly that his suspect was Clarence and the denial ten years later have made it possible to doubt his veracity but it seems that some of his contentions continue to cause disquiet. Caroline Acland's statement naming her father as the famous doctor in the Lees story might be dismissed on the grounds of Stowell's unreliability but if Mrs Acland did relate the incident to him, it constitutes remarkable testimony.

Lees can be discredited on the grounds that he was a Victorian medium and of necessity, a fake and a charlatan – which has never been proved or even strongly suggested – but authors who doubt the story have not gone so far as to allege that Stowell invented Mrs Acland's apparent corroboration of it. For example, in *Jack the Ripper: Anatomy of a Myth*, published in 1995, the author William Beadle dismisses the Lees story for the traditional reason that the medium was a fake, but makes no mention of Caroline Acland or, in that connection, of Stowell. Martin Fido tackled the problem by acknowledging the probable truth of the story but suggesting that Gull, as a kindly person – probably as a bad a description of him as there could be – didn't like to disappoint his two visitors and was pulling their legs. If so, Lady Gull must have anticipated her husband's reaction with uncanny accuracy because, if her part in the incident is as reported, she set the whole thing up for him. Gull would have been far more likely to order the men out and then make an official complaint to the Inspector's superiors.

Although Stowell seems to have been dishonest in his letter of denial to *The Times*, I doubt that he would have attributed an entirely false statement to Caroline Acland. If, as Stephen Knight believed, he was trying to incriminate Gull in an oblique way because loyalty to the Freemasons and the Acland family prevented him from making a direct accusation, he probably sent his letter to *The Times* because his plan had gone wrong. Far more attention was being paid to Clarence as the Ripper suspect than Gull. Stowell's denial that he had suspected Clarence is actually the only proven example of out and out dishonesty on his part. He might be excused for that because there is considerable doubt that he actually believed Clarence to have been the Ripper.

It has to be admitted that the manner of Mrs Acland's alleged disclosure seemed to have been a little too compatible with the tenor of other parts of Stowell's article. If she really failed to realise the significance of all that was said when the two men visited her parents' home, she was being as amazingly ingenuous as Stowell seemed to have been in his reporting of the incident. Possibly she did suspect some connection with the Ripper murders and told Stowell of the incident in the hope that he might set her mind at rest. If she went so far as to confide fears about her father to him, Stowell would again have been showing loyalty to the family by withholding that part of the story.

Gull could have done almost everything that Sickert's story alleges. He would have had the power to confine and certify Annie Elizabeth Crook and quite possibly the medical knowledge to operate on her and impair her mental faculties, although not as specifically as Stephen Knight imagined when he suggested that Gull had set out to destroy her memory. An operation on her brain could certainly have brought about the epilepsy which afflicted her towards the end of her life and finally, the insanity which was apparent when she died. From what we know of Gull, it's likely that he would have relished the opportunity to carry out such an operation experimentally to see what effect it might have. At his age he could not have murdered the final victim because she was obviously overpowered and held down on her bed before her throat was cut but as the Sickert story has it, he would have had two accomplices to assist him when he went to her room to complete the murders.

If Lees was right in saying that a fake burial with a coffin filled with stones was held when the death of the famous doctor was announced, there might still be evidence that the doctor was Gull. The remark of the sexton to Stephen Knight, "Some say more than two are buried there. It's big enough for *three*, that grave", could be followed up by opening Gull's grave. The coffin would have long since disintegrated but if a large number of stones were to be found, perhaps with a fragment of the coffin plate, it would suggest that a fake burial had indeed taken place. Such an excavation would naturally need permission – which would almost certainly be refused.

Sir Arthur Conan Doyle, the creator of Sherlock Holmes, was himself an expert criminologist and he was almost certainly speaking his own mind when, in *The Speckled Band*, he had Holmes telling Dr Watson,

"When a doctor does go wrong he is the first
of criminals. He has nerve and he has
knowledge."

Sir William Withey Gull had knowledge, some of his deeds show that he also had nerve which, used in persuance of his personal creed of the infallibility of his own judgement and standards, could often amount to reckless arrogance. It will never be proved to everyone's satisfaction but it's very easy to imagine him as Jack the Ripper who, in many ways, will always be "the first of criminals".

CHAPTER 14

Macnaghten

Sir Melville Macnaghten completed his memoranda, speculating over the identity of Jack the Ripper in 1894, three years after the head of his Scotland Yard department, Sir Robert Anderson, had definitely established it – at least to his own satisfaction. That is not the only strange fact concerning Macnaghten's enterprise.

When Lady Aberconway revealed her transcript of her father's notes it was hailed as an important breakthrough, with one important fact emerging. Jack the Ripper had killed "five times and five times only". Until then, there had been speculation that there had over ten murders. Macnaghten took up his appointment at Scotland Yard in 1889, some months after the last Ripper murder. Consequently, he must have obtained his information, including the names of the three men suspected by the Yard at the time of the murders and the true number of victims, from colleagues who had been there during the investigation.

A relevant question that arises is why Elizabeth Stride was accepted as a victim. As more than one author has pointed out, other women who would have appeared to be more likely victims of the man who killed Nichols, Chapman and, on the same night, Eddowes, were quickly rejected. Of the five official victims, Stride was the only one who escaped mutilation and whereas the other four were killed in the area of Spitalfields and Aldgate, she was murdered in Berner Street, to the south of the main Whitechapel High Street, some way away from the others. Add to that the evidence of Israel Schwartz suggesting that two men were involved and the fact that Stride was killed by a different knife to the one used on the other victims, and the whole thing becomes stranger.

The police could not have been infuenced by the second "Jack the Ripper" message claiming Stride as the first victim of his "Double

Event" because the Littlechild Letter makes it clear that Scotland Yard always regarded both messages as part of a journalistic hoax. How, then, did they reach their firm and apparently immediate conclusion? The reason, perhaps too simple for some and unacceptable to those who automatically reject anything that might be suggest a "conspiracy theory" is probably that they knew.

What adds weight to that suspicion is that although they never believed the Ripper messages to be genuine, the police made no attempt to denounce them as fakes. Those messages must have increased the feelings of horror and panic in Whitechapel, as well as undermining confidence in the police – but they might also have been seen to restore the public conception of the lone murderer, which might have changed if Israel Schwartz had given his evidence. Schwartz could be precluded from the inquest and his evidence suppressed but he could still talk. If he had told friends and relations that he had seen two men at Dutfield's Yard that night and they had repeated what he had said to others, the generally accepted view of the murderer might have been questioned. When the Jack the Ripper messages were published, apparently from the gloating murderer, anything that Schwartz had said would instantly have been forgotten.

It's possible that in their handling of that part of the investigation, Scotland Yard made a colossal error of judgement and missed a good opportunity to save themselves a lot of embarrassment. Knowing that Stride was, in effect, one of the Ripper victims, they immediately began to investigate her murder as such, as journalists covering the case could see. Schwartz made his statement to Swanson in Whitechapel and when news of it reached the Yard, it would have caused consternation, and probably so much so that a potential solution was overlooked.

Warren or Anderson could have issued a statement to the press, saying that the Jack the Ripper messages were fakes, because the second one claimed Stride as his victim, when they were certain that she had not been. The evidence for that would have been the lack of mutilation and the different knife. Schwartz and Matthew Packer could then have testified at the inquest and with the evidence of PC Smith also given, it would have been decided that the man who spent so much time with Stride had been luring her to a convenient spot where his accomplice could rob her. Like so many street crimes at that time, it had ended in the death of the victim. The robbery motive would have been all the more acceptable when it was reported that Stride had had no money on her when she was found.

As it was, the police stuck to their original line – Stride was a victim of the man then known as Jack the Ripper and any evidence to the contrary suppressed. Packer had to be dismissed as unreliable and Schwartz was virtually hidden, with the possibiltiy that at any time, he might cause embarrassment – which he probably did when he gave his newspaper interview. The Clarence-Masonic theory was once disparagingly described by a rival author as "a lot of people going to unnecessary lengths to keep a secret", but that was the Victorian way.

In earlier times some former mistresses of the aristocracy were no doubt installed in well appointed houses in fairly remote areas, where they could spend the rest of their lives in comfort, with the freedom to indulge in other relationships when the chance arose. The Victorians, however, had a publicly proclaimed if phoney code of strict morality and the threat of a Royal scandal would have caused panic throughout the Establishment. Years after she had revealed her father's notes, Lady Aberconway gave a broad hint that such a panic had arisen over the Jack the Ripper murders.

It might be assumed that having gone to Scotland Yard after the murders, Sir Melville Macnaghten was not involved in any cover-up activities and in 1894, compiled his memoranda in good faith. If any of this colleagues had been aware that Kosminski had been put up for identification three years earlier, they could not have told him about it when he was seeking information from them. Neither did they correct him when he wrote that Montague Druitt was "thought to be a doctor". In 1972, however, two years before her death, Lady Aberconway made a remark to a friend, Michael Thornton, that suggested that her father might not have been the recipient of incomplete or inaccurate information. Writing in the *Sunday Express* in 1992, Thornton disclosed revealed that she had said that in accusing Druitt, her father had simply "followed the official line" and that the truth "could cause the Throne to totter."

What exactly did she mean by that? Did Macnaghten know "the truth" all along and reveal it in some other document that remained with his family with his original notes – did she mean that he had been influenced by the Scotland Yard and Home Office statements pointing to Druitt but found out "the truth" at some later time – or was it simply surmise on her part? Lady Aberconway was still alive when Thomas Stowell published his famous *Criminologist* article and when Joseph

Sickert made his television appearance, telling the story of Clarence's secret marriage, which she may already have known about. Knowing of her father's connection with the case, both of those events would have commanded her interest, and perhaps she drew her own conclusions from them. On the other hand, if the statements of Stowell and Sickert were compatible with something her father had said or written many years ealier, did she feel it was finally safe to make a further revelation about a family secret?

We can only speculate why it was that in 1965, six years after she had revealed her father's memoranda, that Lady Aberconway gave her permission for the names of her father's three suspects to be revealed – or why, indeed, she had originally withheld that permission. One obvious conclusion from that would be that, as her later remark to Michael Thornton suggested, she somehow knew that none of them had actually been guilty and didn't want an innocent man to be implicated. If so, she may have felt that some proof of the Ripper's true identity would soon be revealed when she finally allowed Druitt, Kosminski and Ostrog to be named. It was also in 1965 that the American author Tom Cullen published his book, *Autumn of Terror* in which, basing his case on Macnaghten's memoranda, he accused Druitt. Perhaps Lady Aberconway relented simply to be accommodating to Cullen – or possibly she believed that evidence would soon be produced to clear Druitt's name and no lasting damage would be done.

Yet again, the Ripper mystery causes conjecture and contradiction. Macnaghten, in his later years, said that he had destroyed the various papers that the had amassed during his years at Scotland Yard – Lady Aberconway denied this. Why would her father have made a false statement – or why would she have felt it necessary to contradict him? The act of destroying papers might be considered suspicious, perhaps Lady Aberconway thought it might point to secrets being kept. If so, her remark to Michael Thornton when she was eighty-two might suggest that after a long life, she had come to believe that the time for secrets was over and in any case, they were usually revealed, sooner or later. Once again a possible solution to the Ripper mystery simply adds to it.

CHAPTER 15

At The End Of The Day

When the murder of Polly Nichols was discovered there was doubt as to whether she had actually been killed at the place in Buck's Row where her body was found. Surveying the crime scene a few hours after she had been taken to the mortuary, Inspector Helson said that it was difficult to believe that she had received her fatal wounds at that place. Giving evidence at the inquest a few days later, he said that he was quite sure that she had been murdered there. We don't know what removed his doubts. It could not have been the evidence of the police surgeon Dr Llewellyn, who remarked on the marked lack of blood at the scene and was of the opinion that she was already dead when her throat was cut.

The question of when Annie Chapman was murdered has never been properly resolved but the evidence of John Richardson proves that she was not in the yard at Hanbury Street when according to Dr Phillips' instinctive and probably accurate estimate, she would have been dead for over half an hour. The sudden haste of the usually meticulous coroner prevented a proper consideration of the sequence of events but there seems little doubt that Albert Cadosche heard the unexplained sounds from the yard of No 29 *before* 5.30, when Mrs Elizabeth Long saw the woman she believed to have been Chapman.

The suddenly amenable Dr Phillips could have challenged Mrs Long's evidence on the grounds that there would not have been time between 5.30 and 5.50, when the body was probably discovered, for the mutilation of it to have been completed. Instead, he admitted to a possible error of judgement which would have meant that Chapman had been dead for less than half the time he had suggested when he saw her.

At the inquest on Elizabeth Stride, Dr Phillips went out of his way to say that the deceased had not eaten any grapes immediately prior to her

165

death, but there can be little doubt that she had. Less than half an hour before she was murdered, Stride and a companion bought grapes from Matthew Packer's shop. Packer's identification of her was accurate – as accurate in fact as his identification of her companion who was clearly the man seen with her by PC Smith and then by Israel Schwartz – but his evidence was dismissed on grounds that he was unreliable.

Apparently carried away by his sudden importance, he had made voluntary statements to the press, claiming that he had seen Stride's companion on other occasions, after the murder. This did not, of course, make his description of the man any the less accurate, as the police must have known, and his absence from the inquest meant that the Coroner had no reason to question Dr Phillips' denial that Stride had eaten grapes on the night of the murder.

Packer's statement, given under strange circumstances to Sir Charles Warren, was altered at the request of the police so that the time of Stride's visit to his shop was put back by an hour. From the evidence of Constable Smith and Israel Schwartz, however, Packer must have been correct in what he said. Schwartz, the only man who ever witnessed an attack on a Ripper victim – as, rightly or wrongly, Stride was regarded at the time – never gave evidence at the inquest. Following the murders of Stride and Eddowes on the same night, the "Jack the Ripper" messages were released to the Press, although the police never regarded them as genuine. If Schwartz's newspaper interview or anything he told friends or relations of what he had seen in Berner Street had altered the accepted picture of the lone, opportunist assassin, publication of those messages immediately restored it.

The extensive mutilation of Catharine Eddowes was apparently carried out within the five minutes between police patrols in and around Mitre Square but Dr Brown's post mortem report suggested that all of that time would have been occupied by one small part of the facial mutilation. Brown also said that Eddowes was laying on her back when her throat was cut but found no evidence of a struggle, which would surely have been needed to put her in that position. The police accepted Joseph Lawende's very doubtful identification of the body of Eddowes as that of the woman he had seen near Mitre Square, only nine minutes before the murder was discovered, although Dr Brown's evidence proved that she could not have been alive at the time of the sighting.

The inquest on Mary Jane Kelly was legal in the sense that the coroner, Dr Roderick MacDonald, was entitled to preside over it, but he made no attempt to explain the circumstances which gave him jurisdiction when a juror complained at being called and another said that he lived in different district. He threatened the first juror and contradicted himself in a way that strongly suggested that he was uneasy at the matter of jurisdiction being raised.

Later, after telling the jurors that they would hear the full medical evidence of Dr Phillips at a later session, he called for a verdict *without* recording that evidence. In doing so, he failed to meet the legal requirements of an inquest. Closing the hearing, he said that there was other evidence that could have been heard but, "if we at once make public every fact brought forward in connection with this terrible murder, the ends of justice might be retarded", which closely echoed one of the arguments put forward by Dr Phillips when he tried to withhold his evidence at the Chapman inquest. He had conferred, in private, with Phillips before the inquest began.

Individually, all these thing can be explained but it must be a remarkable coincidence that they all occurred during the same investigation – and the irregularities continued. On the evening of the inquest on Kelly, George Hutchinson went to the police and told them of his meeting with the victim, shortly before the murder, and how the strangely dressed man had approached her and then accompanied her into Millers Court. Abberline thought his description of the man was important and had it circulated to all police stations in the area – but he made no attempt to follow up the lead he had been given as he left Whitechapel almost immediately and took no further interest in the investigation.

In 1894, Sir Melville Macnaghen compiled his memoranda on the case, in which he suggested that of three men – Aaron Kosminski, Michael Ostrog and Montague Druitt – who had been suspected by Scotland Yard at the time of the murders, Druitt was the most likely. Many years later, the discovery of the Swanson Marginalia showed that during Macnaghten's time at the Yard – probably in 1891 – Kosminski was almost certainly identified as Jack the Ripper. The identification, which took place in mysterious circumstances at a police convalescent home on the coast, must therefore have been held without Macnaghten's knowledge, and yet he was a senior member of the Criminal Investigation Department, headed by Sir Robert Anderson, who definitely knew about it and probably attended it.

In 1972 Macnaghten's daughter, Lady Christabel Aberconway, cast doubt on his motives, saying that in accusing Druitt, he had followed the "official line" and that the truth "could cause the Throne to totter." Perhaps she was influenced by the fact that Thomas Stowell had by then published his *Criminologist* article apparently accusing Clarence – or did she know something else? In 1973, the Scotland Yard official sent the BBC to Joseph Sickert, saying that he could give them the "definitive version" of Jack the Ripper. Did he feel that as Clarence had been implicated, the full story might has well be told – and why was he able to supply the BBC with Sickert's telephone number a few days later?

Following Joseph Sickert's television appearance in 1973, Stephen Knight obtained permission to examine the then closed case files and three years later, published his *Final Solution*. In the years following, several writers, including myself, noticed flaws in Knight's evidence and while this prompted some authors to write as though the theory is conclusively discredited, two facts emerge. One is that there were actually no discrepancies in the story that could not be attributed to the inevitable inaccuracies that would affect account handed down only by word of mouth over a period of years. The other is that the process of disparagement continued long after Knight's death and it often included nit-picking, often on a childish level.

Joseph Sickert told Stephen Knight that Annie Crook came from the Midlands but was of Scottish descent. One author, dismissing the whole story as nonsense, still found it necessary to trace the Crook family tree back to Berwick Upon Tweed and state that as Berwick has officially been in England since 1482, Annie could not have been of Scottish descent. As any reasonably experienced genealogist could have told him, however, the nineteenth century census returns show that English towns on the Welsh and Scottish borders were full of people born in Wales and Scotland. Many of them had children born in England – who obviously would have claimed Welsh or Scottish descent.

When Stephen Knight reported in 1976 that among the personal belongings found by the body of Annie Chapman were coins, he was only saying what most authors at that time would have said. He suggested that the coins had been removed with the other objects because an initiage into the Freemasons is divested of all metal. Later research into the police and witness statements, caused some doubt as to whether there were coins by the body, but *The Jack the Ripper A–Z*, while mentioning conflicting reports, state that there were "almost certainly two farthings" there. Another author, in what is in many respects an excellent book, states that the coins were necessary to support Knight's "Masonic fantasy".

Later in the book, while describing the body of Catharine Eddowes he admitted that while he had previously dismissed the possibility of any ritual having been enacted during the murder, the markings on Eddowes' face certainly suggested it. It would have been fairer to Knight – as well as covering all possibilities – to include at that point his theory as to what those markings meant. They were, of course, the nicking of the lower eyelids, which is shown in the Hogarth etching "The Reward of Cruelty" and the two triangles – one on each side of the face – which Knight contended were the symbol of the altar top of the Freemasons' Holy Royal Arch.

There is, of course, no doubt that Mitre Square, where Eddowes was found, had long Masonic associations and nobody has disproved Stephen Knight's claim that 29 Hanbury Street, where Annie Chapman's body was found, was between two buildings previously used for Masonic meetings. There is no doubt that the victims' intestines were placed over their shoulders in the manner of the execution of the three apprentices who, in the Masonic legend, murdered Hiram Abiff, the Master Mason. It's also true that Eddowes could have been said to have received the most "Masonic" treatment of all the victims, which might have been because it was believed that she was Mary Kelly who, within that scenario, had triggered off the whole thing with her blackmail attempt.

Neither of the authors I've quoted has ever nominated a suspect, so it would be unfair to say that they have disaparaged Knight's theory because it differed from their own. It's possible, however, that there is now a pronounced tendency to shy away from anything that can be labelled a Conspiracy Theory and, of course, even the most objective observer can get too close to a subject. It can be useful, therefore to consider the opinions of the less committed and those approaching for the first time. In 1988, the centenary of the murders was marked by a television mini-series starring Michael Caine as Abberline, in which Gull was shown as the murderer. One of the final shots was of his death certificate, signed by his son-in-law Theodore Dyke Acland. It was suggested, without following every facet of the Lees story, that Gull was put into an asylum and his death announced.

The series was criticised for its verdict and also for a lack of realism. Among other things, the Whitechapel prostitutes were far too clean, well-dressed and attractive. Some of the faults were no doubt due to the almost inevitable forfeiting of complete authenticity in the interest of presentation and entertainment value – and, of course, the virtual impossibility of gaining a proper empathy with the subject in the time that it takes to produce a television series. There was, however, value in the opinions of the programme makers.

Coming to the subject "cold", the producers obviously recognised the significance of Acland's signature on the death certificate, and it's probably safe to say that if this were put to any disinterested party, it would be agreed that there was something very odd about it. During his final illness, Gull was attended by two other doctors and although Acland would obviously have been interested, as a surgeon he would not have treated Gull in any way. He was, therefore, unqualified to attest to the cause of death, as well as being unorthodox in signing the certificate. Nobody has given any plausible reason for Acland to have ignored medical convention in the way that he did, mainly because nobody has tried. No author, not even one of those apparently most determined to discredit Knight, has made any mention of it. The second and third editions of the *Jack the Ripper A–Z* – which is very objective in its treatment of authors and theories – does not give Acland an individual entry but he is mentioned twice, very much "in passing", in entries relating to Gull and Thomas Stowell. The question of the death certificate is not mentioned and consequently, no explanation of Acland's departure from medical protocol is attempted.

I experienced another example of a disinterested opinion being of value after I appeared on the BBC's *Mastermind* programme in 1995. In the heat, my specialist subject was "The Whitechapel Murders of 1888" and after the semi-final, which I reached as one of the highest scoring runners-up, I talked with Elizabeth Salmon of the BBC, who researched the subject for the programme. I said that to be valid, any theory would have to explain how Catharine Eddowes was apparently murdered in Mitre Square in five minutes, when the post mortem report had stated that all of that time would have been taken up by the nicking of the lower eyelids. Her response was, "So there were two people involved?"

Ms Salmon had completed her research a few months earlier and, having found some aspects of the subject a little hard to take, had probably done her best to forget it. Consequently, as far as theories were concerned, she was completely unbiased. Her opinion was formed purely on the evidence presented, and the logic of it was obvious. Eddowes could not have been murdered in Mitre Square and whoever was responsible would have needed somebody to help him take her body there. Against this, it has been argued by aspiring experts, horrified at the idea of a Conspiracy Theory, that the victims must all have been murdered where they were found because a coach or cart to transport them to those places "would have been heard". In the case of Eddowes, this is a very lame argument as it's really saying that although she *couldn't* have been murdered in Mitre Square, she *must* have been – and nobody, after all, can say with any certainty that a vehicle of any kind *would* have been heard.

The truth is that you would have had a similar situation to one that occurs in one of G. K. Chesterton's *Father Brown* stories. A man is murdered in a building and the killer could only have entered in one way. The police are able to narrow down the time in which he came and went to a few minutes. There are witnesses, however, who could see the entrance for all of that time and they are all certain that nobody went in. In fact, they all saw the murderer enter and leave – but as he was wearing a postman's uniform, they all dismissed him from their minds.

A coach might certainly have been heard at night in the streets of Whitechapel, but it's unlikely that anyone would have taken any notice of it. The Whitechapel Murderer was thought to be somebody like "Leather Apron", the man who had been terrorising the local prostitutes by jumping out at them from alleyways and around street corners, shouting, "I'm going to rip you up!" – which quite possibly prompted the writer of the original Jack the Ripper letter to choose that name and mention "ripping" in his message. Nobody would have thought of anyone like Leather Apron riding in a coach. Most people hearing one would probably have assumed that it was some "toff" passing through on his way home and promptly forgotten about it.

Stephen Knight has been criticised for suppressing evidence but I think that in some instances, he may simply have been careless. He did, after all, faithfully report Joseph Sickert's claim that Mary Kelly fled from Cleveland Street in April 1888, but proudly reproduced witness statements that he had found, which showed that she could not possibly have been there at that time. He made no attempt to hide that evidence. What he did do, was establish four basic questions that any theory must answer if it is to be considered valid. Why were the murders committed in the way that they were? How were they carried out so quickly? Why was there a cover-up? Why did the murders stop? His theory remains the only one that answers all those questions, but there were points which he missed, that might have strengthened that theory. In the next chapter I've applied some imagination to those points. Some may call it empty theorising but I don't think that any of the suggestions that I've made can be completely dismissed. They should, therefore, as Hamlet says, "give us pause".

CHAPTER 16

A Little Imagination

In an earlier chapter I defended Stephen Knight against charges of suppressing evidence on the grounds that he was sometimes careless, in once instance to his own disadvantage. He actually included in his book witness statements taken by Inspector Abberline on the morning of the final murder, which disproved his assertion that the liaison between the Duke of Clarence and Annie Elizabeth Crook was ended by the authorities in April 1888. Knight may also have been careless in dismissing some evidence that he could have used to support his theory that Kelly and the other women were not random but intended victims. This was in another of the statements taken by Abberline, which Knight found in what was then the Greater London Record Office in Northampton Road, Clerkenwell. It was given by Mrs Caroline Maxwell, the wife of a deputy in a lodging house in Dorset Street, almost opposite John McCarthy's. Mrs Maxwell said –

> "I have known the deceased woman during the past
> four months, she was known as Mary Jane, and that
> since Joe Barnett left her she had obtained her
> living as an unfortunate. I was on speaking
> terms with her although I had not seen her for
> three weeks until Friday morning, 9th instant,
> about half past 8 o'clock. She was then standing
> at the corner of Millers Court in Dorset Street.
> I said to her, 'What brings you up so early?'
> She said, 'I have the horrors of drink upon me as
> I have been drinking for some days past.'
> I said, 'Why don't you go to Mrs Ringer's (meaning

the public house at the corner of Dorset Street
called The Britannia) and have half a pint of
beer?'

She said, 'I have been there and had it, but I
brought it all up again.' At the same time she
pointed to some vomit in the roadway.
I then passed on and went to Bishopsgate on an
errand and returned to Dorset Street about 9 a.m.
I then noticed deceased standing outside Ringers'
public house. She was talking to a man, age I
think about 30, height about 5ft 5in, stout,
dressed as a Market Porter. I was some distance
away and am doubtful whether I could identify him.
The deceased wore a dark dress, black velvet body
and coloured wrapper round her neck."

In his *Final Solution*, Knight wrote –

"Mrs Maxwell's assertion that she saw Kelly
at nine o'clock when medical evidence shows
that she had been dead five or six hours is
one of the enduring mysteries concerning the
Ripper case. Whether Mrs Maxwell was lying,
mistaken or drunk has never been explained.
The only certainty is that she was wrong."

That summing up was echoed by Philip Sugden in his *Complete History
of Jack the Ripper* in 1994, but other experts have felt that Mrs Maxwell's
detailed account of her alleged conversation with Kelly was too detailed
to be dismissed out of hand. One attempted explanation has been that
the witness might have mistaken the time or the day, and a *Times* report
on the day after the murder suggests that this was suspected at the time
as Mrs Maxwell was quizzed on that point. Stating that as a result of
her statement there was "great difference of opinion" as to the time of
the murder, the report went on to say that when she was asked how
she could "fix" the time of the meeting, she had said that after leaving
Kelly she had gone to a shop where she had not been for some time
and bought some milk. The police had been to the shop and her visit

on that morning had been confirmed. Although it was not mentioned in *The Times*, Mrs Maxwell had also told the police that when she met Kelly that morning, she had been collecting some plates from the lodging house where her husband worked and had taken them back to their house. The possibility that she had mistaken the time or the day is any case remote. Abberline is said to have taken her statement on the morning of the murder which, at the most, would only have been two or three hours after the alleged meeting.

The "difference of opinion" mentioned by *The Times* was because Dr Phillips had been of the opinion that the murder had occurred at around 4 o'clock in the morning. He had obviously been told of Mrs Maxwell's statement because the same report quoted him as saying that with two windows broken, the room would have been very cold and having been "cut all to pieces", the body would have lost heat far more quickly than if the wound to the throat had been the only one. This was, of course, similar to his non-committal response at the Chapman inquest when the evidence of Mrs Long challenged his opinion as to the time of death. As in that earlier case, his original assessment was probably correct. It would have been an amazing coincidence if the cry of "Murder", heard at around 4 o'clock by Elizabeth Prater and Sarah Lewis, had not been connected with the murder. Also, it was generally agreed that the mutilation of the body would have taken in excess of two hours, so there would have been insufficient time between Mrs Maxwell's second alleged sighting of Kelly at around 9 o'clock and Bowyer's discovery of the murder at 10.45.

A possibility which Knight failed to notice was that with the body in Kelly's room disfigured beyond recognition, the victim might have been somebody else, which would explain how Kelly came to be seen alive, some five hours after the murder took place. If so, Kelly must have been quite content for it to be thought that she was dead – and the most likely explanation for that would be that she knew that she had been the intended victim. In favour of such a theory is one piece of scientific evidence. Melvin Fairclough's *The Ripper and the Royals* has probably done more to discredit Stephen Knight's *Final Solution* than the many outright attacks that it has received, as it shows the source of information to be totally unreliable. Consequently, any valid points made by Knight are now apt to be disregarded. Fairclough's book does, however, contain one of two conclusions which are born of sensible appraisal of evidence, and one of them concerns the Millers Court victim. Fairclough says –

"It may be worth noting that in the police photograph purporting to be of Kelly the blood appears
black because the orthochromatic photographic
plates used in 1888 were not red sensitive (pan-
chromatic film emulsion was invented in 1906).
The hair, which can just be seen, appears much
lighter than the blood. If this was a photograph
of Kelly, whose hair was dark red, the hair would
reproduce as dark as the blood. Clearly this is
not a photograph of Kelly."

This evidence is quite startling but not completely conclusive. The parts
of the photograph mentioned by Fairclough are not as clear as he says
and his statement about the colour of Kelly's hair might be disputed.
His point, however, is still well made. Coupled with Mrs Maxwell's
statement it must raise a reasonable doubt as to whether the body found
in her room was Kelly's – and the question of the final victim's identity
is not the only one which has been too easily dismissed. Parts of George
Hutchinson's description of the man who went into Millers Court with
Kelly have been doubted as he gave them in press interviews, and the
possibility that that man might have murdered her has been discounted
merely on the grounds that had he intended to murder her, he would not
have approached her while Hutchinson was watching him.

It's quite possible that Hutchinson remembered some details of the
man only after he gave his statement to the police, which does not
necessarily mean that they were inaccurate, and if the man was anxious
to stop Kelly getting away from him as she began to hurry off down the
road again, he would probably have taken the risk of Hutchinson seeing
him. He could not, after all, have anticipated that Hutchinson would
wait around to take a closer look at him. The facts are that he met Kelly
that night, went into the lodging house with her and remained there at
least until an hour before the probable time of the murder. There are
good grounds to believe that Kelly invited him to spend the night in her
room and if so, he would still have been there when the murder took
place.

Who was that man? Stephen Knight believed that he was Walter
Sickert, who had used the skill at make-up that he had acquired as
an actor to disguise himself. He based this suggestion largely on

Hutchinson's assertion that the man had a red handkerchief, which he gave to Kelly because she had lost her own. As we know, Sickert had a red handkerchief which his friend Marjorie Lilly remembered as an important aid to him when he created his "Camden Town Murder" series of paintings. It's particularly significant that he would wear round his neck as he acted out the part of a street ruffian, then tie it to a peg or doorknob, so that he could focus his thoughts on it as he worked on his painting.

Knight pointed out that the man seen near Mitre Square with the woman so doubtfully identified as Eddowes, ten minutes before her body was found, also wore a red handkerchief round his neck. He thought that the man was Sickert and that the memory of that night prompted him to use the red handkerchief in later years, as he created the paintings which were inspired by a murder which in some ways was similar to that of Mary Kelly. The victim was a prostitute, murdered early in the morning and found some hours later, laying on her bed with her throat cut. Knight was naturally eager to point out the significance of the red handkerchief worn by the man at Mitre Square, but he overlooked or ignored an inconsistency with his main theory, and missed the chance to make a strong point in favour of it.

Catharine Eddowes was released from Bishopsgate Street police station at around 1 o'clock in the morning and Knight's contention was that she was picked up in the coach by Gull, Sickert and Netley, murdered and mutilated, then dumped in Mitre Square at some time between PC Watkins' patrols at 1.30 and 1.45 a.m. In that case, she would hardly have been walking with Sickert in Duke's Place, near the square, at 1.35. In *The Ripper Legacy*, Keith Skinner and Martin Howells said that the police were "clutching at straws" in accepting the woman as Eddowes on the very flimsy evidence of Joseph Lawende. Knight could have made the same point, and he could also have said that although the woman could not have been Eddowes, the man might have been involved in the murder.

Unless PC Harvey failed to spot it at "eighteen or nineteen minutes to two" as he put it at the inquest, the body of Eddowes could not have been in Mitre Square at 1.35. Lawende's man was not therefore making his escape after helping to place the body, but he might have been walking around the square, seeing how many people were about and assessing the right entrance to use when it was brought there. It's possible that a similar thing happened in Hanbury Street, when Annie Chapman was murdered.

Chapman could not have been alive when Mrs Long saw the couple standing at the front of the house but the man – whose description was similar to those of the men seen by Hutchinson, Lawende, Packer the greengrocer and PC Smith – might just have emerged from the back yard where, as heard by Cadosche a few minutes earlier, he and an accomplice had left her body. With so many prostitutes offering their services at all hours in the East End, it would hardly have been beyond coincidence if on both occasions he was approached by one and seeing other people coming towards him, decided to engage her in conversation until they had gone past. If he had known that area and the women who walked the streets there, he would have realised that to refuse outright the services of one of them would quite possibly provoke an outburst of drunken abuse from her and draw attention to him.

As far as the final murder is concerned, there is support for Knight's solution in the evidence of George Hutchinson. Joseph Sickert told Knight that Mary Kelly had lived at Cleveland Street, first as an assistant in the tobacconist's shop with Annie Crook, and then, at Walter Sickert's instigation, as nanny to Annie's baby. The way in which Kelly and Hutchinson's man greeted each other – the man touching her on the shoulder and both of them bursting into laughter when he spoke – suggests that they knew each other but Kelly did not realise who he was until she heard his voice. When she did, they both laughed because his appearance was so bizarre – as Knight put it, like a typical stage villain of that era. If the man was Walter Sickert and it was true that Kelly had been associated with him before, she would have known of his love of eccentric disguise and would not have asked him *why* he was dressed in that peculiar manner.

In the previous chapter I've suggested that Walter Sickert was the man who left the piece of Catharine Eddowes's apron in the entrance of Wentworth Dwellings – having seen the first police patrols go by because he was lodging in the vicinity. He was known to have lodging places all over Whitechapel. While I believe that he would probably have stayed away after the murder of Eddowes I also think that he would have been able to find lodgings in the Goulston Street area, if not the same room then one near it, on the night of the final murder. He could then have put on his exaggerated disguise there before setting out on what was only a few minutes walk to Dorset Street where he expected to find Mary Kelly – and was lucky enough to encounter her on the way to Aldgate.

Joseph Sickert claimed that the man was Lord Randolph Churchill, who gave Gull his orders, but this was shown as a ludicrous suggestion by Martin Fido. Querying Hutchinson's description in which he said that the man wore gaiters, Fido pointed out that gaiters or spats were strictly for morning wear. If Churchill was so hide-bound to formal dress that he would have invited a mugging by wearing it in the East End at night, he would hardly have made that error. Spats, however, might well have been part of an over the top disguise used by somebody like Walter Sickert.

Fido, who doubted the accuracy of Hutchinson's description, also made the point that if Wynne Baxter had been the coroner at the inquest, he would probably have asked him how he could see the tie pin and other trinkets that the man wore. The answer was obviously that the man's coat was open. That was strange on what must have been a cold night, so he may have worn it like that to draw attention to those things, rather than his face. If he was Sickert, who was well over the average height for a man at that time, he might also have left the coat open to make him look less tall and recognisable. As an artist and an expert in things like form and proportion, he would have known that from even a fairly short distance, the open coat would have made him look broader and therefore a little shorter in height.

Something else which may be a pointer to that man having been Sickert is the "parcel" carried by the man with Stride, then wrapped in newspaper, which seemed to have been similar in dimension to the object which Hutchinson's man had in his hand. Hutchinson said –

"He also had a small parcel in his left hand
with a kind of strap round it."

In a newspaper interview, he said that it was covered with "dark American cloth", another name for oil cloth, which at that time was often used by artists to wrap paintings. Hutchinson's reference to the "kind of strap" suggests that the object was in fact some sort of case, although it would have been a very small one. Walter Sickert often went to Whitechapel to paint the local scenes and was probably a familiar figure there. If he had a case in which he carried crayons or pencils to make his preliminary sketches, it would also have been familiar, so if he was the man seen with Stride and Kelly, he probably wrapped it to prevent it from being recognised. He may have used oil cloth on that second occasion because it was waterproof – it rained on the night of Stride's murder and the newspaper might have gone soft and then disintregrated. The reason that he risked taking it with him could have been that on the nights of the murders it contained grease paints, kept from his theatrical days, or some other means of changing his appearance quickly, if the need arose.

It's possible that Sickert had gone to Spitalfields to see Kelly on previous occasions. Like Jean Overton Fuller, I believe that he was the victim of Kelly's blackmail attempt. If so, he might have panicked and reported it, and in doing so triggered off the murders. Later, when he saw the result of his action, he would have regretted it and it's possible that he found Kelly and resolved their differences, then did whatever he could to help her to escape the fate of the other women. There is evidence in support of this idea in the statement of John McCarthy. He said that she had been renting her room at 4s 6d (22½p) per week, and that it was several weeks in arrears at the time of her death. Stephen Knight said that the amount she was paying was almost twice what a whole family would have paid for such a room, and that she could not have afforded it. He asked, "Who was paying to keep her in hiding?"

Knight was correct in saying that Kelly would have been safer in permanent lodgings than using the local doss houses but he was wrong about the rent. Contemporary sources indicate that an average rent for a furnished room in that area was around eight old pence a day. For seven days that would be 56 pence, or 4s 8d but McCarthy had obviously rounded it down to 4s 6d – 54 pence – or four and a half shillings as a weekly rent. What was unusual was that he had allowed Kelly to stay in the room when according to his statement, she owed him 29 shillings in rent – which amounted to arrears of over six weeks. Most lodging house keepers would have evicted defaulting tenants after a fortnight at the most, so McCarthy may have had some special reason for letting Kelly remain there which, following the murder, he was probably anxious to conceal.

In his statement to the police and in others that he made to the press, he seemed to go out of his way to claim that he had had no idea that Kelly had been a prostitute, or that she and Barnett had not been married. In one newspaper, he was quoted as saying that he had let the room to "a coal porter named Kelly and his wife", and as everyone else in the immediate neighbourhood knew the couple's true names, their circumstances and that Barnett had actually been a fish porter when he was last employed, these errors were probably deliberate ones, made to imply ignorance of the victim and her affairs.

Some authors have suggested that McCarthy allowed Kelly to stay on because she was actually working for him, which would certainly have accounted for him claiming to know nothing of her activities. Prostitutes were an accepted part of the East End scene but the police and magistrates could be very hard on pimps. What makes such a theory unlikely, however, is that Barnett was known to dislike Kelly going out on the streets to earn money for them and would probably have stopped her if he had known that McCarthy was taking some of her earnings. Therefore, the more likely explanation for McCarthy's dubious pleas of ignorance about Kelly and Barnett seems to be that he had entered into an agreement about her rent with some third party and when she was murdered, he sensed that there had been more to the arrangement that he had thought. With that in mind, he decided that the less he knew about her, the safer for him it would be.

When Thomas Bowyer looked into Kelly's room and saw the body on the bed, he immediately went back to McCarthy's shop and told him that there had been a murder. McCarthy accompanied Bowyer back to the lodging house and looked into the room. Having satisfied himself that Bowyer had been right, he sent the man to the police station, as he put it "following myself". He arrived at Commercial Street station a few minutes later, and found Bowyer talking to the duty Inspector, Walter Beck. Having seen the terrible sight in the room McCarthy might have needed a little time to recover, or possibly he went back to his shop to tell his wife that he would be away for a while and to keep an eye on things – but it could also have been because there was somebody nearby who, he thought, should know what had happened.

If Kelly's rent had been guaranteed by somebody who seemed reliable and appeared to have more money than most people in that area, McCarthy would have regarded her as a good investment. Consequently, when she fell behind with it, he would have been prepared to wait, which he would not have done with ordinary tenants. The money would obviously have been given to Kelly and not to him direct and it may be more than coincidence that the period of arrears was roughly the same as the interval that elapsed between the murder of Eddowes and the final killing at Millers Court.

Giving Kelly the money to pay her rent would have been one reason for Sickert to have gone to Whitechapel that night but within Stephen Knight's theory, there could have been a more sinister reason on that particular night. In the original story, as given to Knight by Joseph Sickert, Catharine Eddowes was murdered in error because she sometimes used the name Mary Ann or Mary Jane Kelly. When Knight came to believe that Walter Sickert was involved in the murders, he reasoned that the killing of Eddowes could not have been accidental – Sickert had known Kelly and would not have mistaken Eddowes for her. The fact that Masonic ritual could be particularly applied to the murder of Eddowes adds weight to the suggestion that she was believed to be Kelly.

Knight thought that Sickert had tried to save Kelly by allowing the killers to believe that Eddowes was her, but later assisted with her murder when his ploy was discovered. That would not have taken very long, because if only a few personal details of Kelly had been known, it would have been obvious that she had not been the Mitre Square victim, almost as soon as Eddowes was identified. Sickert, however, might have decided to stop going to Whitechapel after the murder of Eddowes in case he was followed, and so she was unable to pay her rent to McCarthy.

If Sickert did go to Millers Court on the night of the murder it would probably have been because somebody else had managed to trace Kelly, and he had been sent there to keep her in her room until his accomplices arrived. That, of course, would have been achieved by him asking her if he could stay in her room for the night – so up to that point, everything would have gone according to plan. Sickert had met Kelly – luckily it seems, because had he not come up Commercial Street while she was talking to Hutchinson she would probably have spent the rest of the night looking for clients around Aldgate, where she is said to have had her regular beat – and he had gained access to her room. With the trap set, all that remained was for the killers to arrive and finally silence her, as they thought they had done over five weeks earlier. How, then, would she have escaped them and been in the street a few hours later, when she met Caroline Maxwell?

It might have happened if at the last moment, Sickert felt that he could not help to murder a woman who knew and trusted him, and told Kelly to go. When the others arrived he would have said that he had been unable to find her – and it would probably have been decided that they should stay nearby, to see if she returned. Barnett told the police that he had left Kelly ten days before the murder because she had allowed another prostitute who he seemed to have known only as "Julia" to stay in their room. In the week of the murder, Kelly had also allowed another woman, Maria Harvey, to sleep in the room. Perhaps there were others who she had helped in that way, and it's possible that during her absence, one of them came there looking for a bed for the night.

Julia, or perhaps another woman who had stayed there, would have known how to manipulate the lock, which Kelly and Barnett had done when the key was lost, by reaching through a broken window pane, near the door.   Seeing her enter, one of the killers might have approached her, believing her to be Kelly, and pretended to be a would-be client. If the woman was not averse to poaching some of Kelly's business she would have stripped down to her chemise – the only garment found on the body – which was the way of the Whitechapel prostitutes when they entertained a client in the privacy of a room. The cry of "Murder!" heard by the neighbours, would then have been her's, because she had seen the knife and realised the real purpose of the man's approach.

If that or something similar had happened, Sickert would have had to let Kelly go off alone and it's quite possible that he would have been unable to find her again before she came back to Millers Court and found the horribly mutilated corpse in her room. This could have been at around 8 o'clock in the morning because *The Times* report which mentioned Mrs Maxwell's statement also said that a tailor named Maurice Lewis had claimed to have seen Kelly at that time. Lewis said that she had come out of the lodging house and gone back inside again – which might indicate that she was in a state of bewilderment and uncertain of what she should do. Nauseated with shock and horror at what she had seen in her room and feeling the effects of having been drunk the night before, it would not have been surprising if she had been sick as she wandered out into the street again, still trying to decide on her best course of action. Meeting Mrs Maxwell might have concentrated her thoughts enough for her to attribute her early presence in the street and her sickness to her hangover. It would have been later that she thought of letting it be assumed that she was the victim – or that the idea was suggested to her – or she would not have remained in the street for another half an hour or so.

It would probably have been Sickert who realised that the murder of the other woman and the complete disfigurement of her face had given Kelly the chance to escape further attempts on her life. When they met again later that morning and she told him of her conversation with Mrs Maxwell he would have had to think of a way of countering any danger to their plan that it might have caused. In her statement and at the inquest, Mrs Maxwell described the clothes that Kelly was wearing when they met, including a red or maroon woollen cross-over shawl. The police found the shawl in Kelly's room and this, together with Mrs Maxwell's statement, caused the original speculation, as mentioned in *The Times*, that the murder had taken place at some time after 9 o'clock in the morning. As an artist, Sickert would probably have anticipated that Kelly's brightly-coloured shawl would be the garment that Mrs Maxwell particularly remembered and he may have taken it back to the room, later that morning. What he would not have realised was that two women had heard the victim' screams during the night, so establishing the real time of the murder, or that Mrs Maxwell's evidence would be brushed aside in the coroner's haste to close the inquest.

Commenting on the scene when the police finally entered Kelly's room, some authors have mentioned the harrowing sight, in among the carnage, of the victim's clothes, neatly folded on a chair beside the bed, where she had apparently left them. Surprisingly, there seems to have been no mention of anyone seeing bloodstains on the clothes. This may have been a simple omission in reporting but in the statements made at the time and in later years, those involved have rarely missed an opportunity to include any explicit details. With the Ripper moving about the room distributing pieces of the body – although not to the extent that some of the early reports suggested – some blood would surely have found its way onto the clothes. One of the first officers to enter the room was Walter Dew, then a Detective Constable with the local police. In later years he recalled slipping on the blood or as he put it, the "awfulness" on the floor, which shows the extent to which it was scattered around. If he did take the shawl back, Sickert might also have removed the victim's clothes in case they provided some clue to her identity, then replaced them on the chair by the bed with some of Kelly's – which would not have been bloodstained.

The police found that some clothing had been burnt in the grate and a widely accepted explanation has been that it was done by the murderer to provide light – an opinion which really should have been contested by those authors who believe that the Ripper could have removed the kidney of Catharine Eddowes and accurately mark her face in almost complete darkness behind a building in Mitre Square. Among the ashes were remnants of some clothing which was recognised as having belonged to Kelly, and from this it was assumed was that all the burnt garments had been her's. This may have been the intention. Kelly's clothes could have been put on the fire when the flames had died down so that enough of them would have remained for them to be identified. The police said that the ashes in the grate were still warm when they examined them, which would probably have been some seven hours after the murderer left. Ashes can retain heat and even flare up again after some time, but it hardly seems likely that there would have been any warmth left after such a long time in that ice-cold room. If the fire had been lit at some time after 9 o'clock, however, it might still have retained some heat.

Re-entering the room and planting the clothes there would have been a very unpleasant task and with the risk of being discovered, a dangerous one – and there were what could have been indications of an understandable haste. It was reported that the fire in the room was a "fierce" one, as it destroyed the spout of a kettle hanging above it. This could have been because the victim's clothes were all piled on together, in an effort to destroy them quickly, with the result that the fire flared up and reached the kettle. A pair of boots, assumed to have been Kelly's, were lying nearby, perhaps because they were gathered up with rest of the victim's clothing and taken over to the grate but left there because it was realised that they would not burn quickly. It would have been better to have put them back by the bed where the victim would have left them with the rest of her clothes but in such a situation not every move would have been coolly thought out.

If the victim was not Mary Kelly, her real identity will never be known. Apart from Maria Harvey, who was definitely alive after the murder, the only woman known to have slept in Kelly's room was Julia. This was at around 30 October, when Barnett left, so there could well have been others before Mrs Harvey spent the two nights there during the week of the murder. It has been claimed that the police interviewed Julia after the murder but there is no record of this. Another of McCarthy's tenants was a Mrs Julia Venturney or Van Teurney, who made a statement to Abberline and may have been confused with the other Julia.

Some authors have, in fact, suggested that Mrs Venturney was Barnett's "Julia", but it's difficult to see why. Mrs Venturney lived in the same lodging house as Kelly and Barnett and from her statement, seemed to be on good terms with both of them. She enjoyed Kelly's confidences about her relationships with different men and she referred to Barnett as "Joe". He would almost certainly have known her full name, although clearly he had no idea of the other Julia's, and there is no evidence at all that she was a prostitute. Her statement made it clear that she had been a resident in the lodging house for some weeks and that although a widow, she was living with a man named Harry Owen. She would have had no need to share Kelly's room, as the other Julia did.

Julia Venturney was certainly not the woman who was murdered in Mary Kelly's room – but if Walter Sickert really was involved, he might have believed that she was. If he was in the habit of seeing Kelly to give her the money to pay her rent they would have talked together, and Kelly would probably have mentioned her friends at the lodging house – including Mrs Venturney. If another woman was murdered in her place and Kelly told Sickert that it was her friend "Julia", he may well have thought she meant Julia Venturney. "Van Teurney" could actually have been her name or in Kelly's Limerick accent, the first syllable of her name may have sounded like "Van" – from which Sickert assumed that she was Dutch.

One of the paintings which Stephen Knight believed to have reflected Sickert's memories of the Ripper murders was "La Hollandaise" (The Dutch Woman) which he created in 1905. Knight said –

"It depicts a large-limbed nude reclining
awkwardly on a bed in a melancholy room.
Her face is quite unrecognizable, and the
difficulty presented in trying to discern
her features is similar to that experienced
in studying the Scotland Yard photograph of
Kelly's mutilated face. The nose of 'La
Hollandaise' seems to have been cut off, like
Kelly's, her eyes are blurred and the whole
effect is that she had the head of an animal
rather than a human. The same nauseating
feeling is gained from the picture of Kelly."

Was this Walter Sickert's cryptic way of saying what he mistakenly believed – that "the victim was the Dutch Woman"? The idea may seem fanciful in the extreme, and the whole theory is built on a chain of mere possibilities, all of which would have had to come together to make it in the least viable – but can we dismiss it? Read again the statement of Caroline Maxwell, made on the morning of the murder – could she have imagined it all or mistaken the person, the time or the day?

The relevant points, made before but which cannot be over-emphasised, are that if the woman who was murdered in McCarthy's lodging house was *not* her, Mary Kelly was obviously quite happy for it to be believed that she was dead, and if so, the most likely reason is that she thought that she was the intended victim. So far, the only reasonable explanation for that belief that has been suggested, is in the story that Joseph Sickert told the BBC, when a Scotland Yard contact, a man of unquestionable reliability, had sent them to him – a story which has received corroboration from Jean Overton Fuller and may have been hinted at in the enigmatic statement by Lady Christabel Aberconway. The final word goes to Inspector Abberline, in what is said to have been his last recorded statement on Jack the Ripper –

"You'd have to look for him not at the bottom
of London society but a long way up."

CHAPTER 17

Epilogue

When the doctors had completed their examination of the body in John McCarthy's lodging house, it was removed to the Shoreditch mortuary. It was mid-afternoon on that cold November day and the light would already have been fading when a cart, drawn by a single horse, came up to the entrance of Millers Court. On it, under a tarpaulin, was a battered coffin or "shell", which was often used when the bodies of murder or accident victims were moved.

The arrival of the cart was the signal for people to come out from the nearby "courts" and stand in the street, waiting for the body to be brought out from the lodging house. *The Times*, reporting the scene, remarked that those people were among the poorest in London but they showed no lack of propriety – "Cloth caps were doffed – slatternly looking women wept."

In the courts or "rookeries" as they were also called, whole families often shared a single room and many of the neighbours who came out to pay their respects to Mary Jane Kelly would have lived in the utmost squalor. One of the better facets of human nature is that extreme adversity can sometimes produce the sort of fellow feeling that brought the people out into the street that afternoon. From the statements of witnesses, it's possible to tell that the respectable women of Whitechapel lived side by side with the local prostitutes with no feeling of hostility or disapproval towards them. It was probably a realisation that "There but for the grace of God go I" which produced this tolerance – mere survival was difficult in those days and the term "unfortunate" for prostitute was more apt than many Victorian euphemisms. Few of them would have chosen that way of life.

As we look back on the Ripper saga, that scene in Dorset Street seems to have a fitting air of finality about it. What Tom Cullen aptly called the "Autumn of Terror" was over. Nobody then knew that but it's likely that they soon sensed it. The ordinary people of Whitechapel would not have known of Abberline's swift departure when the final inquest had been completed but they would have noticed the sudden reduction in the police presence in the district. The sense of finality, quite unintentionally, is also in the statement of Elizabeth Prater, one of the witnesses who heard what were almost certainly the screams of the final victim. After being awakened by her pet kitten jumping on her bed, Mrs Prater heard a woman's voice scream, "Murder!" but as she often heard search cries from the direction of the lodging house on the other side of Millers Court and as it was not repeated, she went back to sleep. Her statement continued –

"I was up again and downstairs in the court
at 5.30 a.m. but saw no one except two or
three carmen harnessing their horses in
Dorset Street."

The night was over and Whitechapel was preparing for a new day. Later that morning there would be the horrific discovery of the body, followed by the police and the press converging on Dorset Street but in a sense, Jack the Ripper – if he ever existed – was already on his way into the history books. Having got up, Mrs Prater went to the nearby pub, the Three Bells, and had a drink of rum. It was probably while she was imbibing that the malign presence actually emerged from that cold, shabby little room in the lodging house, leaving behind him a scene of almost unimaginable carnage, and disappeared into the chill early winter dawn.

Most of the Whitechapel of those days has also disappeared but one or two landmarks remain. If you walk up the left hand side of Commercial Street towards Shoreditch, you'll come to the stretch of road where George Hutchinson met Mary Kelly, about two hours before the final murder took place. Hutchinson said –

"I was coming up by Thrawl Street, Commercial
Street, and just before I go to Flower and Dean
Street, I met the murdered woman Kelly…"

Flower and Dean Street has gone but Thrawl Street, a turning off Commercial Street on the opposite side to where Hutchinson was walking, is still there. It was from Thrawl Street that Polly Nichols set out when she was ordered from the doss-house there, and she would have made her way down Commercial Street, hoping that her "jolly" bonnet would soon attract a client.

Go further up Commercial Street, past White's Row, and you come to a multi-storey car park. This is where Dorset Street, Millers Court and "The Britannia", the pub on the corner, used to be. Dorset Street was almost opposite Hanbury Street, which does still exist. It was named after the brewers Truman, Hanbury and Buxton, and what was the Truman's Brewery has expanded over the site of No. 29, where Annie Chapman's body was found by John Davis in the backyard. Dutfield's Yard, where the body of Long Liz Stride frightened Louis Diemschutz's horse, has also disappeared and Berner Street, where it was situated, has now become Henriques Street. Two of the murder sites do remain, however.

Buck's Row, where it all began, became Durward Street in deference to it residents, who were embarrassed by its association with the Ripper murders. It can still be seen, a little way from Whitechapel High Street and only a short walk from the junction with Osborne Street, where Polly Nichols told her friend Ellen Holland that she would soon join her, back at the Thrawl Street doss-house. Not surprisingly, there's nothing to show us of where Charles Cross saw what he thought was a tarpaulin, laying by the gates of a stable, and found himself looking at the body of Polly Nichols.

Mitre Square, a small, irregular-shaped space between building, still exists, with its aspect improved by some large, built-up flower beds. It still has cobbles, but not the originals on which Catharine Eddowes' blood flowed. The warehouses, including the one in which George Morris was on duty when Constable Watkins sought his help, are long gone. The square is now a quiet little backwater behind modern office blocks and bordered on one side by the historic Sir John Cass school. There is still a police station on the original sight in Bishopsgate but a more modern building has replaced the one from which Eddowes set out in the last hour of her life, having bid Constable Hutt, the duty gaoler, a cheerful, "Goodnight, old cock."

Until fairly recently it was possible to see the ornamental façade to the tenement building in Goulston Street where the piece of Eddowes' bloodstained apron but of the building itself, only the entrances and some of the staircases behind them remained. They were blocked off when the building was demolished and so remained like caves. A street market functioned in that part of the street and, provided with stout wooden doors, some of those entrances were used as storerooms by the stallholders. One of them was converted into a tiny fast food shop, selling burgers and coffee. Now, even that part of the old building has gone.

In modern Whitechapel, then, there are still glimpses of Jack the Ripper's prowling ground. Time and the aura of mystery may add a little undeserved romance to him and his story – a story of terrible deeds in foul, dirty, disease-ridden surroundings – but there is still the recollection of that group of sad, shocked people who gathered in the now non-existent Dorset Street to mourn an Irish girl who had lived among them and who they had accepted as one of their own.

Nothing can ever lessen the horror of what happened in those terror-stricken months in Whitechapel but in a tale of brutality and almost certainly corruption, that spontaneous demonstration of respect stands out as at least on manifestation of genuine sympathy and of the generosity of the human spirit.

ALSO AVAILABLE FROM
AMBERLEY PUBLISHING

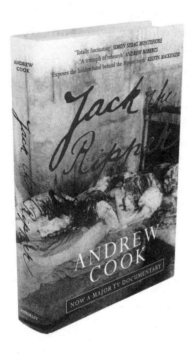

JACK THE RIPPER
Andrew Cook

(Available in hardback and paperback)

HARDBACK:
Price: £18.99
ISBN: 978-1-84868-327-3
Extent: 256 pages

PAPERBACK:
Price: £9.99
ISBN: 978-1-84868-522-2
Extent: 256 pages

Available from all good bookshops or order direct
from our website www.amberleybooks.com